T. Hopp, N. Ruiter, J. C. Bamber, N. Duric, K. W.A. van Dongen (Eds.)

International Workshop on Medical Ultrasound Tomography

1.- 3. Nov. 2017, Speyer, Germany | Proceedings

International Workshop on Medical Ultrasound Tomography

1.- 3. Nov. 2017, Speyer, Germany | Proceedings

Edited by
Torsten Hopp
Nicole Ruiter
Jeffrey C. Bamber
Neb Duric
Koen W.A. van Dongen

KIT Scientific Publishing

Impressum

Karlsruher Institut für Technologie (KIT)
KIT Scientific Publishing
Straße am Forum 2
D-76131 Karlsruhe

KIT Scientific Publishing is a registered trademark
of Karlsruhe Institute of Technology.
Reprint using the book cover is not allowed.

www.ksp.kit.edu

Print on Demand 2018 – Gedruckt auf FSC-zertifiziertem Papier

ISBN 978-3-7315-0689-8
DOI 10.5445/KSP/1000071328

Preface

Ultrasound Tomography is an emerging technology for medical imaging that is quickly approaching realization. Multiple research groups around the globe are engaged in research spanning theory to practical clinical applications and commercialization. In order to bring together the growing community we organized the first International Workshop ond Medical Ultrasound Tomography (MUST), which was held from 1st to 3rd November 2017 in Speyer, Germany.

The purpose of this workshop was to discuss and exchange ideas and research results in order to boost Ultrasound Tomography. The workshop provided a setting for discussing recent developments in a wide variety of topics including theory and practical application of image reconstruction and calibration algorithms, signal and image processing, image analysis and evaluation as well as system and transducer design and clinical application of ultrasound tomography.

The program of the three day workshop included eight invited talks, which covered the history and possible future trends of Ultrasound Tomography (*J. Greenleaf*), the clinical motivation (*P. Littrup*) and status of breast imaging (*H. Madjar*), the connection to seismics (*A. Fichtner*) and geophysics (*G. Pratt*), the latest trends in ultrasound transducers (*N. de Jong*) as well as the aspects of commercialization of photoacoustic imaging systems (*C. Wiest*). Additionally 29 oral presentations were given and 11 posters were presented. In dedicated discussion sessions the current challenges and future directions of ultrasound tomography were discussed with the audience. 59 participants from 10 countries attended and actively contributed to a very successful workshop.

Oral and poster presenters were asked to submit a one-page abstract before the workshop, which was reviewed by the scientific committee. Authors of accepted abstracts as well as the invited speakers were asked to submit a full paper. This book comprises the written versions of most of the contributions presented during the workshop and thereby provides an overview of the state of the art in medical ultrasound tomography.

We would like to sincerely thank all the colleagues involved in the scientific and local committee for their commitment. We are furthermore grateful for the support by Deutsche Forschungsgemeinschaft (DFG), the city of Speyer and Pepperl + Fuchs GmbH.

Karlsruhe, Dec. 2017 – *J. Bamber, K.W.A. van Dongen, N. Duric, T. Hopp, N.V. Ruiter*
(Scientific organizing committee)

Organization

Scientific Committee

Jeffrey Bamber
Institute of Cancer Research, London, UK

Koen van Dongen
Technical University Delft, Netherlands

Neb Duric
Delphinus Medical Technologies, Detroit, US

Torsten Hopp
Karlsruhe Institute of Technology, Germany

Nicole V. Ruiter
Karlsruhe Institute of Technology, Germany

Local Organizing Committee

Torsten Hopp
Karlsruhe Institute of Technology, Germany

Nicole V. Ruiter
Karlsruhe Institute of Technology, Germany

Saskia Baier
Karlsruhe Institute of Technology, Germany

Christiane Buchwald
Karlsruhe Institute of Technology, Germany

Antje Martin
Karlsruhe Institute of Technology, Germany

Session Chairs

T. Azuma	*The University of Tokyo*
J. Bamber	*The Institute of Cancer Research*
J. Camacho	*Spanish National Research Council*
N. Duric	*Delphinus Medical Technologies*
A. Fichtner	*ETH Zurich*
H. Gemmeke	*Karlsruhe Institute of Technology*
J. Greenleaf	*Mayo Clinic*
J. Hesser	*Heidelberg University*
T. Hopp	*Karlsruhe Institute of Technology*
P. Huthwaite	*Imperial College London*
P. Lasaygues	*Aix Marseille University CRNS*
P. Littrup	*Delphinus Medical Technologies*
F. Natterer	*University of Münster*
R. Prager	*University of Cambridge*
N. Ruiter	*Karlsruhe Institute of Technology*
G. Sandhu	*Delphinus Medical Technologies*
J. van der Neut	*Delft University of Technology*
K. van Dongen	*Delft University of Technology*
M. Zapf	*Karlsruhe Institute of Technology*

Table of Contents

Current challenges in Breast Screening and Diagnosis: From Molecules to Peritumoral Regions and Radiomics – The Emerging Imaging of Whole Breast Stiffness 1
P. Littrup, N. Duric, C. Li, M. Sak, G. Sandhu, K. Bergman, M. Boone, D. Chen

Imaging and inversion I

One-dimensional Marchenko inversion in stretched space 15
J. van der Neut, J. Fokkema

Ultrasound imaging from reflection data 25
F. Natterer

Using a 2-D approximation of the 3-D incident field for Born inversion 33
U. Taskin, L. Heijnsdijk, L. Hoogerbrugge, K. van Dongen

Imaging and inversion II

USCT Image Reconstruction: Acceleration using Gauss-Newton Preconditioned Conjugate Gradient 41
H. Wang, H. Gemmeke, T. Hopp, J. Hesser

Efficient simulation of ultrasonic waves using an extended spectral element method 53
C. Boehm, N. Korta Martiartu, M. van Driel, L. Krischer, M. Afanasiev, A. Fichtner

Imaging and inversion III

Medical ultrasound tomography: lessions from exploration geophysics 65
G. Pratt

Non-linear Ultrasonic Computed Tomography (USCT) for soft and hard tissue imaging 77
P. Lasaygues, J. Rouyer, S. Mensah, E. Franceschini, G. Rabau, R. Guillermin, S. Bernard, V. Monteiller, D. Komatitsch

Imaging and inversion IV

Real-Time Ultrasound Transmission Tomography based on Bézier Curves 89
M. Perez-Liva, J. Udias, J. Camacho, J. Herraiz

3D imaging of the breast using full-waveform inversion 99
O. Calderon Agudo, L. Guasch, P. Huthwaite, M. Warner

Ultrasound tomography systems

Ultrasound Computed Tomography: Historically Guided Musings 111
J. Greenleaf

A Multi-Modal Ultrasound Breast Imaging System 119
J. Camacho, J. Cruza, N. González-Salido, C. Fritsch, M. Pérez-Liva, J. Herraiz, J. Udias

First steps towards the Delft Breast Ultrasound Scanning System (DBUS) 131
L. Heijnsdijk, E. Jansen, H. den Bok, E. Bergsma, E. Noothout, N. de Jong, K. van Dongen

System design

Upper Bound of Accuracy for Self-Calibration of an 3D Ultrasound Tomography System without groundtruth 137
W. Tan, T. Steiner, N. Ruiter

Ultrasound transducers

Manufacturing Technologies for Ultrasonic Transducers in a Broad Frequency Range .. 147
S. Gebhardt, K. Hohlfeld, P. Günther, H. Neubert

Dice-and-fill single element octagon transducers for next generation 3D USCT 159
M. Zapf, P. Pfistner, C. Imbracio Liberman, K. van Dongen, N. de Jong, B. Leyrer, H. Gemmeke, N. Ruiter

Clinical applications I

Challenges in Breast Ultrasound 179
H. Madjar

Ultrasound Tomography for Breast Cancer Screening 189
N. Duric, P. Littrup, C. Li, M. Sak, Y. Sandhu, K. Bergman, M. Boone, D. Chen

3D Ultrasound Computer Tomography for Breast Cancer Diagnosis at KIT: an Overview 205
N. Ruiter, T. Hopp, M. Zapf, A. Menshikov, C. Kaiser, H. Gemmeke

Breast Tissue Characterization with Sound Speed and Tissue Stiffness 217
C. Li, G. Sandhu, M. Boone, N. Duric, P. Littrup, M. Sak, K. Bergman

Image processing

Postprocessing workflow of 3D-USCT: bridging the gap to the clinic 229
T. Hopp, M. Zapf, H. Gemmeke, N. Ruiter

Tissue Characterization with Ultrasound Tomography Machine Learning 241
G. Sandhu, P. Littrup, M. Sak, C. Li, N. Duric

Challenges and applications of registering 3D Ultrasound Computer Tomography with conventional breast imaging techniques 253
P. Cotic Smole, N. Ruiter, N. Duric, T. Hopp

Clinical applications III

A simple method for acoustic properties determination of cancerous tissue and its implementation into the clinical workflow 263
F. Wolfram, T. Lesser

The New Generation of the KIT 3D USCT 271
H. Gemmeke, L. Berger, T. Hopp, M. Zapf, W. Tan, R. Blanco, R. Leys, I. Peric, N. Ruiter

Poster papers

Comparison of two ray tracing methods for sound speed imaging 283
X. Fang, Y. Wu, M. Ding, M. Yuchi

Contrast resolution enhancement of Ultrasonic Computed Tomography using a wavelet-based method – Preliminary results in bone imaging 291
P. Lasaygues, R. Guillermin, K. Metwally, S. Fernandez, L. Balasse, P. Petit, C. Baron

Fast reflectivity imaging in 3D using SAFT 303
N. Ruiter, M. zapf, T. Hopp, H. Gemmeke

Minimum-variance beamforming for ultrasound computer tomography imaging 315
S. Wang, J. Song, L. Zhou, P. Yang, M. Ding, M. Yuchi

Piezofibre composite transducers for next generation 3D USCT 323
M. Zapf, K. Hohlfeld, P. Pfistner, C. Imbracio Liberman, K van Dongen,
H. Gemmeke, N. Ruiter, A. Michaelis, S. Gebhardt

Improved temperature measurement and modeling for 3D USCT II 339
M. Zapf, A. Patel, A. Menshikov, N. Ruiter

Visualisation of Ultrasound Computer Tomography Breast Dataset 349
N. Tan Jerome, Z. Ateyev, V. Lebedev, T. Hopp, M. Zapf, S. Chilingaryan,
A. Kopmann

Comparison of registration strategies for USCT-MRI image fusion: preliminary results 361
T. Hopp, P. Cotic Smole, N. Ruiter

Measurement of the speed of sound, attenuation and mass density of fresh breast tissue 369
L. Keijzer, M. Lagendijk, N. Stigter, C. van Deurzen, C. verhoef,
W. van Lankeren, L. Koppert, K. van Dongen

The USCT reference database 385
N. Ruiter, M. Zapf, T. Hopp, H. Gemmeke, K. van Dongen, J. Camacho,
C. Fritsch, J. Cruza, J. Herraiz, M. Perez Liva, J. Udías

Object Classification and Localization with an Airborne Ultrasound Imaging System 395
W. Tan, G. Erbacher, T. Steiner, N. Ruiter

Current challenges in Breast Screening and Diagnosis: From Molecules to Peritumoral Regions and Radiomics – The Emerging Imaging of Whole Breast Stiffness

Peter J. Littrup[1-4], M.D., Nebojsa Duric[2,3], PhD, Cuiping Li[3], PhD, Mark Sak[3], PhD, Gurshuran Sandhu[3], PhD, Ken Bergman[3], Michael Boone[3], M.S., and Di Chen[3]

Prof. of [1]Radiology and [2]Oncology, Wayne State University, Detroit, Michigan, USA. Co-founder and Medical Advisor, [3]Delphinus Medical Technologies, Inc., Novi, Michigan, USA. Director Tumor Ablation Program, [4]Crittenton Hospital, Rochester, MI;
E-Mail: PLittrup@gmail.com

Abstract

Current advances in breast imaging technologies have been improved breast cancer screening and diagnosis. In parallel, advances in the molecular understanding of underlying tissue biology has highlighted complex interactions between glandular and surrounding adipose tissue. This in turn has emphasized the role of tissue stiffness in the extracellular matrix, from progression of the individual cancer cell to the stiff invading margins of the peri-tumoral region around breast cancers. While advances in magnetic resonance imaging and ultrasound elastography can provide both diagnostic and prognostic information for an isolated mass region, whole breast evaluations of stiffness are needed for screening. Ultrasound tomography provides unique whole-breast imaging of tissue stiffness, thereby better characterizing the highest risk region at the interface between fibroglandular and adipose tissue, as well as peri-tumoral regions. Further work is needed on whole breast analyses that include emerging and highly promising work with radiomics of quantitative UST data.

Keywords: Ultrasound tomography, stiffness, elastography, density, radiomics, breast, cancer

1 The importance of adjacent fat for breast cancer initiation and imaging

To better understand the role of imaging for breast cancer screening and diagnosis, this paper broadly addresses some of the biological underpinnings of cancer initiation and development. Moreover, the role of ultrasound tomography (UST) as a new breast imaging technology needs to be placed in perspective with strengths and weaknesses of current breast imaging modalities for screening and/or diagnosis. But before an overview of imaging specifics will be covered, insights into emerging concepts of cancer initiation may provide better understanding of the diversity and spectrum of breast cancer types. Opportunities for imaging surrogate biomarkers, such as tissue stiffness, can be placed in better context. Finally, improved localization of cancer initiation near the interface of fibroglandular and adipose tissue (IFGA) will be covered.

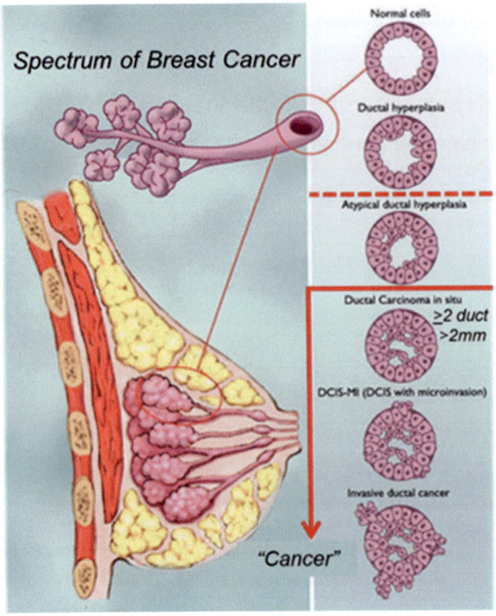

Figure 1: (adapted from [1]): The spectrum of breast cancer extends from high risk lesions, such as atypical ductal hyperplasia (ADH) to multiple forms of DCIS and invasive cancer.

Figure 1 shows a graphic representation of the progression by cells lining a normal duct to invasive ductal carcinoma [1]. Cancer development can be considered as a progression from a single layer of epithelial cells lining a normal duct to multiple layers beginning to fill a duct, with associated increased cancer risk, or atypical ductal hyperplasia (ADH). In fact, if two separate ducts are involved or extent of ADH is >2 mm, low-grade ductal carcinoma in situ (DCIS) is noted [2]. In addition, a spectrum of DCIS types may not imply imminent clinical cancer since occult DCIS has been noted in ~9% of autopsy studies [3]. A complex "conversation" between tissues of intracellular, extracellular, ductal and surrounding stroma regions appears to control the development of different types of DCIS and their risk for cancer progression [4]. This cellular cross-talk is further supported by genetic expressions and interactions within the extracellular matrix (ECM) [4, 5]. Cancer of greater prognostic significance appears to begin with high-grade DCIS, since it is more likely to progress to invasive cancer and/or develop recurrence following definitive treatment. For these reasons, over 95% of DCIS is treated aggressively by some form of surgery [6, 7], despite the lack of associated mortality reduction benefits from treating DCIS. Concurrent with aggressive treatment, continued diagnostic and imaging dilemmas emerge for the entire spectrum of ADH, DCIS and invasive breast cancer.

The most common risk assessment for breast cancer is the relative density on mammogram. However, correlations of mammographic density with breast cancer risk suffers the conundrum of decreased mammographic performance in women with dense breasts. Mammographic breast density, associated risk and prognostic significance has been thoroughly reviewed, confirming the role of ECM components, lysyl oxidase (LOX) enzymes and multiple forms of collagen [8]. Greater aromatase immunoreactivity has been noted in dense tissue, leading to the greater conversion of estrogens and association with developing breast cancer [9, 10]. Perhaps more importantly, cancers arising in dense breast tissue have been associated with larger tumor size, higher histologic grade, more advanced stage, higher local recurrence and risk of secondary breast-cancer, let alone worse survival [11]. Tissue interactions at the boundary of dense tissue also need to be considered.

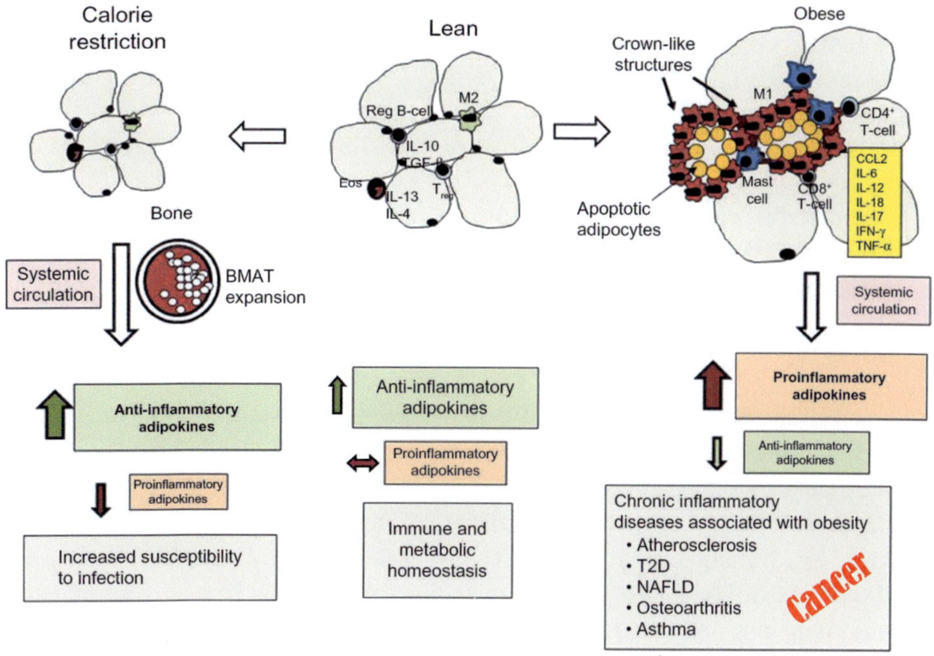

Figure 2: (adapted from Mancuso) [12]: The complex role of adipocytes and the associated balance of adipokines in multiple diseases. Lean body habitus gives rise to an optimal balance that likely leads to disease prevention and improved immunity, whereas starvation and obesity lead to infection susceptibility and an array of obesity-associated diseases, respectively.

In most women, fat cells make up more of the breast than dense tissue. The human fat, or adipose, layer may be the largest endocrine gland in the body, mediating blood pressure, reproductive function, appetite, glucose homeostasis, angiogenesis and immune function [12]. The link between obesity and multiple diseases on the rise (figure 2) appears to include breast cancer. When the balance of adipokines tip toward an excessive pro-inflammatory state, multiple adipokines, such as leptin, have been implicated in the initiation of cancer via aromatase expression [13, 14]. Tumor growth of cancer cell lines become markedly accelerated in the presence of adipocytes [13]. Moreover, a bidirectional crosstalk between cancer cells and adipocytes lead to the formation of cancer-associated adipocytes (CAA). These CAA's secrete the adipokine, fibronectin, along with collagen alterations, to generate a phenotypic change in fibroblast-like cells known as adipocyte-derived fibroblasts (ADF). When tumor cells are cultivated with these ADF's, cancer cells now demonstrate increased invasive ability. CAA's also display overexpression of collagen VI and ECM-related molecules that contribute to breast cancer progression. This entire progression leads to the presence of a dense collagenous stroma, the so-called *desmoplastic reaction* around breast cancers. This is the etiology of a clinically palpable mass and an imaging opportunity for displaying *stiffness*.

2 Tissue stiffness and cancer

Breast cancer detection has relied upon using palpable stiffness for hundreds of years. Imaging has predominantly relied upon assessment tissue stiffness using elastographic techniques by either ultrasound or MR [15-18]. In addition, mammography has also recently used tissue deformation as a surrogate of stiffness, noting improved breast cancer risk delineation beyond breast density alone [19]. A brief overview of imaging signs found with breast cancer will be presented prior to considering the adjunctive value of imaging stiffness.

2.1 Imaging for whole breast screening and targeted diagnosis

By mammography, the dominant signs of breast cancer relate to a focal mass or asymmetry, a "cluster" of microcalcifications and/or a region of architectural distortion. Newly diagnosed cancers by mammography were noted as a mass or asymmetry in over 2/3, by calcifications in 29% and by architectural distortion in only 4% [20]. Masses or persistent asymmetry by mammography are generally then evaluated by ultrasound, which predominantly identifies a cyst or solid mass for follow-up or biopsy, respectively. A suspicious group of calcifications, or cluster, usually consists of a heterogeneous, branching and/or fine group of $\geq$4 calcifications within an estimated 1 cm^3 of breast tissue. However, most isolated calcifications (i.e., no discrete associated mass or architectural distortion) going on to biopsy are generally noninvasive (i.e., DCIS) and smaller size [20].

Breast tomosynthesis, or 3-D mammography, has shown improved detection of architectural distortion [21, 22]. Moreover, 3-D mammography better characterizes focal asymmetries and mass margins, which helps account for reduced screening callbacks and improved biopsy positive predictive value (PPV). Thereby, the significantly improved 3-D mammography performance of ~4/1000 additional cancer detection, with less call-backs and biopsies, over 2-D digital mammography provides a good example for new additional screening modalities to deliver BOTH sensitivity and specificity improvements, or "more bang for the buck".

Whole breast evaluation by additional screening with magnetic resonance imaging (MRI) and ultrasound (US) has already been thoroughly covered [23-29]. MRI has become the "gold standard" of breast imaging, demonstrating significantly greater detection of mammographically occult breast cancers, particularly in the highest risk groups [23-25]. However, MR imaging costs, patient/imaging-center access and the use of intravenous contrast agents preclude its broad use for the general population. Whole breast ultrasound has also demonstrated significantly greater detection of mammographically occult cancers, ranging between 1.9-4.3 cancers/1000 depending upon overall technique and patient population [26-29]. However, unlike 3-D mammography, the significantly greater callbacks and resultant lower biopsy PPV emphasized the need for additional specificity. Nevertheless, the concept of evaluating the whole breast remains paramount.

2.2 Stiffness and elastography - the need for whole breast imaging?

US elastography has become more commonplace in nearly all US units used specifically for breast imaging, but only targets a grayscale region of interest. This can improve the specificity of mass detection, but lacking visualization of the whole breast ignores the potential for increased detection, or improved cancer sensitivity. US elastography has evolved from strain imaging [15-16] and the BI-RADS-like Tsukuba score, to shear wave imaging (SWI) and quantitative measures of the shear wave in kilopascals (kPa) or sound speed (m/s)[17]. Yet, similar to the strain artifact seen with cysts (i.e., the Blue-Green-Red (BGR) sign), shear waves do not travel through a liquid.

MR elastography more readily displays the whole breast [18], but remains predominantly a research technique limited to few imaging centers. Combining the strengths of MRI and US elastography can produce better localization of focal MR abnormalities by second-look US [30, 31]. More importantly, cancers noted by both qualitative US elastographic strain images [32] and quantitative SWI measurements [33] have also been used for tumor histology comparisons and prognostication. Both quantitative stiffness (kPa) and elasticity ratios [32, 34] have shown that high stiffness corresponded with adverse prognostic factors such as tumor size, node involvement, histologic grade, vascular invasion and Ki-67 expression. Greater stiffness was also noted in tumors that were ER negative, PR negative, p53 positive, high nuclear grade, and high histologic grade. Finally, stiffness has been used to better predict pathologic complete response (pCR) or residual cancer burden to neoadjuvant chemotherapy (NAC) [35, 36].

US elastography has also helped define the underlying molecular etiologies of stiffness, extending into the peritumoral region. Indeed, quantitative SWI assessments of the peritumoral area [37] also led to using computer-aided diagnostic possibilities [38-39]. Interestingly, tumor response to NAC was also noted as changing stiffness of the peritumoral region [36], leading to the suggestion that abnormal collagen of the ECM was likely involved. Moreover, collagen cross-linking of the cancer-associated stroma and abnormal collagen has been defined up to a centimeter beyond breast cancers [40]. Recent efforts with 3-D elastography [41] perhaps better define the extent of peritumoral stiffness and look similar to 3-D vascular patterns [42]. Coincidentally, analyses of 3-D vascular patterns also varies with different tumor types [43] and show response to NAC by decreasing tumoral and peri-tumoral vascularity [44]. Perhaps the increased, tortuous "feeder" vascularity surrounding malignant tumors also contributes to stiffness from their tubular and collagenous architecture.

Correlations of current elastography and/or 3-D Doppler with clinically significant tumor, underlying molecular/cellular stiffness, and potential for improved *specificity* remains *diagnostic* – limited to localized masses detected by standard grayscale. Without whole breast evaluation, US elastography and/or 3-D Doppler lack the potential for tumor detection and improved *sensitivity* for breast cancer *screening*.

3 Ultrasound tomography (UST), stiffness and radiomics

Presentations at this conference will cover additional SoftVue details. The significant and ongoing UST imaging improvements that have gone into launching a multicenter trial of SoftVue as an adjunct to mammographic screening is beyond the scope of this paper.

Whole breast UST offers the potential for multi-parametric evaluation of breast tissue types by quantitative analyses that can eventually be used for radiomics. Extensive work has gone into the development of a UST prototype [45], now called SoftVue (Delphinus Medical Technologies, Inc.; Novi, Michigan). SoftVue has been thoroughly evaluated for volumetric breast density measurements, stiffness, comparison with clinical outcomes, MRI correlation and early experience with region of interest evaluations for radiomics [46-53]. UST imaging is acquired and displays optimal resolution in the coronal plane, allowing a symmetric comparison of central fibroglandular tissue with surrounding subcutaneous fat in each breast (figure 3).

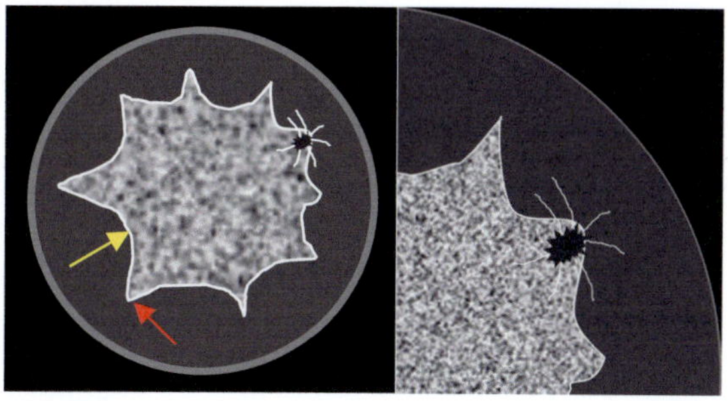

Figure 3: Graphic representation shows coronal format of UST allowing easy recognition of the IFGA (yellow arrow): the Interface of FibroGlandular (central speckled) and Adipose tissue (darker surrounding). Red arrow denotes a Cooper's peak, frequently noted by standard US. Magnified view (right) denotes irregular black focus of cancer at a Cooper's peak with radiating spicules of architectural distortion (white lines).

The coronal plane best shows a tissue retraction phenomenon, or spiculation, surrounding some cancers, which has been clearly associated with improved mass characterization and important molecular subtypes of cancer (e.g., triple negative vs. luminal A) [54]. The circumferential visualization of each breast by UST in the coronal plane emphasizes an under-recognized localization of cancer origin at the **I**nterface of **F**ibro**G**landular and **A**dipose tissue (IFGA) [55]. The IFGA localized 99% of cancers (N=291/294) by MRI [55] and nicely correlates with the biological importance of cancer initiation in proximity to fat [12-14]. Figure 3 graphically shows "*where to look for cancer*" in UST - at the IFGA, as well as the potential association with so-called Cooper's peaks that can produce false positive shadowing (i.e., greater attenuation) by standard US. Greater stiffness by circumferential UST has also been noted at some of these Cooper's peaks, but the additional reflection and SS image stacks generally can exclude dense parenchyma flowing from slice-to-slice from any underlying 3-D mass effect at the IFGA, especially if that mass is associated with spiculation.

The basic concept of UST stiffness relates more to the bulk modulus than any of the previously discussed strain or shear wave elastography provided by standard US units. UST data sets consist of reflection and quantitative transmission images of sound speed (SS) and attenuation (ATT). SoftVue combines these in a fusion format, which overlays stiffness upon an underlying reflection image [48]. The following images show the adjunctive benefit of whole breast stiffness in conjunction with reflection and SS for optimal detection and characterization.

Figures 4-6 demonstrate the synergy of viewing three stacks of UST images simultaneously. Figure 4 and 6 show the potential for improved mass detection by a focal area of stiffness for both benign and malignant masses, respectively. The benign cyst at 6:00 in figure 4 likely contains thick, or inspissated, proteinaceous material with unusually high sound speed. Conversely, the stiffer area associated with the spiculated mass in figure 6 corresponds well with the anticipated cancer extension beyond the central tumor nidus into the peritumoral region with mild architectural distortion. Note that these masses lie on the IFGA, whereas most cysts in figure 4 are surrounded by parenchyma and don't have a fat interface.

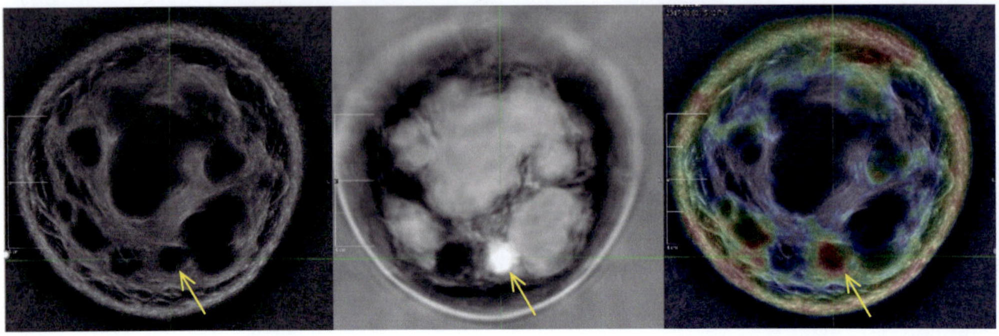

Figure 4: CYSTS - Coronal reflection, SS and stiffness images of a woman with dense breasts and the multiple cysts. Yellow arrow denotes a probable inspissated, or complicated, cyst at the 6 o'clock position that has even higher SS than all the other cysts (middle), and high focal stiffness (red-right). Yet, reflection (left) shows it still retains a sharp boundary, or capsule, with subtle homogeneous internal echoes. Despite relatively high sound speed of all other cysts, they showed no stiffness and relatively sharp margins with minimal central echoes on reflection. While it is unusual for any mass to have such focal high SS, the stiffness image shows the potential for better conspicuity IF this had been a cancer encountered during screening.

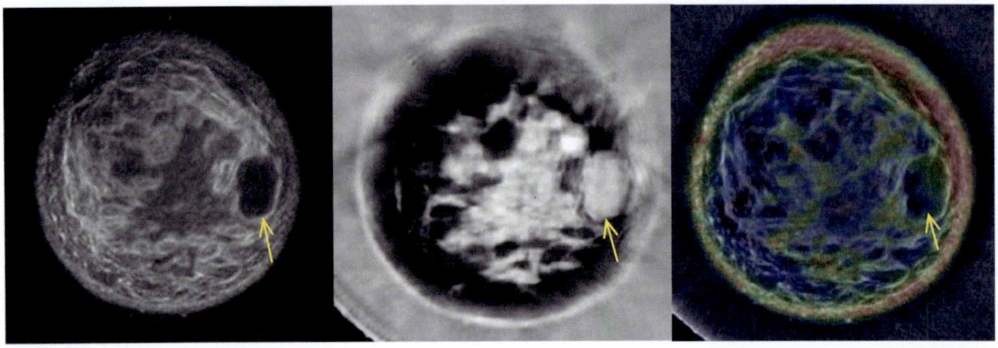

Figure 5: FIBROADENOMA - Coronal reflection, SS and stiffness images show a 2 cm fibroadenoma in the 3:00 position (yellow arrows). Reflection (left) and SS (middle) show well-defined margins, or capsule. Stiffness image (right) shows minimal stiffness (blue-green).

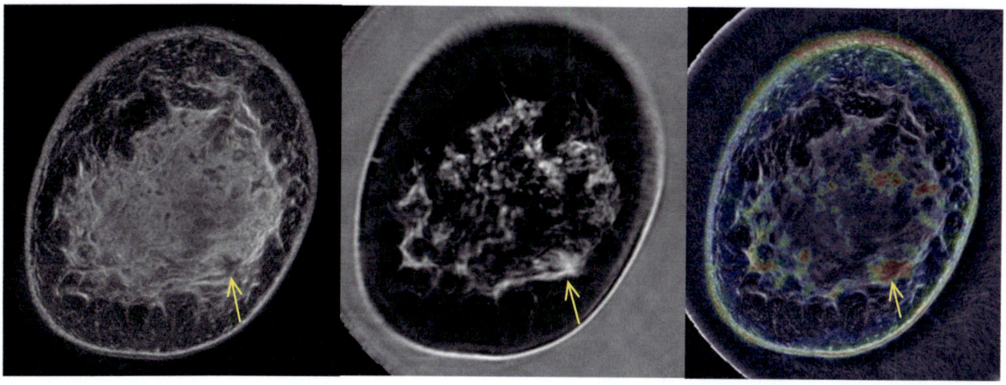

Figure 6: CANCER - Coronal reflection, SS and stiffness images show a 1 cm cancer in the ~4:00 position (yellow arrows). Reflection (left) and SS (middle) show spiculated margins, extending well beyond the central tumor margin. Stiffness image (right) shows stiffness (red) extending beyond the size of the central hypoechoic nodule on reflection. Other regions of red are better dismissed on viewing this stack as the stiffer parenchyma near the IFGA flows more from slice to slice and also tracked with non-masslike regions on reflection and SS.

UST has attained sufficient image quality to allow more detailed assessment of *mass margins*, with associated characterization differences between the three image stacks. However, additional characterization benefits may be obtained by computer-aided assessment of pattern recognition of both *mass contents* and surrounding *peritumoral regions* [51, 53]. As a brief insight to the radiomics paper to follow, some of these mass patterns are already apparent to a radiologist's perception by cross-referencing the 3 dominant imaging stacks. For example, cysts generally have a homogeneous central pattern on SS and reflection, whereas cancer is much more heterogeneous and irregular. Moreover, similar patters analyses are already being applied for improved risk analyses for simple breast density assessments [56]. Radiomic analyses of UST patterns, using multiple SoftVue image stacks, *within* and *surrounding* any breast mass can provide improved tumor characterization well beyond the already improved image resolution of mass margins and BI-RADS criteria alone.

Finally, more work needs to be done with pattern analyses of stiffness to provide perhaps the most comprehensive breast mass assessment by UST, which may lie beyond the limits of current human perception.

References

[1] https://cancerwall.com/dcis-breast-cancer/

[2] Tozbikian G, Brogi E, Vallejo CE, Giri D, Murray M, Catalano J, Olcese C, Van Zee KJ, Wen HY. Atypical Ductal Hyperplasia Bordering on Ductal Carcinoma In Situ: Interobserver Variability and Outcomes in 105 Cases. Int J Surg Pathol 2017; 25:100-107.

[3] Welch HG, Black WC. Using autopsy series to estimate the disease "reservoir" for ductal carcinoma in situ of the breast: how much more breast cancer can we find? Ann Intern Med 1997; 127:1023–8.

[4] Boghaert E, Radisky DC, Nelson CM. Lattice-based model of ductal carcinoma in situ suggests rules for breast cancer progression to an invasive state. PLoS Comput Biol. 2014 Dec 4;10(12):e1003997. doi: 10.1371/journal.pcbi.1003997.

[5] Gorringe KL, Fox SB. Ductal carcinoma in situ biology, biomarkers, and diagnosis. Front Oncol 2017; 7:248. doi: 10.3389/fonc.2017.00248

[6] Stuart KE, Houssami N, Taylor R, Hayen A, Boyages J. Long-term outcomes of ductal carcinoma in situ of the breast: a systematic review, meta-analysis and meta-regression analysis. BMC Cancer 2015; 15:890. doi: 10.1186/s12885-015-1904-7.

[7] Ozanne EM, Shieh Y, Barnes J, Bouzan C, Hwang ES, Esserman LJ. Characterizing the impact of 25 years of DCIS treatment. Breast Cancer Res Treat 2011;129:165-73.

[8] Sherratt MJ, McConnell JC, Streuli CH. Raised mammographic density: Causative mechanisms and biological consequences. Breast Cancer Res 2016; 18(1):45. doi: 10.1186/s13058-016-0701-9.

[9] Ghosh K, Brandt KR, Reynolds C, Scott CG, Pankratz VS, Riehle DL, et al. Breast Cancer Res Treat 2012; 131(1):267-75. doi: 10.1007/s10549-011-1727-4.

[10] Vachon CM, Sasano H, Ghosh K, Brandt KR, Watson DA, Reynolds C, Lingle WL, Goss PE, Li R, Aiyar SE, Scott CG, Pankratz VS, Santen RJ, Ingle JN. Aromatase immunoreactivity is increased in mammographically dense regions of the breast. Breast Cancer Res Treat 2011; 125(1):243-52. doi: 10.1007/s10549-010-0944-6.

[11] Huo CW, Chew GL, Britt KL, Ingman WV, Henderson MA, Hopper JL, Thompson EW. Mammographic density-a review on the current understanding of its association with breast cancer. Breast Cancer Res Treat 2014; 144(3):479-502. doi: 10.1007/s10549-014-2901-2.

[12] Mancuso P. The role of adipokines in chronic inflammation. Immunotargets Ther. 2016; 5: 47–56.

[13] Dirat B, Bochet L, Dabek M, Daviaud D, Dauvillier S, Majed B, Wang YY, Meulle A, Salles B, Le Gonidec S, Garrido I, Escourrou G, Valet P, Muller C. Cancer-associated adipocytes exhibit an activated phenotype and contribute to breast cancer invasion. Cancer Res. 2011; 71(7):2455-65.

[14] Bochet L, Lehuédé C, Dauvillier S, Wang YY, Dirat B, Laurent V, Dray C, Guiet R, Maridonneau-Parini I, Le Gonidec S, Couderc B, Escourrou G, Valet P, Muller C. Adipocyte-derived fibroblasts promote tumor progression and contribute to the desmoplastic reaction in breast cancer. Cancer Res 2013; 73(18):5657-68.

[15] Itoh A, Ueno E, Tohno E, et al. Breast disease: Clinical application of US elastography for diagnosis. Radiology. 2006;239:341–50.

[16] Barr RG. Sonographic breast elastography: a primer. J Ultrasound Med 2012; 31:773-83.

[17] Berg WA, Cosgrove DO, Dore CJ, Schafer FKW, Svensson WE, Hooley RJ, Ohlinger R, Mendelson EB, Balu-Maestro C, Locatelli M, Tourasse C, Cavanaugh BC, Juhan V, Stavros AT, Tardivon A, Gay J, Henry JP, Cohen-Bacrie C. Elastography improves the specificity of breast US: The BE1multinational study of 939 masses. Radiology 2012;262:435–449.

[18] Hawley JR, Kalra P, Mo X, Raterman B, Yee LD, Kolipaka A. Quantification of breast stiffness using MR elastography at 3 Tesla with a soft sternal driver: A reproducibility study. J Magn Reson Imaging 2017; 45(5):1379-1384.

[19] Boyd NF et al. Evidence that breast tissue stiffness is associated with risk of breast cancer. PLoS One. 2014; 9:e100937.

[20] Venkatesan A, Chu P, Kerlikowske K, Sickles EA, Smith-Bindman R. Positive predictive value of specific mammographic findings according to reader and patient variables. Radiology. 2009; 250(3):648-57.

[21] Partyka L, Lourenco AP, Mainiero MB. Detection of mammographically occult architectural distortion on digital breast tomosynthesis screening: initial clinical experience. AJR Am J Roentgenol 2014; 203:216–222.

[22] Bahl M, Lamb LR, Lehman CD. Pathologic outcomes of architectural distortion on digital 2-d versus tomosynthesis mammography. AJR Am J Roentgenol 2017; 209(5):1162-1167.

[23] Niell BL, Freer PE, Weinfurtner RJ, Arleo EK, Drukteinis JS. Screening for Breast Cancer. Radiol Clin North Am 2017; 55(6):1145-1162.

[24] Kuhl CK, Schrading S, Bieling HB, et al. MRI for diagnosis of pure ductal carcinoma in situ: a prospective observational study. Lancet 2007; 370(9586):485–92.

[25] Lehman CD, Gatsonis C, Kuhl CK, et al. MRI evaluation of the contralateral breast in women with recently diagnosed breast cancer. N Engl J Med 2007;356(13):1295–303.

[26] Kolb TM, Lichy J, Newhouse JH. Comparison of the performance of screening mammography, physical examination, and breast US and evaluation of factors that influence them: an analysis of 27,825 patient evaluations. Radiology. 2002 Oct;225(1):165-75.

[27] Kelly KM, Dean J, Comulada WS, Lee SJ. Breast cancer detection using automated whole breast ultrasound and mammography in radiographically dense breasts. Eur Radiol 2010; 20(3):734-42.

[28] Berg WA, Zhang Z, Lehrer D, Jong RA, Pisano ED, Barr RG, Böhm-Vélez M, Mahoney MC, Evans WP 3rd, Larsen LH, Morton MJ, Mendelson EB, Farria DM, Cormack JB, Marques HS, Adams A, Yeh NM, Gabrielli G; ACRIN 6666 Investigators. Detection of breast cancer with addition of annual screening ultrasound or a single screening MRI to mammography in women with elevated breast cancer risk. JAMA. 2012 Apr 4;307(13):1394-404.

[29] Brem RF, Tabár L, Duffy SW, Inciardi MF, Guingrich JA, Hashimoto BE, Lander MR, Lapidus RL, Peterson MK, Rapelyea JA, Roux S, Schilling KJ, Shah BA, Torrente J, Wynn RT, Miller DP. Assessing improvement in detection of breast cancer with three-dimensional automated breast US in women with dense breast tissue: the SomoInsight Study. Radiology 2015; 274(3):663-73.

[30] Plecha DM, Pham RM, Klein N, Coffey A, Sattar A, Marshall H. Addition of shear-wave elastography during second-look MR imaging-directed breast US: effect on lesion detection and biopsy targeting. Radiology 2014; 272(3):657-64

[31] Park SY, Choi JS, Han BK, Ko EY, Ko ES. Shear wave elastography in the diagnosis of breast non-mass lesions: factors associated with false negative and false positive results. Eur Radiol 2017; 27(9):3788-3798

[32] Grajo JR and Barr RG. Strain elastography for prediction of breast cancer tumor grades. J Ultrasound Med 2014; 33:129–134.

[33] Youk JH, Gweon HM, Son EJ, Kim, J-H, and Jeong J. Shear-wave elastography of invasive breast cancer: correlation between quantitative mean elasticity value and immunohistochemical profile. Breast Cancer Res Treat 2013; 138:119–126.

[34] Choi WJ, Kim HH, Cha JH, Shin HJ, Kim H, Chae EY, and Hong MJ. Predicting prognostic factors of breast cancer using shear wave elastography. Ultrasound in Med. & Biol 2114; 40:269–274.

[35] Hayashi M, Yamamoto Y, Ibusuki M, Fujiwara S, Yamamoto S, Tomita S, Nakano M, Murakami K, Iyama K, Iwase H. Evaluation of tumor stiffness by elastography is predictive for pathologic complete response to neoadjuvant chemotherapy in patients with breast cancer. Ann Surg Oncol. 2012; 19:3042-9. Epub 2012 Apr 3.

[36] Evans A, Armstrong S, Whelehan P, Thomson K, Rauchhaus P, Purdie C, Jordan L, Jones L, Thompson A, Vinnicombe S. Can shear-wave elastography predict response to neoadjuvant chemotherapy in women with invasive breast cancer? Br J Cancer 2013; 109:2798-802.

[37] Xiao Y, Zeng J, Qian M, Zheng R and Zheng H. Quantitative analysis of peri-tumor tissue elasticity based on shear-wave elastography for breast tumor classification. Conf Proc IEEE Eng Med Biol Soc 2013; 1128-1131.

[38] Xiao Y, Zeng J, Niu L, Zeng Q, Wu T, Wang C, Zheng R, Zheng H. Computer-aided diagnosis based on quantitative elastographic features with supersonic shear wave imaging. Ultrasound Med Biol 2014; 40:275-86.

[39] Zhang X, Xiao Y, Zeng J, Qiu W, Qian M, Wang C, Zheng R, Zheng H. Computer-assisted assessment of ultrasound real-time elastography: Initial experience in 145 breast lesions. Eur J Radiol. 2014; 83:e1-7. doi: 10.1016/j.ejrad.2013.09.009.

[40] Lewis RA, Rogers KD, Hall CJ, Towns-Andrews E, Slawson S, Evans A, Pinder SE, Ellis IO, Boggis CR, Hufton AP, Dance DR. Breast cancer diagnosis using scattered X-rays. J Synchrotron Radiat. 2000; 7(Pt 5):348-52.

[41] Youk JH, Gweon HM, Son EJ. Shear-wave elastography in breast ultrasonography: the state of the art. Ultrasonography. 2017; 36(4):300-309

[42] Chang YC, Huang YH, Huang CS, Chang RF. Vascular morphology and tortuosity analysis of breast tumor inside and outside contour by 3-Dpower Doppler ultrasound. Ultrasound Med Biol 2012; 38(11):1859-69.

[43] Chang YC, Huang YS, Huang CS, Chen JH, Chang RF. Intrinsic subtypes and tumor grades in breast cancer are associated with distinct 3-D power Doppler sonographic vascular features. Eur J Radiol. 2014; 83(8):1368-74.

[44] Shia WC, Chen DR, Huang YL, Wu HK, Kuo SJ. Effectiveness of evaluating tumor vascularization using 3D power Doppler ultrasound with high-definition flow technology in the prediction of the response to neoadjuvant chemotherapy for T2 breast cancer: a preliminary report. Phys Med Biol 2015; 60(19):7763-78.

[45] Duric N, Littrup PJ, Poulo L, et al. Detection of breast cancer with ultrasound tomography: First results with the Computed Ultrasound Risk Evaluation (UST) prototype. Med. Phys. 2007; 34: 773-785

[46] Glide-Hurst CK, Duric N, Littrup P. Volumetric breast density evaluation from ultrasound tomography images. Med Phys 2008; 35(9):3988-3997.

[47] Li C, Duric N, Huang L. Comparison of ultrasound stiffness tomography techniques for breast cancer diagnosis. Proc. SPIE 6920, 6920-49 (2008).

[48] Ranger B, Littrup PJ, Duric N, Chandiwala-Mody P, Li C, Schmidt S, Lupinacci J. Breast ultrasound tomography versus MRI for clinical display of anatomy and tumor rendering: Preliminary results. AJR Am J Roentgenol 2012; 198:233-9.

[49] Duric N, Boyd N, Littrup P, Sak M, Myc L, Li C, West E, Minkin S, Martin L, Yaffe M, Schmidt S, Faiz M, Shen J, Melnichouk O, Li Q, Albrecht T. Breast density measurements with ultrasound tomography: A comparison with film and digital mammography. Med Phys 2013; 40(1):013501

[50] Duric N, Littrup P, Li C, Roy O , Schmidt S, Cheng X, Seamans J, Wallen A. Breast imaging with SoftVue: initial clinical evaluation. SPIE Medical Imaging 2014, 90400V-90400V-8

[51] Littrup PJ, Duric N, Brem RF, Yamashita MW. Improving specificity of whole breast ultrasound using tomographic techniques. Paper SSA02-05. Presented at Radiology Society of North America, 11/27/2016.

[52] Sak M, Duric N, Littrup P, Bey-Knight L, Ali H, Vallieres P, Sherman ME, Gierach GL. Using Speed of Sound Imaging to Characterize Breast Density. Ultrasound Med Biol 2017; 43(1):91-103.

[53] Sandhu G, Littrup PJ, Sak M, Li C and Duric N. The importance of peritumoral comparisons by ultrasound tomography: Radiomics and breast mass discrimination. Abstract ID: 17013805; Radiology Society of North America 11/28/17.

[54] van Zelst JCM, Balkenhol M, Tan T, Rutten M, Imhof-Tas M, Bult P, Karssemeijer N, Mann RM. Sonographic Phenotypes of Molecular Subtypes of Invasive Ductal Cancer in Automated 3-D Breast Ultrasound. Ultrasound Med Biol 2017; 43(9):1820-1828.

[55] Zhu W, Harvey S, Macura KJ, Euhus DM, Artemov D. Invasive Breast Cancer Preferably and Predominantly Occurs at the Interface Between Fibroglandular and Adipose Tissue. Clin Breast Cancer. 2017 Feb;17(1):e11-e18.

[56] Gastounioti A, Conant EF, Kontos D. Beyond breast density: a review on the advancing role of parenchymal texture analysis in breast cancer risk assessment. Breast Cancer Res. 2016 Sep 20;18(1):91. doi: 10.1186/s13058-016-0755-8.

One-dimensional Marchenko inversion in stretched space

J. van der Neut and J. T. Fokkema

Department of Applied Sciences, Delft University of Technology, Delft, the Netherlands
E-mail: j.r.vanderneut@tudelft.nl

Abstract

In acoustic inversion, we aim to retrieve the density and compressibility of an unknown medium from single-sided reflection data. The relationship between the desired medium properties and the acquired data is intrinsically nonlinear and can be described by an integral representation, which is often referred to as the Lippmann-Schwinger equation. If the wavefield were known throughout the medium, this equation simplifies as a linear map between the medium properties and the reflection data. To acquire the wavefield inside the medium, we propose to use a Marchenko equation. This equation has recently been derived in order to compute a wavefield at an arbitrary location in the medium directly from a single-sided reflection response. To solve the Marchenko equation in physical space, the propagation velocity of the medium must be known *a priori*. If we transform the wavefields and medium properties to a stretched spatial coordinate system in which the wave speed is constant, we can solve the Marchenko equation in stretched space instead. This solution can be obtained without any information on the medium other than its single-sided reflection response. By substituting this solution into an integral representation in stretched space, we can establish an exact and linear map between the medium properties in stretched space and the reflection data. We demonstrate that this map can be used for linear inversion in stretched space without involving any approximation. Our theory is derived for a one-dimensional medium only. In the future, we aim to investigate if this formulation can be extended to higher dimensions.

Keywords: Inverse problems, Inverse scattering

1 Introduction

The retrieval of the density and compressibility of an unknown medium from single-sided reflection data is a long-standing problem with applications at a range of scales [1, 2]. To solve this problem, we often make use of an integral representation, which is known as the

Lippmann-Schwinger equation. This equation relates the desired medium properties to the acquired data through an operator that depends on the wavefield in the medium. Since the wavefield in the physical medium is typically unknown, it is common practice to approximate this quantity by the wavefield in a background model, leading to the so-called Born approximation [3]. Alternatively, the wavefield inside the medium and the medium properties can be iteratively updated in a nonlinear inversion framework [4].

Recently, it was shown that the wavefields inside an unknown medium can also be retrieved by solving a multi-dimensional Marchenko equation [5]. This equation has recently been derived as an extension of its one-dimensional equivalent [6, 7]. If the solutions of the Marchenko equation can be substituted in the Lippmann-Schwinger equation, we may establish a linear map between the medium contrasts and the acquired reflection data. Unfortunately, a model of the propagation velocity is required in order to solve the Marchenko equation in physical space. Hence, constructing the desired map in space requires knowledge of the (exact) velocity. Without knowledge of the velocity, the Marchenko equation can still be solved as a function of the focal time [8], which is defined as the direct propagation time of a wave traveling from the acquisition location to the (unknown) location of observation.

In this contribution, we relate solutions of the Marchenko equation in a one-dimensional medium to wavefields in a stretched coordinate system. We start with a definition of the stretched coordinates and we present an integral representation, which has been derived recently in this coordinate system [9]. We show how the solutions of the Marchenko equation can be substituted directly into this representation. This substitution leads to a linear map between the medium properties in stretched space and the recorded reflection data. We demonstrate that this map can indeed be realized in a one-dimensional medium without any information other than the reflection data. Finally, we show that the map can be used to retrieve the medium properties by linear inversion.

We are not the first to derive a linear map from the Marchenko equation. In the past, several others have used this equation to resolve the medium parameters of a one-dimensional medium from its single-sided reflection response [10, 11, 12, 13]. For a long time, these works could not be extended to higher dimensions. Recently, it has been shown that the medium parameters of a three-dimensional layered medium can be retrieved directly from the solutions of the multi-dimensional Marchenko equation by solving a linear inverse problem [14]. In this contribution, we present an alternative inverse problem for the same purpose by substituting the solution of the Marchenko equation into an integral representation in stretched space.

2 Stretched coordinates

We consider a 1D medium with a specific velocity $c(x)$ and density $\rho(x)$ profile. An example of such a medium is shown in figure 1. In this figure, we also show the impedance $Z(x) = \rho(x)c(x)$. We can stretch the spatial coordinates x to stretched coordinates ξ through the the following (stretching) transform:

$$\xi(x) = \int_{x'=0}^{x} \frac{c_0}{c(x')} dx' \tag{1}$$

The medium parameters and wavefield quantities can be stretched accordingly. While waves propagate in the original coordinates with a variable (and unknown) velocity $c(x)$, they propagate with a constant velocity c_0 in the stretched coordinates. Since we are free to choose this velocity ourselves (even though we may not know the velocity in the original coordinate system), c_0 is known by definition.

Quantities in the stretched coordinate system are indicated by a bar. In figure 2a, we show the stretched impedance $\overline{Z}(\xi)$ of the medium that was shown earlier in figure 1. Note that the yellow high-velocity layers have been squeezed in the stretched coordinates. Since $c(x) = c_0$ in the other layers, their thicknesses have not been altered.

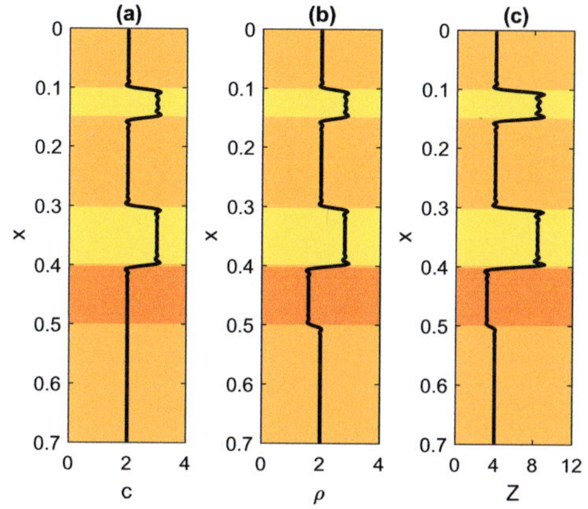

Figure 1: Example of a 1D medium: (a) velocity $c(x)$ (in $10^3\ m \cdot s^{-1}$), (b) density $\rho(x)$ (in $10^3\ kg \cdot m^{-3}$) and (c) acoustic impedance $Z(x)$ (in $10^6\ kg \cdot m^{-2} \cdot s^{-1}$) (with x in m), At $x < 0$ and $x > 0.7$, all medium parameters are constant. The colors indicate the different layers in the model.

3 Stretched integral representation

The following integral representation has been derived to express wavefields in the stretched coordinate system [9]:

$$\overline{p}(\xi,s) - \overline{p}^{inc}(\xi,s) = \int_{\mathbb{D}} \frac{\partial \overline{G}(\xi - \xi', s)}{\partial \xi} \overline{p}(\xi',s)\, \overline{\chi}_r(\xi')\, d\xi'. \tag{2}$$

Here, $\overline{p}(\xi,s)$ is the wavefield at the stretched coordinate ξ, expressed in the Laplace domain, where s is the transform parameter of time t. Further, $\overline{G}(\xi,s) = \frac{c_0}{2s} \exp\left(-\frac{s}{c_0}|\xi|\right)$ is a Green's function in a reference medium with constant velocity c_0 and $\overline{p}^{inc}(\xi,s) = q(s) \exp\left(-\frac{s}{c_0}\xi\right)$ is the incident wavefield in the same reference medium (here, $q(s)$ is the source wavelet).

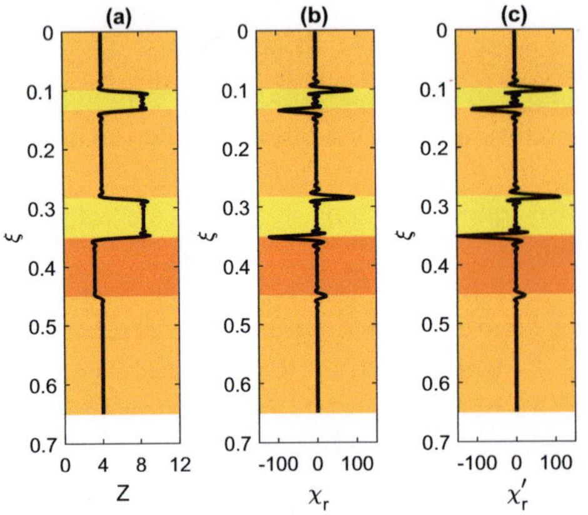

Figure 2: (a) Stretched impedance $\overline{Z}(x)$, (b) reflectivity contrast $\overline{\chi}_r(\xi) = \frac{1}{\overline{Z}(\xi)} \frac{\partial \overline{Z}(\xi)}{\partial \xi}$ and (c) rescaled reflectivity contrast $\overline{\chi}'_r(\xi) = \sqrt{\frac{\overline{Z}(\xi)}{\overline{Z}(0)}} \overline{\chi}_r(\xi)$ of the medium in figure 1.

The reflectivity contrast $\overline{\chi}_r(\xi)$ has been defined in terms of the impedance in the stretched coordinates, according to

$$\overline{\chi}_r(\xi) := \frac{1}{\overline{Z}(\xi)} \frac{\partial \overline{Z}(\xi)}{\partial \xi}. \tag{3}$$

In figure 2b, we show the reflectivity contrast of the medium that we discussed before. Our aim is to retrieve this contrast function from recorded reflection data $R(s) = \overline{p}(0,s) - \overline{p}^{inc}(0,s)$ at the acquisition level $\xi = 0$. Before we discuss this problem, we show how the wavefield $\overline{p}(\xi,s)$ can be computed throughout the medium if the contrast $\overline{\chi}_r(\xi)$ is known. This is done by inverting equation 2 for the wavefield $\overline{p}(\xi,s)$, given $\overline{\chi}_r(\xi)$, $\overline{p}^{inc}(\xi,s)$ and $\overline{G}(\xi,s)$. We have solved this equation by a Neumann series, leading to the wavefield in figure 3a.

4 Inversion

If the wavefield $\overline{p}(\xi',s)$ is known throughout the medium, the following modeling operator can be designed:

$$\mathscr{L}\{\overline{\chi}_r\}(\xi,s) := \int_{\mathbb{D}} \frac{\partial \overline{G}(\xi-\xi',s)}{\partial \xi} \overline{p}(\xi',s)\, \overline{\chi}_r(\xi')\, d\xi'. \tag{4}$$

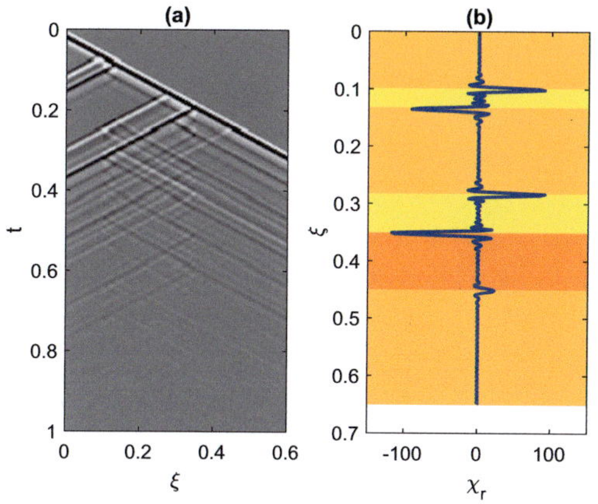

Figure 3: (a) Wavefield $\overline{p}(\xi,s)$ (converted to the time domain) as retrieved by inversion of equation 2. (b) Retrieved reflectivity contrast $\overline{\chi_r}(\xi)$ by inversion of equation 5, given that the wavefield $\overline{p}(\xi,s)$ is known.

Through operator $\mathscr{L}$, we can establish a linear map between the reflectivity contrast $\overline{\chi}_r(\xi)$ and the scattered wavefield in the medium, following $\overline{p}(\xi,s)-\overline{p}^{inc}(\xi,s)=\mathscr{L}\{\overline{\chi}_r\}(\xi,s)$ (i.e. equation 2). By evaluating this wavefield at $\xi=0$, we find the following linear relation between the reflectivity contrast and the recorded data $\overline{R}(s)$:

$$\overline{R}(s)=\mathscr{L}\{\overline{\chi}_r\}(0,s). \tag{5}$$

We can solve this equation for $\overline{\chi_r}$. In figure 3b, we show the result of such inversion, where we have used a conjugate gradient scheme. As expected, this response matches the reflectivity profile in figure 2b. However, to realize this inversion, we required the wavefield $\overline{p}(\xi,s)$, which is generally unknown in practice.

5 Marchenko operator

Recently, it has been shown that a wavefield at location x in the medium can be retrieved by solving a Marchenko equation [5, 8]. To obtain this solution, one requires knowledge of the single-sided reflection response $R(s)$ and the traveltime $t_d(x)$ of the direct wave to propagate from the acquisition location to the observation location x. This traveltime is given by

$$t_d(x)=\int_{x'=0}^{x}\frac{1}{c(x')}dx'. \tag{6}$$

Since the velocity of the medium is typically unknown, we prefer to solve the Marchenko equation as a function of t_d rather than as a function of x [8]. If we compare equations 1 and 6, it is clear that $\xi(x) = c_0 t_d(x)$. Hence, the solution of the Marchenko equation at t_d can also be interpreted as the wavefield at the stretched coordinate $\xi = c_0 t_d$. This interpretation allows us to compute the wavefield in the stretched coordinates without knowledge of the velocity. We refer to these wavefields as $\overline{p}^m(\xi,s)$, where superscript m has been added to denote the solution of the Marchenko equation. To solve the Marchenko equation, we have scaled the wavefields with respect to powerflux, following a particular normalization that has recently been proposed [15, 16]. The wavefields that are obtained in this way are related to the quantities as they occur in equation 2, according to

$$\overline{p}^m(\xi,s) = \sqrt{\frac{\overline{Z}(0)}{\overline{Z}(\xi)}}\,\overline{p}(\xi,s). \tag{7}$$

To validate equation 7, we have solved the Marchenko equation with powerflux normalization for the model that was shown in figure 1. We emphasize that no information other than the reflection response has been used to obtain this solution. The retrieved wavefield $\overline{p}^m(\xi,s)$ is shown in figure 4a. According to equation 7, this wavefield is related to the wavefield $\overline{p}(\xi,s)$, which we have computed in figure 3a, after multiplication with $\sqrt{\frac{\overline{Z}(0)}{\overline{Z}(\xi)}}$. We applied this multiplication to the wavefields in figure 3a and show the result in figure 4b. As expected, the wavefields in figures 4a and 4b are very similar, which becomes even more evident after subtraction, see figure 5.

To create the desired map between the reflectivity and the reflection data at $\xi = 0$, we substitute equation 7 into equation 2, leading to

$$\overline{p}(\xi,s) - \overline{p}^{inc}(\xi,s) = \int_{\mathbb{D}} \frac{\partial \overline{G}(\xi-\xi',s)}{\partial \xi}\,\overline{p}^m(\xi',s)\,\overline{\chi_r}'(\xi')\,d\xi'. \tag{8}$$

In this representation, we have defined a rescaled reflectivity contrast $\overline{\chi_r}'(\xi)$, according to

$$\overline{\chi_r}'(\xi) := \sqrt{\frac{\overline{Z}(\xi)}{\overline{Z}(0)}}\,\overline{\chi}_r(\xi) = \sqrt{\frac{1}{\overline{Z}(\xi)\overline{Z}(0)}}\,\frac{\partial \overline{Z}(\xi)}{\partial \xi}. \tag{9}$$

In figure 2c, we show the rescaled reflectivity of the medium that we studied before. Based on equation 8, we can define the following Marchenko modeling operator:

$$\mathscr{M}\{\overline{\chi_r'}\}(\xi,s) := \int_{\mathbb{D}} \frac{\partial \overline{G}(\xi-\xi',s)}{\partial \xi}\,\overline{p}^m(\xi',s)\,\overline{\chi_r}'(\xi')\,d\xi'. \tag{10}$$

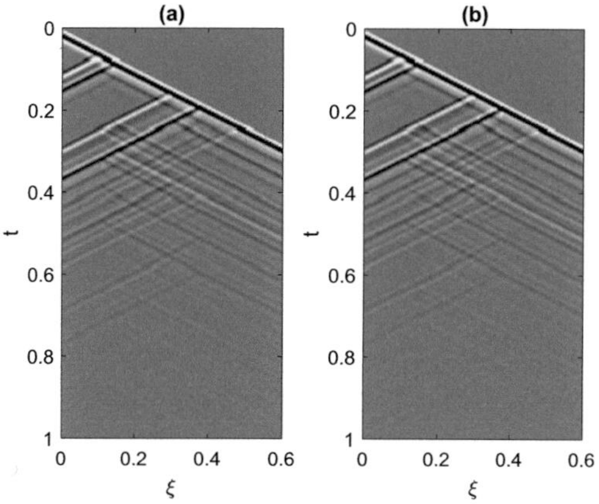

Figure 4: (a) Wavefield $\overline{p}^m(\xi,s)$ as retrieved by the Marchenko equation (converted to the time domain). (b) Rescaled wavefield $\sqrt{\frac{\overline{Z}(0)}{\overline{Z}(\xi)}}\overline{p}(\xi,s)$ (converted to the time domain).

Since $\overline{p}^m(\xi',s)$ can be computed directly from the reflection data by solving the Marchenko equation, this operator can be realized without direct access to the medium properties. By evaluating $\mathscr{M}\{\overline{\chi_r'}\}(\xi,s)$ at $\xi=0$, we propose the following inverse problem akin to equation 5:

$$\overline{R}(s)=\mathscr{M}\{\overline{\chi_r}'\}(0,s). \tag{11}$$

This linear problem can be solved for the rescaled reflectivity contrast $\overline{\chi_r}'$. This is demonstrated in figure 6a. Note the close match with the reflectivity profile in figure 2c. Now that the reflectivity contrast is known, we can compute the wavefield $\overline{p}(\xi,s)$ throughout the medium by evaluation of $\mathscr{M}\{\overline{\chi_r}'\}(\xi,s)$ (given the retrieved values of $\overline{\chi_r}'(\xi)$). The constructed wavefield $\overline{p}(\xi,s)$ can be compared with $\overline{p}^m(\xi,s)$. If we deconvolve these wavefields at each stretched coordinate ξ individually, an estimate of $\sqrt{\frac{\overline{Z}(0)}{\overline{Z}(\xi)}}$ can be obtained, see equation 7. By squaring the estimated values of $\sqrt{\frac{\overline{Z}(0)}{\overline{Z}(\xi)}}$, dividing by $\overline{Z}(0)$ and taking the inverse, the acoustic impedance $\overline{Z}(\xi)$ can be found. In figure 6b, we show that this procedure does indeed allow us to find the impedance profile of the medium in stretched space. Finally, we note that the retrieved reflectivity $\overline{\chi_r}'(\xi)$ and impedance $\overline{Z}(\xi)$ profiles in stretched space can be transformed to reflectivity and impedance profiles in physical space if an estimate of the velocity $c(x)$ is available.

6 Discussion

The extension of the proposed methodology to three-dimensional media remains an open question. For laterally invariant media, it is relatively straightforward to decompose wavefields in

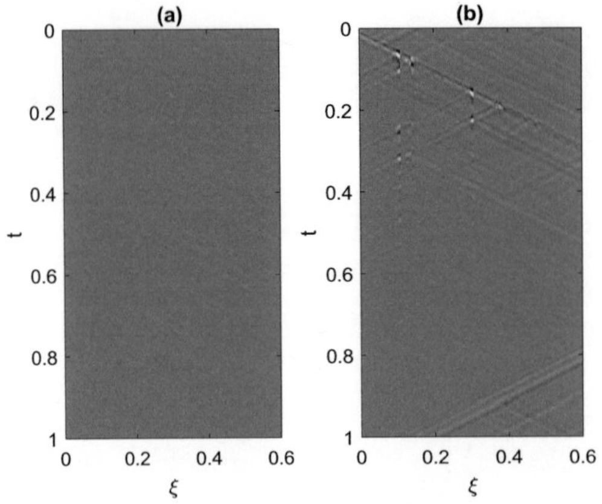

Figure 5: Difference between figures 4a and 4b, plotted (a) at the same colorscale and (b) after amplification with a factor 10.

terms of rayparameters and to solve a one-dimensional Marchenko equation for each rayparameter individually [8]. For laterally varying media with smoothly curved interfaces, the Marchenko equation can be solved in physical space [5], given that the velocity model (or an estimate thereof) is known *a priori*. The need for a velocity model is two-fold. First, the velocity is required to impose the causality conditions that undergird the Marchenko equation. Second, the velocity is required to project the solutions of the Marchenko equation into physical space. From practical experience, we have realized that the causality conditions can often still be successfully applied without accurate velocity information [17]. However, these estimates can no longer be projected to the correct spatial coordinates in this case.

Stretched coordinates may provide a useful framework to solve the Marchenko equation in the future. As we have demonstrated, the one-dimensional Marchenko equation projects its solutions directly to the stretched coordinates of a one-dimensional medium. If a proper three-dimensional extension of the stretching transform could be developed, it might be possible to formulate a multidimensional Marchenko equation that projects its solutions into these stretched coordinates with no or limited information on the propagation velocity. The development of such a stretching transform is the main direction of our current research.

7 Conclusion

Wavefields in a one-dimensional acoustic medium can be retrieved in a stretched coordinate system by solving a Marchenko equation. This solution requires no information other than a single-sided reflection response of the medium. The retrieved wavefields are related to the pressure fields that are found in a stretched integral representation, apart from a scaling factor ($\sqrt{Z(0)/Z(\xi)}$). By substituting the solutions of the Marchenko equation into the stretched

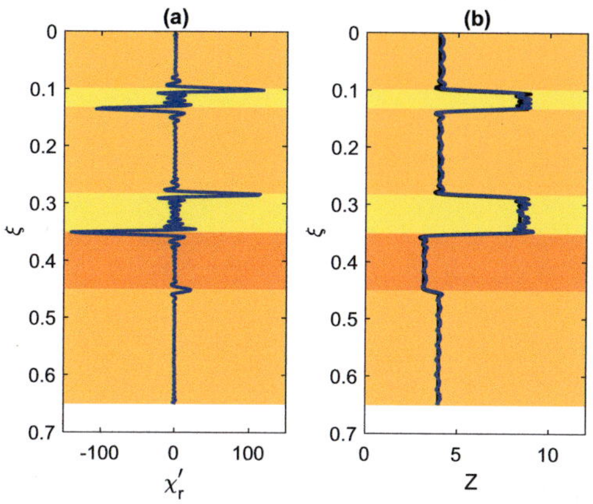

Figure 6: (a) Retrieved (rescaled) reflectivity contrast $\overline{\chi_r}'(\xi)$ (in blue) by inversion of equation 5, using the wavefields that were retrieved from the reflection response by solving the Marchenko equation. (b) Retrieved impedance $\overline{Z}(\xi)$ (in blue) versus the true impedance values in the medium (in black).

integral representation, we establish a linear relation between the reflectivity in stretched space and the recorded data. This relation can be used to invert for the reflectivity. Once the reflectivity is found, the pressure field can be computed throughout the medium by evaluating the integral representation. By comparing the result with the original solution of the Marchenko equation, the scaling factor ($\sqrt{\overline{Z}(0)/\overline{Z}(\xi)}$) can be found. From this scaling factor, one can easily compute the impedance in stretched space, as we have demonstrated.

8 Acknowledgments

We acknowledge Evert Slob and Peter van den Berg (Delft University of Technology) for fruitful discussions, which have contributed to this paper.

References

[1] N. Ozmen, R. Dapp, M. Zapf, H. Gemmeke, N. V. Ruiter, K. W. van Dongen: Comparing different ultrasound imaging methods for breast cancer detection. IEEE Transactions on ultrasonics, ferroelectrics and frequency control 62 (2015) 637-646

[2] J. Virieux, S. Operto: An overview of full-waveform inversion in exploration geophysics. Geophysics 74 (2009) WCC127-WCC152

[3] A. Tarantola: Linearized inversion of seismic reflection data. Geophysical Prospecting 32 (1984) 998-1015

[4] P. M. van den Berg and R. E. Kleinman: A constrast source inversion method. Inverse Problems 13 (1997) 1607-1620

[5] K. Wapenaar, F. Broggini, E. Slob, R. Snieder: Three-dimensional single-sided Marchenko inverse scattering, data-driven focusing, Green's function retrieval, and their mutual relations. Physical Review Letters 110 (2013) 084301

[6] R. Burridge: The Gel'fand-Levitan, the Marchenko and the Gopinath-Sondhi integral equations of inverse scattering theory, regarded in the context of inverse impulse-response problems. Wave Motion 2 (1980) 305-323

[7] J. H. Rose: Singe-sided autofocusing of sound in layered materials. Inverse Problems 18 (2002) 1923-1934

[8] E. Slob, K. Wapenaar, F. Broggini, R. Snieder: Seismic reflector imaging using internal multiples with Marchenko-type equations. Geophysics 79 (2014) S63-S76

[9] J. T. Fokkema, P. M. van den Berg: Stretched backgrounds for acoustic scattering models. Journal of Computational Physics 231 (2012) 1728-1742

[10] J. G. Berryman: Inverse methods for elastic waves in stratified media. Journal of Applied Physics 50 (1979) 6742-6744

[11] R. G. Newton: Inversion of reflection data for layered media: A review of exact methods. Geophysical Journal of the Royal Astronomical Society 65 (1981) 191-215

[12] S. Coen: The inverse problem of the shear modulus and density profiles. Journal of Geophysical Research 86 (1981) 6052-6056

[13] A. M. Bruckstein, B. C. Levy, T. Kailath: Differential methods in inverse scattering. SIAM Journal of Applied Mathematics 45 (1985) 312-335

[14] E. Slob, K. Wapenaar: Data-driven inversion of GPR surface reflection data for lossless layered media. The 8th European Conference on Antennas and Propagation (2014) 3378-3382

[15] J. Brackenhoff: Rescaling of incorrect source strength using Marchenko redatuming. MSC dissertation, Delft University of Technology (2016)

[16] J. van der Neut, J. Brackenhoff, M. Staring, L. Zhang, S. de Ridder, E. Slob, K. Wapenaar: Single- and double-sided Marchenko imaging conditions in acoustic media. IEEE Transactions on Computational Imaging *(in press)*

[17] F. Broggini, R. Snieder, K. Wapenaar: Data-driven wave field focusing and imaging with multidimensional deconvolution: numerical examples for reflection data with internal multiples. Geophysics 79 (2014) WA107-WA115

Ultrasound imaging from reflection data

Frank Natterer

Department of Mathematics and Computer Science, University of Münster, Münster, Germany

Abstract

This paper is concerned with wave equation reflection imaging for source pulses that do not have low frequencies. It is well known that the lack of these low frequencies causes serious difficulties in the image reconstruction. We show that under favorable circumstances good images can be obtained nevertheless by a data completion procedure.

Keywords: Reflection imaging, Spectrally incomplete data, Analytic continuation

1 Introduction

One of the biggest difficulties in seismic reflection imaging is the lack of low frequencies in the source pulses. As is well known (see e. g. [1], [5]) and well understood in a mathematical context (see [12], [6], [10]) this makes it impossible to quantitatively recover the the velocity distribution. Recently much effort has been put into using sources which have a relevant amount of low frequencies [3]. Corresponding problems occur in medical ultrasound if it is based on reflection measurements only.

In the present note we study a purely mathematical approach which does not require extra measurements at low frequencies. We rather use a data completion procedure to synthesize the missing low frequency data. Our method is some sort of analytic continuation in the spirit of the work of Landau, Slepian and Pollak [11]. It is clear that one can't expect miracles from such an approach due to the inherent instabilty of analytic continuation. However, we shall demonstrate by numerical estimates of the eigenvalues of the extension operator and by numerical simulation that quantitatively correct images can be reconstructed with acceptable stability, provided the range of missing frequencies is not too large. We closely follow [10].

The outline of the paper is as follows. In the next section we solve the inverse scattering problem for the wave equation with sources and receivers on a horizontal plane in the Born approximation. It is shown that the Fourier transform of the velocity distribution is determined

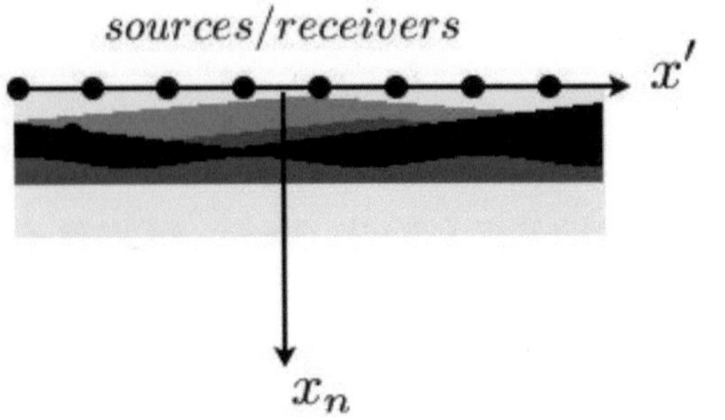

Figure 1: Sources and receivers are sitting on the plane/line x_n=0.

by these reflection data outside a torus of radius k with a circle of radius k around the origin in the horizontal plane as axis. This fact was recognized long ago by Wu and Toksöz [12] and Mora [6]. An elegant way to see this is the plane wave decomposition of the free space Green's function, as was done in [2], [8]. In section 3 we describe the data completion process by a second kind integral equation. The spectrum of the integral operator reveals the same dichotomy as the operators in the Landau-Slepian-Pollak theory [11]. By computing the largest eigenvalue numerically we find the spatial and frequency ranges for which the second kind integral equation can be solved with acceptable stability. In section 5 we present a numerical example from mammography.

2 The inverse scattering problem and Fourier analysis

We study the following inverse problem: Consider the initial value problem of the wave equation

$$\frac{\partial^2 u}{\partial t^2}(x,t) = c(x)^2(\Delta u(x,t) + \delta(x-s)q(t)) \text{ for } t > 0, x \in R^n, \tag{1}$$

$$u = 0 \text{ for } t < 0. \tag{2}$$

Here, $c = c(x)$ is the sought-for speed of sound in the medium which is situated in the half space $x_n > 0$, $n = 2,3$. We assume that with a known constant background speed c_0, $c^2 = c_0^2/(1+f)$ with a certain function f. $s = (s',0)^\top, r = (r',0)^\top$ denote sources and receivers, resp., sitting on $x_n = 0$, and q is the source pulse which vanishes for $t < 0$. The inverse problems consists in finding c, i. e. f, from the measurements of $u(x,t)$ for all s, r on $x_n = 0$, $t > 0$; see Fig. 1.

In the following we make frequent use of the Fourier transform in R^n, for which we use the notation

$$\hat{f}(\xi) = (2\pi)^{-n/2} \int_{R^n} e^{-ix\cdot\xi} f(x)dx \tag{3}$$

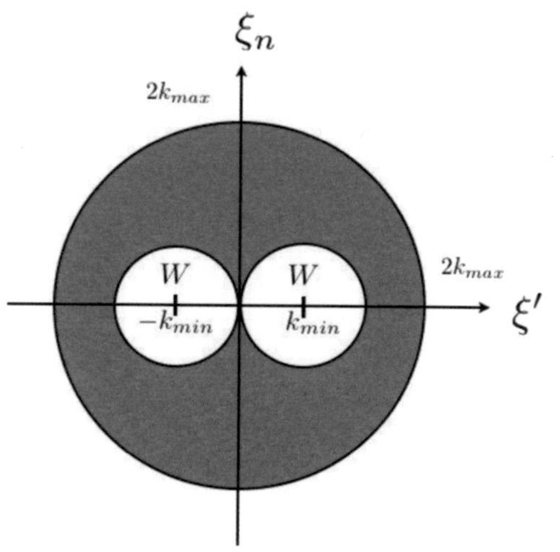

Figure 2: The Fourier transform $\hat{f}$ is determined by the data in the blue domain. For $n = 2$ this domain is the circle of radius $2k_{max}$, except for the two circles of radius k_{min} around $(\pm k_{min}, 0)$, which together make up the domain W. For $n = 3$ one has to rotate this picture around the ξ_n axis.

A 1D Fourier transform with respect to t takes (1,2) into

$$-\Delta u(x,\omega) - \frac{\omega^2}{c(x)^2} u(x,\omega) = \delta(x-s)\hat{q}(\omega) \tag{4}$$

which has to be complemented by the outgoing Sommerfeld radiation condition. For each source position s', each receiver position r' and each frequency ω we put $g_\omega(r',s') = u(r',0,\omega)$. This is our data function. It has been shown in [8] that, after linearisation the inverse problem is solved in the Born approximation by

$$\hat{f}(\rho' + \sigma', a(\rho') + a(\sigma')) = -\frac{c_0^2}{(2\pi)^{n/2}\gamma_n^2} \frac{\hat{g}_\omega(\rho',\sigma')}{\omega^2 \hat{q}(\omega)} a(\rho') a(\sigma') \tag{5}$$

where $a(\xi') = \sqrt{k^2 - |\xi'|^2}$, $k = \omega / c_0$, $\hat{g}$ is the $2(n-1)$ D Fourier transform of the data function with respect to r' and s', and $\gamma_n = 1/4\pi$ for $n = 2$ and $1/8\pi^2$ for $n = 3$. Assuming that $\hat{q}(\omega)$ is significantly different from 0 for $\omega_{min} \leq \omega \leq \omega_{max}$ we find that the nD Fourier transform $\hat{f}$ of f is determined by the data for ξ inside the circle of radius $2k_{max}$ and outside the domain W; Fig. 2. In the present context k_{max} is much bigger than k_{min} and can be considered as infinitely large.

3 Data completion

Let f be a function in R^n whose Fourier transform is known outside a domain W (e. g. the W depicted in Fig. 2). Then, by taking the inverse Fourier transform, we obtain

$$f(x) = (2\pi)^{-n/2} \int_W e^{ix\cdot\xi} \hat{f}(\xi) d\xi + (2\pi)^{-n/2} \int_{R^n \setminus W} e^{ix\cdot\xi} \hat{f}(\xi) d\xi .$$

The second term, which we denote by $f_W(x)$, is known. In the first term we express $\hat{f}(\xi)$ by the Fourier integral, obtaining

$$f(x) = (2\pi)^{-n} \int_{R^n} \int_W e^{i(x-y)\cdot\xi} f(y) d\xi dy + f_W(x).$$

Putting

$$K_W(x) = (2\pi)^{-n} \int_W e^{ix\cdot\xi} d\xi \tag{6}$$

this can be written as the second kind integral equation

$$f = \mathcal{K}_W f + f_W, \; (\mathcal{K}_W f)(x) = \int K_W(x-y) f(y) dy. \tag{7}$$

We consider this integral equation only in a domain B that contains the support of f. It is this integral equation on which our completion process is based. In principle it can be solved by the obvious iteration

$$f \leftarrow \mathcal{K}_W f + f_W . \tag{8}$$

A preliminary study has already been presented in [9]. Integral equations of this type occur in the Landau-Slepian-Pollak theory [11]. In the simplest case n is 1 and W the interval $[-k,k]$. Then $K_W(x) = (k/\pi)\text{sinc}(kx)$ and the integral equation is considered in the interval $B = [-r,r]$. For this case the integral operator has been carefully studied in [11]. Its eigenfunctions turn out to be the prolate spheroidal wave functions, and the eigenvalues are all in $(0,1)$, with about $2kr/\pi$ of them being virtually 1, the other ones virtually 0. From this it is clear that the solution of integral equation such as (7), although unique, is very unstable.

However, due to the special geometry of the set W in Fig. 2 we obtain a much more favorable result. First we compute the kernel function K_W (6) for the set W from Fig. 2. From the formula

$$\int_{|\xi|<k} e^{ix\cdot\xi} d\xi = (2\pi)^{n/2} k^n \frac{J_{n/2}(k|x|)}{(k|x|)^{n/2}}$$

(see e. g. formulas VII.1.2 and VII.1.3 in [7]) we conclude that for $n = 2$

$$K_W(x) = 2(2\pi)^{-1} k_{min}^2 \cos(k_{min} x') \frac{J_1(k_{min}|x|)}{k_{min}|x|} .$$

where J_1 is the first kind Bessel function of order 1.

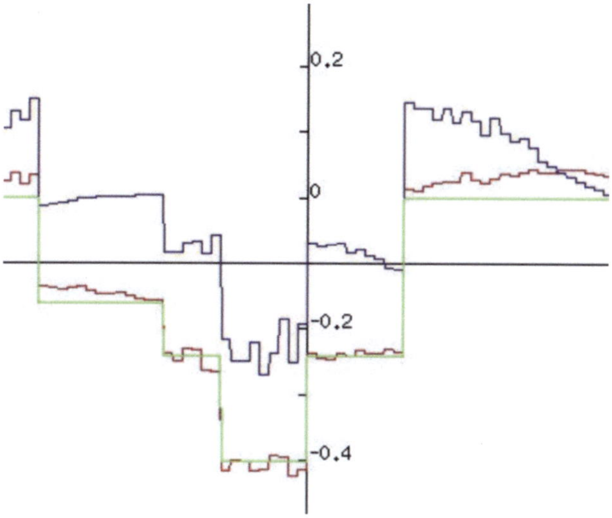

Figure 3: Vertical cross sections through center of original 2D structure from Fig. 1 (green), without completion process (blue), and final result (red) after 15 iterations of the iteration (8).

4 Numerical experiments in seismics

We did some numerical experiments with the 2D seismic structure in Fig. 1 with wavelength 400 m and depth 2 km. We first computed f_W to show what one can obtain without data completion and corrupted it with 10% multiplicative Gaussian noise. With the corrupted f_W we did 15 steps of the iteration (8) using 0 as initial approximation. After 15 steps the iteration became stationary. Cross sections along the vertical axis in Fig. 1 of the original structure f (green), the corrupted structure f_W as obtained without the completion process (blue), and the final result (red) are displayed in Fig. 3. It is obvious that the improvement achieved by the completion procedure is substantial.

5 Numerical experiments in mammography

We created a breast phantom patterned after the Salt Lake City breast phantom [4], adjusted to pure reflection imaging, with the patient in supine position, see Fig. 4. We used 20 sources, with frequencies from 15 kHz to 1MHz. The ambient speed of sound was taken to be 1500 m/sec. Thus the wave length was 1.5 mm, hence the expected resolution 0.75 mm. The tumors have a diameter of 0.75 mm. As can be seen from Fig. 4 the tumors are clearly resolved, even with the correct speed of sound. The reconstruction has been done by the Kaczmarz method with 5 sweeps.

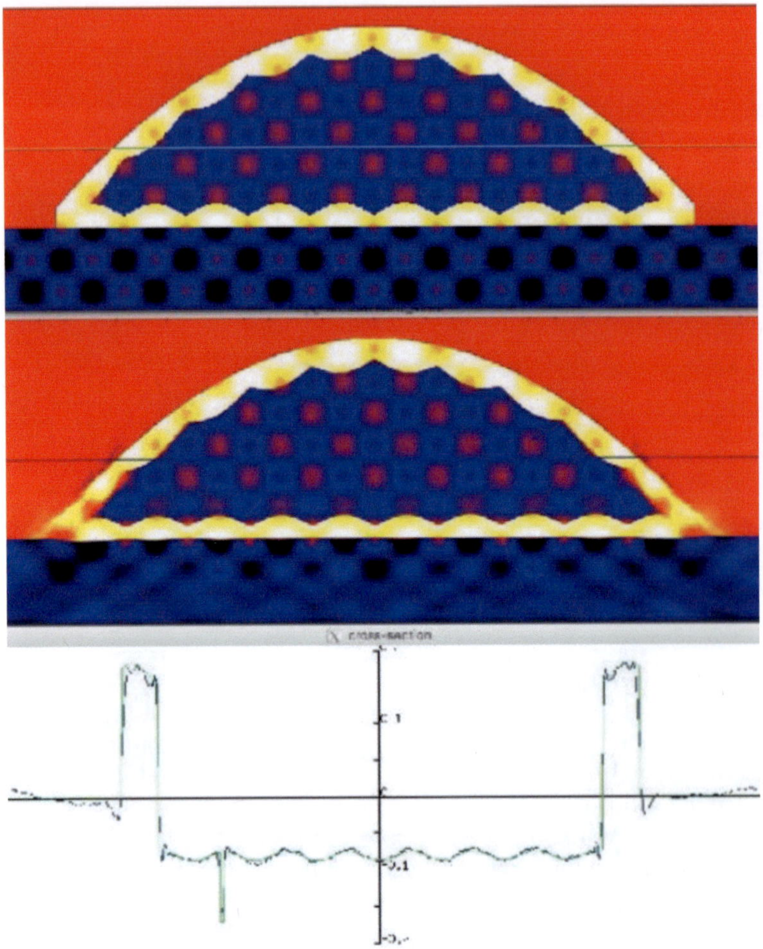

Figure 4: Top: Salt Lake City breast phantom. Middle: Reconstruction. 20 sources are sitting on the top boundary. Bottom: Horizontel cross sections through original (green) and reconstruction (blue). Width 20 cm, height 7.5 cm.

References

[1] Claerbout, J. F.: Imaging the Earth's Interior, Blackwell Sci. Publ. (1985).

[2] Devaney, A. J.: A filtered backpropagation algorithm for diffraction tomography, Ultrasonic Imaging **4**, 336-350 (1982).

[3] Dragoset, B. and Gabitsch, J.: Introduction to this special section: Low-frequency seismic, The Leading Edge **26**, 34-36 (2007).

[4] Duric, N. et al.: Development of ultrasound tomography for breast imaging:Technical assessment. Medical Physics **32**, 1375-1386 (2005).

[5] Jannane, M. et al.: Wavelengths of earth structures that can be resolved from seismic reflection data, Geophysics **54** 906-910 (1989).

[6] Mora, P.: Inversion = migration + tomography, Geophysics **54**, 1575-1586 (1989).

[7] Natterer, F.: The Mathematics of Computerized Tomography. Wiley-Teubner 1986, reprinted as Classics in Applied Mathematics vol. **32**, SIAM 2001.

[8] Natterer, F.: Ultrasound tomography with fixed linear arrays of transducers, Pubblicazioni del CentroDe Giorgi, Proceedings of the Interdisciplinary Workshop on Mathematical Methods in Biomedical Imaging and Intensity-Modulated Radiation Therapy (IMRT), Pisa, Italy, October 2007.

[9] Natterer, F.: Incomplete data problems in wave equation imaging, Inverse Problems and Imaging (IPI) **4**, 685-691 (2010).

[10] Natterer, F. Reflection imaging without low frequencies. Inverse Problems **27**, 035011 (2011).

[11] Slepian, D.: Some comments on Fourier analysis, uncertainty and modeling, SIAM Review **25**, 379-393 (1983).

[12] Wu, R. and Toksöz, M. N.: Diffraction tomography and multisource holography applied to seismic imaging, Geophysics **52**,11-25 (1987)

Using a 2-D approximation of the 3-D incident field for Born inversion

U. Taskin, L. Heijnsdijk, L. Hoogerbrugge, and K.W.A. van Dongen

Delft University of Technology, Delft, the Netherlands
E-mail: u.taskin@tudelft.nl

Abstract

Ultrasound imaging and inversion is successfully used in many biomedical applications. Currently, there is a growing interest for full-wave form inversion for breast cancer detection as it allows for a quantitative reconstruction of the acoustic medium properties of breast tissue. However, it remains a challenge to do inversion on real measurement data. Because 3-D inversion is computationally demanding, the inversion is often limited to 2-D. To overcome problems that occur because of this reduction in dimensions, different approaches are used to compute the incident field which serves often as input for the reconstruction algorithms. In this work, we compute a 2-D approximation of the 3-D incident field and use it for 2-D Born inversion. This approach provides a better reconstruction as compared to commonly used approaches for computing the incident field.

Keywords: Imaging, Born inversion, incident field correction, breast ultrasound

1 Introduction

Ultrasound has shown to be a successful technique for imaging the interior of the human body. Reconstructing the speed of sound profile from the measured wave fields is a nonlinear inverse problem for which there are many solution methods available [1]. Born inversion (BI) is a commonly used method where the nonlinear inversion problem is linearized by making the assumption that the total amount of scattering is limited. This approximation is valid for most biomedical applications and it significantly reduces the computational complexity [2].

In a real ultrasound measurement system, acoustic waves show 3-D propagation characteristics. However, in a majority of recently developed wave based imaging methods, the inverse problem is solved in a 2-D framework due to computational restrictions. This reduction causes problems during the inversion of real data. In this work, we address this problem and propose a new approach to compute the incident field which typically serves as input for inversion. In particular, we use a 2-D approximation for the measured 3-D incident field and show that using this approximated incident field for Born inversion improves the resulting reconstruction.

In section 2 we first explain Born inversion. Next, we formulate a 2-D approximation of the 3-D incident field using Hankel functions. In section 3, we present the results obtained with Born inversion using four different approaches to compute the incident field. Finally, a discussion about the obtained results and a conclusion is provided in section 4.

2 Theory

Let us consider an unknown scattering object embedded in a homogeneous medium as illustrated in Figure 1. The objects are located inside the spatial domain $\mathbb{D}$. This domain is enclosed by receivers located in $\mathbb{S}$ and sources in $\mathbb{S}'$. Acoustic wave fields that propagate in the 3-D spatial domain $\mathbb{D}$ satisfy the Helmholtz equation

$$\nabla^2 \hat{p}(\boldsymbol{x}) + \frac{\omega^2}{c^2(\boldsymbol{x})}\hat{p}(\boldsymbol{x}) = -\hat{S}(\boldsymbol{x}), \tag{1}$$

where $\hat{p}(\boldsymbol{x})$ is the acoustic pressure field, $\hat{S}(\boldsymbol{x})$ is the primary source, ω is the angular frequency, $c(\boldsymbol{x})$ is the speed of sound profile of the medium, and $\boldsymbol{x}$ is the location in Cartesian coordinates. The pressure field $\hat{p}(\boldsymbol{x})$ can be decomposed into an incident field $\hat{p}^{\mathrm{inc}}(\boldsymbol{x})$ which is generated by the source and propagates in the homogeneous embedding, and a scattered field $\hat{p}^{\mathrm{sct}}(\boldsymbol{x})$ which equals

$$\hat{p}^{\mathrm{sct}}(\boldsymbol{x}) = \omega^2 \int_{\boldsymbol{x}'\in\mathbb{D}} \hat{G}(\boldsymbol{x}-\boldsymbol{x}')\chi(\boldsymbol{x}')\hat{p}(\boldsymbol{x}')\mathrm{d}V, \tag{2}$$

where $\hat{G}(\boldsymbol{x}-\boldsymbol{x}')$ is the Green's function and $\chi(\boldsymbol{x}')$ is the contrast function given by

$$\chi(\boldsymbol{x}') = \frac{1}{c^2(\boldsymbol{x}')} - \frac{1}{c_0^2}. \tag{3}$$

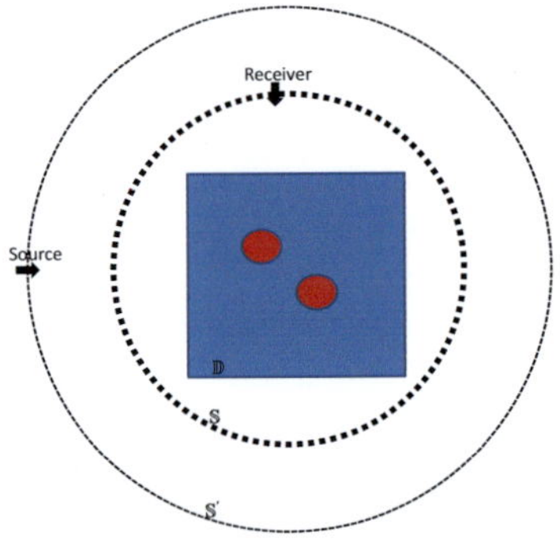

Figure 1: Schematic representation of system geometry.

Under the assumption that the scattering in the domain $\mathbb{D}$ is weak, the total field inside the integral in equation (2) can be approximated by the incident field. This linearization is known as the Born approximation. After the Born approximation, the scattered field equals

$$\hat{p}^{\mathrm{sct}}_{Born}(\boldsymbol{x}) = \omega^2 \int_{\boldsymbol{x}' \in \mathbb{D}} \hat{G}(\boldsymbol{x}-\boldsymbol{x}')\chi(\boldsymbol{x}')\hat{p}^{\mathrm{inc}}(\boldsymbol{x}')\mathrm{d}V, \tag{4}$$

The linearized integral equation (4) can be solved for the unknown contrast function $\chi(\boldsymbol{x}')$ by using iterative solution methods [2, 3].

When the measurement is done in 3-D and the inversion in 2-D, problems occur in the reconstruction due to an erroneous description of the incident field. In the next section, we describe how the incident field is constructed such that the resulting field satisfies the 2-D wave equation while still showing some of the 3-D radiation characteristics.

2.1 Incident field approximation

To describe the incident field in two dimensions, we start with the 2-D Helmholtz equation in polar coordinates, viz.

$$r^2\frac{\partial^2 \hat{p}(r,\phi)}{\partial r^2} + r\frac{\partial \hat{p}(r,\phi)}{\partial r} + r^2\frac{\omega^2}{c_0^2}\hat{p}(r,\phi) + \frac{\partial^2 \hat{p}(r,\phi)}{\partial \phi^2} = 0. \tag{5}$$

As Hankel functions satisfy the 2-D wave equation, the incident pressure field may be approximated as [4]

$$\hat{p}^{inc}_{approx}(r,\phi,\omega) = \sum_{n=-N}^{N} c_n(\omega) H_n^{(1)}\left(\frac{\omega}{c_0}r\right) e^{in\phi}, \tag{6}$$

where $H_n^{(1)}$ are Hankel functions of the first kind with the corresponding coefficients $c_n(\omega)$. To find the coefficients $c_n(\omega)$, we iteratively minimize the L_2-norm of the mismatch Δ between the measured and approximated field, hence

$$||\Delta||^2_{\mathbb{S}} = ||p^{inc}_{3-D}(\omega) - p^{inc}_{approx}(r_m,\phi_m,\omega)||^2_{\mathbb{S}}, \tag{7}$$

with p^{inc}_{3-D} the incident field satisfying the 3-D wave equation, and r_m and ϕ_m pointing to each receiver location. In this way, we may find an incident wave field that satisfies the 2-D wave equation and at the same time shows a large resemblance with the actual 3-D incident wave field. Once the coefficients are found, the approximated 2-D incident field is computed from equation (6) and used for Born inversion.

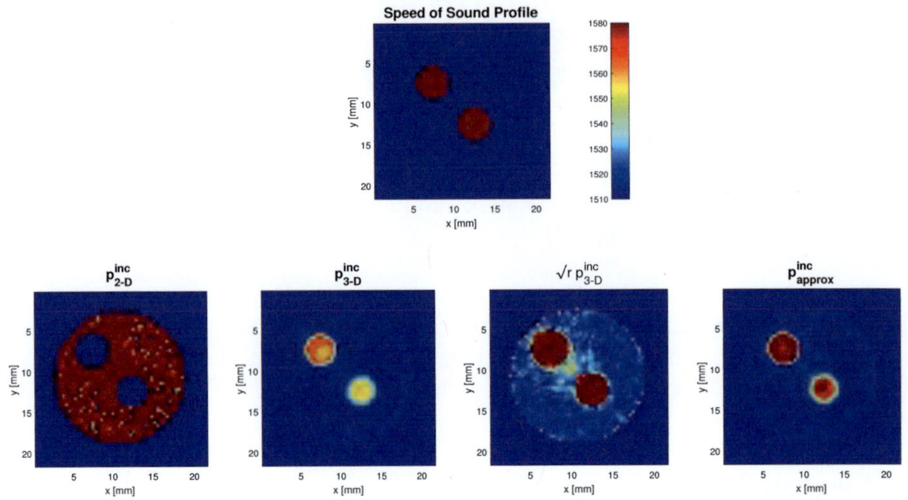

Figure 2: Original (top) and reconstructed (bottom) speed of sound profiles. The reconstructed profiles are obtained with Born inversion using four different incident fields.

3 Results

To test the proposed approach, we first solve the forward problem in 3-D for a circular array, containing point sources and point receivers, scanning a cylindrical and a spherical object. Next, we use a 2-D Born inversion method to reconstruct the acoustic medium properties and compare the resulting reconstructions obtained using four different approaches. These four approaches are based on computing the incident field using (1) an infinite line source (p^{inc}_{2-D}), (2) a point source (p^{inc}_{3-D}), (3) a point source followed by a correction to compensate for geometrical spreading ($\sqrt{r}p^{inc}_{3-D}$), and (4) a point source followed by the proposed method to approximate the field using Hankel functions (p^{inc}_{approx}).

3.1 Configuration

Synthetic 3-D data is obtained by solving the forward problem using the full-wave method proposed in [5]. The outer circular array has a radius of 15 mm and contains 20 point sources equally distributed. The inner circular array has a radius of 10 mm and contains 150 receivers. The spherical object has a radius of 2 mm while the cylindrical object has a radius of 2 mm with 20 mm of height. The spatial computational domain of 20 mm $\times$ 20 mm $\times$ 20 mm is discretized with a grid size of 0.37 mm. Sources and receivers are located in the plane $z = 10$ mm. The speed of sound of the embedding is $c_0 = 1510$ m/s and the contrast is $c = 1580$ m/s.

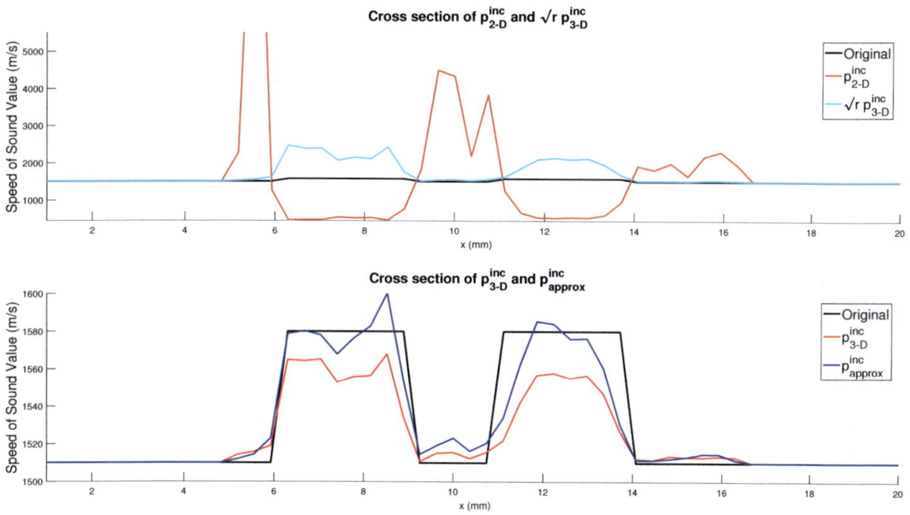

Figure 3: Cross-section of the speed of sound profiles.

The 2-D Born inversion is tested for the four different incident field approximations, using the same measurement data for each case. Two frequencies (0.5 MHz and 0.75 MHz) are used for Born inversion to get accurate results. The reconstruction is done in the plane $z = 10$ mm.

3.2 Born Inversion Results

The applicability of the proposed approach to compute the incident field is investigated by using 2-D Born inversion. The reconstructed speed of sound profiles are displayed in Figure 2. It is shown in the reconstruction results that using the 2-D incident field (p^{inc}_{2-D}) is the worst approach among the other approaches used in this work. With the 3-D incident field (p^{inc}_{3-D}), the cylindrical object is reconstructed successfully but problems occur for the spherical object. Multiplying the 3-D incident field with $\sqrt{r}$ ($\sqrt{r}p^{inc}_{3-D}$) to correct for geometrical spreading gives rise to a noisy reconstruction in which the objects are still clearly recognisable but with wrong amplitudes. Finally, using the proposed formulation for the incident field (p^{inc}_{approx}) gives the best result with respect to amplitude of the contrast and noise in the image.

To show how accurate the reconstructed speed of sound values are, cross-sections of the reconstructed speed of sound profiles along the diagonal is given in Figure 3. With p^{inc}_{2-D} and $\sqrt{r}p^{inc}_{3-D}$ the boundaries and the locations of the objects are determined correctly, but with wrong amplitudes for the speed of sound. The reconstructions improve significantly when using p^{inc}_{3-D} and p^{inc}_{approx}, where p^{inc}_{approx} outperforms p^{inc}_{3-D}.

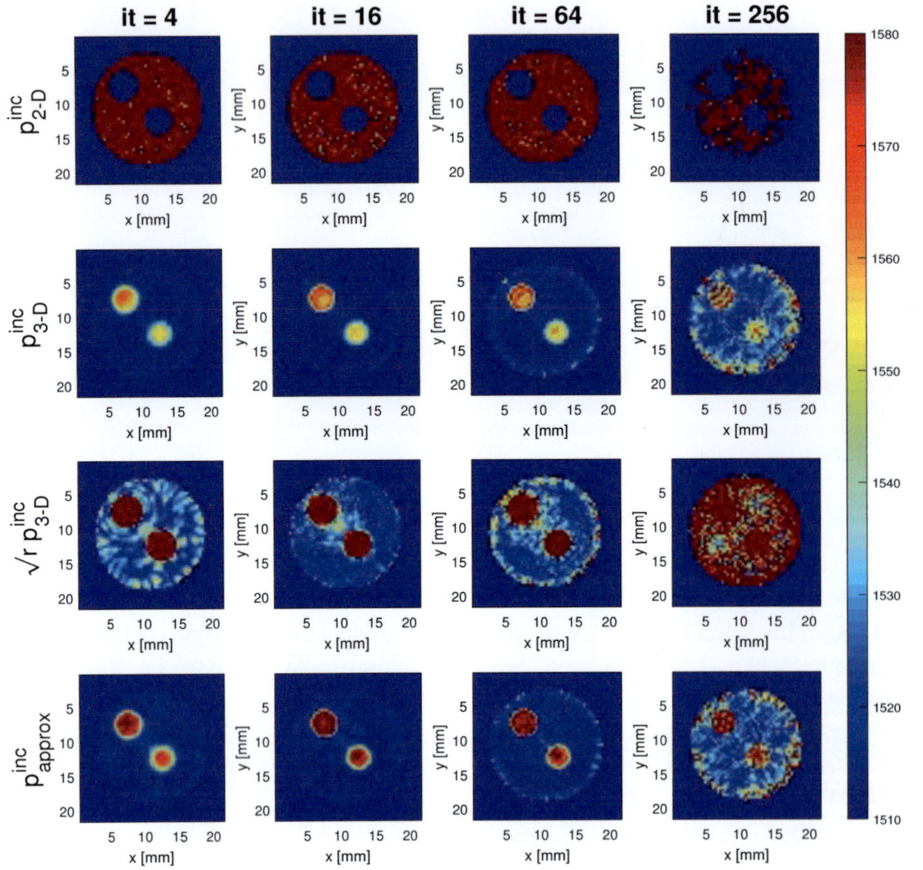

Figure 4: Born inversion results for four different incident fields and for increasing number of iterations.

Finally, Born inversion results at four different iteration numbers (it = 4, 16, 64, and 256) for the four approaches are presented in Figure 4. In general, by comparing the results obtained for different number of iterations, the superiority of the proposed approach is clearly shown. Note that for all methods the reconstruction degrades significantly after a certain number of iterations. The main reason of this problem is that we use a full-wave method to compute the synthetic measurement while the inversion is done within Born approximation. This problem can be solved by using regularization techniques [6] or full-wave inversion methods [7].

4 Conclusion

In this work, a new approach is proposed for applying 2-D inversion on 3-D measurement data. This new approach approximates the incident field from the original 3-D incident field and uses this approximated incident field for inversion. Results with Born inversion show that this new approach provides a better reconstruction compared to the currently applied approaches.The correct speed of sound values can not be reconstructed with the 2-D incident field and the 3-D incident field multiplied by $\sqrt{r}$. The 3-D incident field is a better option compared to the previous ones but it has problems with an object which has 3-D characteristics.

Born inversion is a method with limitations because of the weak scatterer approximation. Problems are expected in the presence of strong scatterers. The proposed method can also be used with other wave based inversion methods. A full-wave inversion method can overcome the limitations one may encounter with Born inversion.

References

[1] N. Ozmen, R. Dapp, M. Zapf, H. Gemmeke, N. V. Ruiter, K.W.A. van Dongen.: Comparing different ultrasound imaging methods for breast cancer detection. IEEE Trans. Ultrason., Ferroelectr., Freq. Control 62(4) (2015) 637-646

[2] A. Abubakar, P. M. van den Berg, S. Y. Semenov.: A robust iterative method for Born inversion. IEEE Trans. Geosci. Remote Sens. 42(2) (2004) 342-354

[3] R. E. Kleinman, P. M. van den Berg.: Iterative Methods for solving integral equations. Radio Sci. 26(1) (1991) 175-181

[4] C. A. Balanis.: Advanced engineering electromagnetics. John Wiley & Sons (1999)

[5] K. W. A. van Dongen, W. M. D. Wright.: A forward model and conjugate gradient inversion technique for low-frequency ultrasonic imaging. J. Acoust. Soc. Am. 120(4) (2006) 2086-2095

[6] A. B. Ramirez, K. W. A. van Dongen.: Sparsity Constrained Born Inversion for Breast Cancer Detection. IEEE Ultrason. Symp. (2015) 1-4

[7] A. B. Ramirez, K. W. A. van Dongen.: Sparsity Constrained contrast source inversion. J. Acoust. Soc. Am. 140(3) (2016) 1749-1757

USCT Image Reconstruction: Acceleration using Gauss-Newton Preconditioned Conjugate Gradient

H. Wang[1], H. Gemmeke[2], T. Hopp[2], and J. Hesser[1]

[1] *Heidelberg University, Mannheim, Germany*
E-mail: hongjian.wang@medma.uni-heidelberg.de
[2] *Karlsruhe Institute of Technology, Karlsruhe, Germany*

Abstract

Ultrasound transmission tomography offers quantitative characterization of the tissue or materials by their speed of sound and attenuation. Reconstruction of such images is an inverse problem which is solved iteratively based on a forward model of the Helmholtz equation by paraxial approximation and thus is time-consuming. Hence, developing optimizers that decrease this time, in particular reducing the number of forward propagations is of high relevance in order to bring this technology into clinical practice. In this paper, we solve the inverse problem of reconstruction in a two-level strategy, by an outer and an inner loop. At each iteration of the outer loop, the system is linearized and this linear subproblem is solved in the inner loop with a preconditioned conjugate gradient (CG). A standard Cholesky preconditioning method based on the system matrix is compared with a matrix-free Quasi-Newton update approach, where a preconditioned matrix-vector product is computed at the beginning of every CG iteration. We also use a multigrid scheme with multi-frequency reconstruction to get a convergent rough reconstruction at a lower frequency and then refine it on a higher-resolution grid. The Cholesky preconditioning reduces the number of CG iterations by approx. 70%~85%; but the computation time for determining the system matrix for the Cholesky preconditioner is dominating, offsetting the gains of the reduction of iterations. The matrix-free preconditioning method saves approx. 30% of the computation time on average for single-frequency and multi-frequency reconstruction. For the robust multi-frequency reconstruction, we test three breast-like numerical phantoms resulting in a deviation of 0.13 m/s on average in speed of sound reconstruction and a deviation of 5.4% on average in attenuation reconstruction, from the ground truth simulation.

Keywords: Ultrasound transmission tomography, Preconditioning, Multigrid reconstruction

1 Introduction

Breast cancer diagnostics based on ultrasound computed tomography (USCT) promises high specificity for early cancer detection. Some 2D or 3D USCT devices [1] measure reflection and transmission tomography at the same time. Transmission tomography offers quantitative characterization of the imaged tissue or materials by speed of sound and attenuation profiles [2]. In this paper, we focus on the image reconstruction of transmission tomography based on the *Karlsruhe USCT* system [1].

For image reconstruction of transmission tomography, we consider the wave equation in the frequency domain. The Helmholtz equation models the wave propagation of ultrasound through an acoustic background medium including refraction, diffraction and multiple scattering as

$$\Delta p + {k_0}^2(1+\eta)^2 p = 0, \tag{1.1}$$

with the frequency dependent pressure field p. The acoustic medium is described by the background wave number $k_0 = \omega/c$ and the refractive index $1+\eta$, where $\omega = 2\pi f$ accounts for the angular frequency for frequency f and speed of sound (SoS) c of the background medium, and η accounts for the deviation of the SoS from the background medium. The full solution of the Helmholtz equation poses a very high computational burden. To mitigate this limitation for medical imaging, the paraxial approximation was chosen [3][4] which is fast enough to be applied for radiological and material diagnosis at the same day. The paraxial approximation describes the ultrasound field via nearly plane waves in forward direction. We use the wide-angle parabolic equation (WAPE) [5] and perform Lie-Trotter splitting [6] to the (formal) solution of the parabolic/paraxial approximation. The forward solution on the computational grid can be calculated by

$$p_{k+1} = e^{i\Delta z k_0 \eta_k} \cdot ifft\left\{e^{i\Delta z\sqrt{k_0^2-\xi^2}} \cdot fft(p_k)\right\}. \tag{1.2}$$

The index k at p and η denote the considered z slice, whereas the indices for the other directions are omitted. The spectral variable is denoted by ξ and the discrete Fourier transformations are denoted by *fft* and *ifft* in 1D or 2D, whether the problem is 2D or 3D respectively.

The image reconstruction consists of determining the distribution of SoS and attenuation which are both derived from η. To be specific, $\eta = a + i\frac{b}{\omega}$, where $Re(\eta) = a = \frac{c_0}{c} - 1$ describes the deviation in the SoS (c is the SoS in the object and c_0 in the background medium), and $Im(\eta) = \frac{b}{\omega}$ accounts for frequency dependent attenuation. Hence, we need to estimate the parameter η according to the forward model (1.2) given the measurements taken by the USCT system. This is known as an inverse problem usually provided as a nonlinear least-squares problem, and it is ill-posed due to the nonlinearity and the extremely large scale of the problem. Therefore, we use Newton type methods to linearize the problem together with preconditioned conjugate gradient (CG) method to solve the linearized system at every Newton iteration.

Iterative methods such as CG [8] and generalized minimal residual (GMRES) [14] are widespread to solve a sequence of linear systems that arise in Newton's framework, without forming the Jacobian matrices explicitly while the Jacobian-vector multiplications are approximated by the finite difference method. A challenge is to determine a preconditioner to accelerate the convergence of the Jacobian-free iterative methods. Existing preconditioning methods [15][16] require the full information of the Jacobian for the first outer iteration and the lower or upper triangular part of the Jacobian for each outer iteration. For large problems, it is still expensive to compute the Jacobian even for the first outer iteration. Moreover, if the Jacobian is dense or has some sparse structure, computing the lower or upper triangular part can be as expensive as computing the whole matrix [16]. On the other hand, few existing preconditioning techniques are truly "matrix-free", where neither the full nor the partial system matrix needs to be formed explicitly [17]. One example can be found in [9], where Morales and Nocedal proposed a preconditioner for CG which has the form of a limited memory Quasi-Newton matrix and is generated using information from CG iterations without requiring explicit knowledge of the system (Jacobian) matrix. Xu et al. [17] proposed an inner-iteration preconditioner based on the weighted Jacobi method, and used it for preconditioning the CGLS [18] and BA-GMRES [19] methods in a trust region framework. In this paper, we adopt the Quasi-Newton updating preconditioning techniques [9][10] for CG in our USCT image reconstruction task.

2 Methods

2.1 Gauss-Newton method

The reconstruction is defined by the least-squares problem on the squared L_2 norm of the residual

$$S(\eta) = \frac{1}{2}\|r(\eta)\|_2^2 , \tag{2.1}$$

where vector $r(\eta): \mathbb{C}^N \to \mathbb{C}^M$, called *residual vector*, is given by $r(\eta) = F(\eta) - p_d$. Here, $p_d \in \mathbb{C}^M$ are the measured pressure field from the USCT system, and $F(\eta): \mathbb{C}^N \to \mathbb{C}^M$ is the predicted pressure field computed according to the forward model of (1.2), i.e., $p = F(\eta)$. The unknowns $\eta \in \mathbb{C}^N$ are the parameters that we want to estimate for reconstruction. The derivatives of $S(\eta)$ can be expressed in terms of the *Jacobian* $J(\eta)$, which is the $M \times N$ matrix of the first partial derivatives of the residuals, defined by

$$J(\eta) = \left[\frac{\partial r_j}{\partial \eta_i}\right]_{\substack{j=1,2,\dots,M\\ i=1,2,\dots,N}} = [\nabla r_1(\eta)^T, \nabla r_2(\eta)^T, \dots, \nabla r_m(\eta)^T]^T. \tag{2.2}$$

The gradient and Hessian of $S(\eta)$ can then be expressed as follows:

$$\nabla S(\eta) = \textstyle\sum_{j=1}^{M} r_j(\eta) \nabla r_j(\eta) = J(\eta)^T r(\eta), \tag{2.3}$$

$$\nabla^2 S(\eta) = \textstyle\sum_{j=1}^{M} \nabla r_j(\eta) \nabla r_j(\eta)^T + \sum_{j=1}^{M} r_j(\eta) \nabla^2 r_j(\eta) = J(\eta)^T J(\eta) + \sum_{j=1}^{M} r_j(\eta) \nabla^2 r_j(\eta). \tag{2.4}$$

To minimize the nonlinear objective function $S(\eta)$ of (2.1), we use the Gauss-Newton (GN) method, which can be viewed as a modified Newton's method [7]. Instead of solving the standard Newton equations $\nabla^2 S(\eta_k) d_k = -\nabla S(\eta_k)$ for a search direction d_k (which can be overdetermined or underdetermined depending on N, M), we solve the following system, i.e. the normal equations, to obtain the search direction d_k^{GN}:

$$J_k^T J_k d_k^{GN} = -J_k^T r_k. \tag{2.5}$$

Here, the use of the approximation $\nabla^2 S_k \approx J_k^T J_k$ relieves us to compute individual residual Hessians $\nabla^2 r_j, j = 1,2, \dots, M$, which are needed in the second term in (2.4).

To solve the linearized system of (2.5), where the system matrix now corresponds to $J_k^T J_k$, we selected the conjugate gradient (CG) method [8] which does not need the system matrix explicitly but only matrix-vector products on both sides of the equation (2.5). Based on the forward model, we can formulate two iterative schemes for the evaluation of the derivative of the forward operator and its adjoint. They are respectively called the *sensitivity* operator F' and the *adjoint* operator F'^* in [4]: the former produces the product of J_k and its input vector while the latter produces the product of J_k^T and its input vector.

After the search direction d_k^{GN} is computed by the CG method, we would like to choose a step length α_k to give a substaintial reduction of S along this direction, but at the same time we do not want to spend too much time making this choice. The ideal choice would be the global minimizer of the univariate function $\phi(\alpha_k) = S(\eta_k + \alpha_k d_k^{GN})$. There is a closed-form solution for α_k if S is a simple quadratic function. In our case, however, S is much more complicated and to find even a local minimizer of ϕ requires many evaluations of S and possibly ∇S. Therefore, we use a practical backtracking line search method [7] to decide the step length α_k along the search direction d_k^{GN}. A general description of the iterative Gauss-Newton method follows.

Algorithm 2.1 (*Gauss-Newton method*)

Given initial solution η_0;
for $k = 0,1,2,\dots$
  Solve $J(\eta_k)^T J(\eta_k) d_k = -J(\eta_k)^T r_k$ for $d_k$by the conjugate gradient method;
  Find the step length α_k for d_k using line search;
  Set $\eta_{k+1} \leftarrow \eta_k + \alpha_k d_k$;
  if $MSE < GNtol$ **then** stop; **endif**   % *MSE stands for mean squared error.*
endfor

2.2 Preconditioners for the conjugate gradient method

For large-scale applications with symmetric system matrices, CG is usually used with preconditioners. A widely used and efficient preconditioner is the incomplete Cholesky preconditioning. The *Cholesky factorization* is a decomposition of a matrix A into the form $A = LL^T$, where L is a lower triangular matrix. Incomplete Cholesky factorization is a variant in which L might be restricted to have the same pattern of nonzero elements as A; other elements of L are ignored [8].

The incomplete Cholesky preconditioning is based on the system matrix while in our forward model computing and storing the Jacobian is expensive both in time and memory consumption. Moreover, when the matrix gets large, factorization is a nontrivial task even though the matrix is sparse. Therefore, matrix-free preconditioning techniques are preferable for our application. An elaborate and recent approach is through limited memory Quasi-Newton update [9][10] given the gradient function without forming the Hessian. This approach approximates the diagonal of the Hessian via Quasi-Newton updates as preconditioners, using information gathered and updated from CG iterations. The preconditioner does not require explicit knowledge of the system matrix and is therefore suitable for our application where only products of the system matrix times a vector can be computed.

Let us denote the problem of (2.5) as $Ax = b$ (i.e., $A = J_k^T J_k$, $x = d_k^{GN}$, $b = -J_k^T r_k$), which we use the preconditioned CG method to solve for the Gauss-Newton search direction x, i.e., d_k^{GN}. It is equivalent to the following optimization problem

$$minimize \quad q(x) = \frac{1}{2} x^T A x - b^T x. \tag{2.6}$$

The Quasi-Newton matrices are updated by means of the Broyden–Fletcher–Goldfarb–Shanno (BFGS) formula,

$$H^{(j+1)} = H^{(j)} + V_j^T H^{(j)} V_j + \theta_j y_j s_j^T \ , \tag{2.7}$$

where

$$V_j = I - \theta_j y_j s_j^T \ , \ \theta_j = 1/y_j^T s_j \ , \ s_j = x^{(j+1)} - x^{(j)} \ , \ y_j = \nabla q\left(x^{(j+1)}\right) - \nabla q\left(x^{(j)}\right). \tag{2.8}$$

The pair of vectors (s_j, y_j) is called a *correction pair*. Practically, we do not form the matrices $H^{(j)}$, but only store the correction pairs and the scalars θ_j, and then use a recursive formula as described in [11] to compute the product of $H^{(j)}$ and the CG residual vector. A general description of the preconditioned CG method with Quasi-Newton update preconditioner (PREQN) follows.

Algorithm 2.2 (*preconditioned CG method with PREQN preconditioner*)

Given $A_k, b_k, x^{(0)}$; *% Note that k means the number of iteration in the outer Gauss-Newton loop.*
$r^{(0)} = b_k - A_k x^{(0)}$;
for $j = 1,2,\ldots$
  Compute $z^{(j-1)} = H_k r^{(j-1)}$ using PREQN preconditioner routine;
  $\rho^{(j-1)} = r^{(j-1)^T} z^{(j-1)}$;
  if $j == 1$ **then** $p^{(1)} = z^{(0)}$;
  else $\beta^{(j-1)} = \rho^{(j-1)}/\rho^{(j-2)}$; $p^{(j)} = z^{(j-1)} + \beta^{(j-1)} p^{(j-1)}$; **endif**
  $\alpha^{(j)} = \rho^{(j-1)}/p^{(j)^T} A_k p^{(j)}$; $x^{(j)} = x^{(j-1)} + \alpha^{(j)} p^{(j)}$; $r^{(j)} = r^{(j-1)} - \alpha^{(j)} A_k p^{(j)}$;
  if $\|r^{(j)}\|_2 < CGtol$ **then** stop; **endif**
endfor

In Algorithm 2.2, only one call to the PREQN preconditioner routine is needed for each CG iteration. The routine is summarized as Algorithm 2.3.

Algorithm 2.3 (*PREQN preconditioner*)

Given $k, j, r^{(j-1)}, (s_{j-1}, y_{j-1})$; *% k is the number of iteration in the outer Gauss-Newton loop.*
% j is the number of iteration in the inner CG loop.
if $j > 1$ **then** decide if (s_{j-1}, y_{j-1}) is to be saved; **endif**
if $k == 1$ **then** $z^{(j-1)} = r^{(j-1)}$; *% No preconditioning for CG at the first outer iteration.*
else { **if** $j == 1$ **then** build preconditioner H_{k+1} ; **endif** } $z^{(j-1)} = H_k\, r^{(j-1)}$; **endif**

2.3 Multi-frequency reconstruction

Convergence for single-frequency reconstruction is only guaranteed if the typical size of the reconstructed object multiplied by the ultrasound frequency is smaller than a given constant [12]. If this condition is not fulfilled, the starting solution must be sufficiently near to the true solution; a simple starting solution like the average SoS in the object fails to converge. Therefore, if we want to reconstruct larger objects at higher frequencies, we can use a multi-frequency method. For each frequency, the problem is solved on a grid resolution that is matching the condition for the used frequency [12]. Firstly, we obtain a convergent rough reconstruction at a lower frequency. From this rough reconstruction with fewer parameters/pixels, we then interpolate a starting solution for the finer reconstruction with more parameters, which corresponds to the reconstruction at higher frequency. This starting solution should be close to the true solution for the high-frequency reconstruction, and hence using it we expect a convergent solution for the high-frequency reconstruction. A general description of our multi-frequency reconstruction follows.

Algorithm 2.4 (*Multi-frequency reconstruction*)

Given initial solution η_0, the starting frequency $f = f_{start}$, the maximum frequency f_{max};
for $i = 1,2,\ldots$
  $\eta_{i-1} = interpolation(\eta_{i-1})$; $\eta_i = reconstruction(\eta_{i-1})$;
  Increase f by $f = f * factor$;
  if $f > f_{max}$ **then** stop; **endif**
endfor

3 Results

In our simulated reconstruction tests, the measurements of pressure field p_d are modeled as $F(\eta_{exact})$ plus additive Gaussian noise characterized by the signal-to-noise ratio (SNR). By minimizing the least-squares problem (2.1), we obtain a solution η that approximates η_{exact}. Considering the robustness of reconstruction with noisy data, we also test Tikhonov regularization where instead of solving (2.5) by CG at every outer iteration (Gauss-Newton iteration), we solve $(J_k^T J_k + \lambda^2 I) d_k^{GN} = -J_k^T r_k$ where I is the identity matrix and λ is the Tikhonov regularization parameter determined by the L-curve method [13].

We firstly test the incomplete Cholesky preconditioning. We use the Matlab build-in function *ichol* to obtain the incomplete Cholesky factorization of the system matrix (Jacobian), as a preconditioner to the Matlab build-in conjugate gradient function *pcg*. We use the sensitivity operator F' to generate the complete Jacobian by giving it a series of input vectors $e_1 = [1,0,\dots]^T, e_2 = [0,1,\dots]^T, \dots, e_N$. Since the computation of the Jacobian is expensive, we do not apply it at every outer iteration, and a preconditioner generated at a given outer iteration is reused for multiple outer iterations. We test five different scenarios denoted as "preconditioner (*re*)", where *re* = {1, 5, 10, 20, and 1000} indicates that the preconditioner is updated after *re* outer iterations. So for example, "preconditioner (5)" means a new preconditioner is generated at every fifth outer iteration. Besides, we also test the situation without preconditioner. For all the six situations, we run four versions of our reconstruction algorithm: (1), (3) no regularization with data of SNR=60dB, SNR=40dB, resp.; (2), (4) Tikhonov regularization with data of SNR=60dB, SNR=40dB, resp. Therefore, we test 24 combinations in total and we report for each combination the sum of outer iterations (S_{outer}), the sum of CG iterations (S_{cg}), and the average CG iterations per outer iteration (S_{mean}), as shown in Figure 1. Note that $S_{mean} = S_{cg}/S_{outer}$. The results show that the incomplete Cholesky preconditioning can reduce about 70%~85% of the CG iterations. It can also reduce outer iterations. The preconditioner update rate, on the other hand, has almost trivial impact on CG iterations.

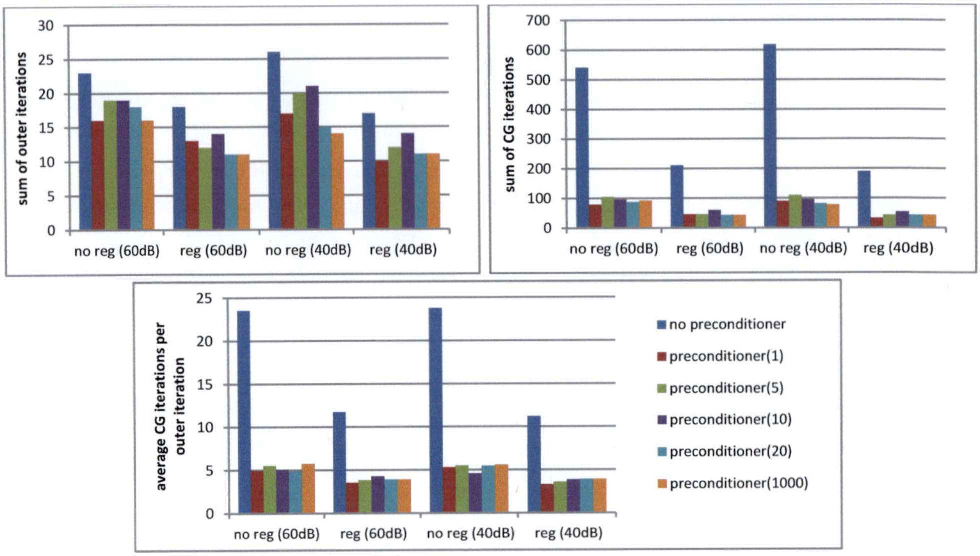

Figure 1: Test results for incomplete Cholesky preconditioning with and without regularization (reg) and at different SNR levels (60dB or 40dB). Upper left: the sum of outer iterations (S_{outer}). Upper right: the sum of CG iterations (S_{cg}). Bottom: the average CG iterations per outer iteration (S_{mean}).

Although the incomplete Cholesky preconditioning reduces CG iterations, it actually does not save computation time in our tests. This is because of the extra computation for forming the Jacobian, especially for large-scale problems where the Jacobian computation is too expensive even though we only have to do it once at the first outer iteration. In contrast, the matrix-free preconditioner PREQN does not need to calculate the Jacobian explicitly. We have rewritten the Fortran PREQN routine[1] [10] into Matlab code and then tested it in our algorithm with several configurations. Specifically, we test six configurations where the main differences are *frequency*, problem *size N* (number of parameters/pixels to be reconstructed), and *CG tolerance* (see the $CGtol$ parameter in Algorithm 2.2). The six tested configurations are:

test1 = (2.5MHz, 48×38, 0.05), test2 = (2.5MHz, 48×38, 0.01),
test3 = (2.5MHz, 96×76, 0.01), test4 = (2.5MHz, 96×76, 0.005),
test5 = (1.5MHz, 104×80, 0.01), test6 = (1.5MHz, 104×80, 0.005).

We set the stop condition of the Gauss-Newton reconstruction (see the $GNtol$ parameter in Algorithm 2.1) to 1e-5. The sum of outer iterations, sum of CG iterations, average CG iterations per outer iteration, and the computation time are reported in Figure 2. The program was executed under *MATLAB R2017a* on a laptop equipped with *Intel Core i7-6700HQ* (4

[1] http://users.iems.northwestern.edu/~nocedal/preqn.html

cores, 2.6GHz) CPU and 16 GB RAM. As shown from the last chart of Figure 2, the PREQN preconditioning does save computation time for all the tests. For smaller problems or larger CG tolerances, the time saved by PREQN preconditioning is not impressive. This implies that the cost of applying preconditioner is similar to the time saved by the reduction in the number of CG iterations. However, for larger problems such as test5 and test6, the PREQN preconditioner saves about 50% computation time. On average, the computation time saved is about 30% for the six tests.

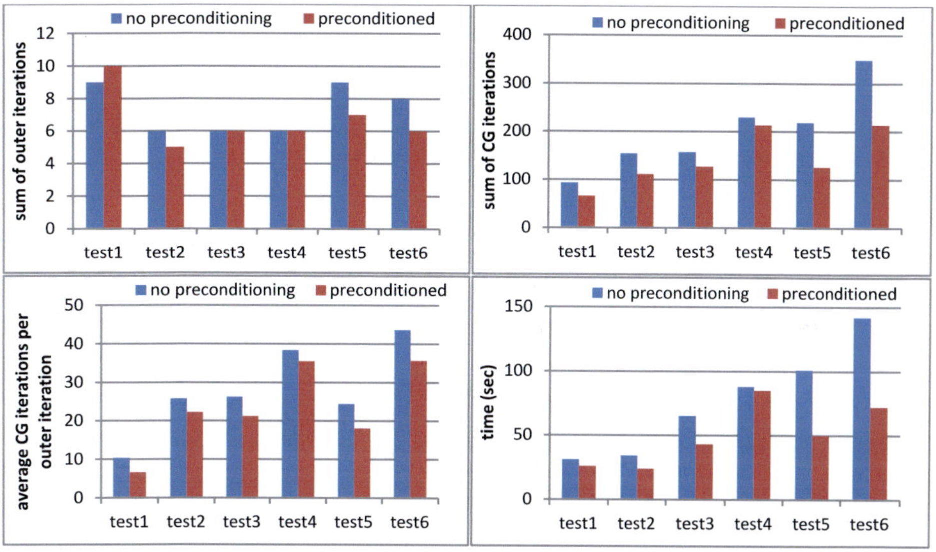

Figure 2: Results of PREQN preconditioning.

The above six reconstruction tests we have reported are for small objects, where the radius of region of interest (ROI) is about 10~20 mm. The radius of measuring device for *Karlsruhe USCT II* is 130 mm, and we have used scaling factors of 0.14 and 0.25 for the previous tests. For reconstruction without scaling, we use the multi-frequency reconstruction method. We start at 250kHz and increase the frequency with a factor of 1.1 each time, reaching the max. frequency 2.5MHz after 26 frequency steps. For all the frequencies before the final one, we use a relatively loose tolerance for reconstruction, in order to get a quick approximate solution which is then interpolated as the starting solution of the next higher frequency. We test multi-frequency reconstruction with three numerical phantoms under *MATLAB R2016a* running on a standard node of *bwForCluster*[2], which is equipped with 2×*Intel Xeon E5-2630v3* (Haswell) (8 cores, 2.4 GHz) CPU and 64 GB Memory. The phantom 1 is a simple simulation of a breast where the background is water, and from outside to inside are skin, fat,

[2] https://www.bwhpc-c5.de/wiki/index.php/Main_Page

gland, and tumor. The phantom 2 is with more shapes allowing identifying sharp edges. The phantom 3 contains the structure of a breast as segmented from a clinical MRI image. The results are reported in Figure 4, where the values are accumulated values of 26 frequencies from 250kHz to 2.5MHz. The PREQN preconditioning reduces both the outer iterations and the CG iterations for multi-frequency reconstruction. The computation time saved is about 30% on average for the three tested phantoms. At the final frequency of 2.5MHz, the number of parameters/pixels is 344×270 with the pixel size of 0.59 mm (also the ultrasound wavelength).

As for visualized results, we report in Figure 3 the Matlab program (running on the laptop used before) snapshots for phantom 3. The multi-frequency reconstruction begins from a starting frequency of 0.5MHz, reaching the final frequency 2.5MHz after 8 frequencies, where the number of parameters/pixels is 110×68 at the final frequency. In Figure 3, the top row 2D images are reconstructed SoS and attenuation respectively. The bottom row 1D profiles focus on the parameters/pixels at the pink dotted lines, where the reconstructed profiles are given in red and their simulated reference in blue. For the 1D profiles, the standard deviation from the simulation for SoS is 0.001 m/s, while the standard deviation for attenuation is 3.4%.

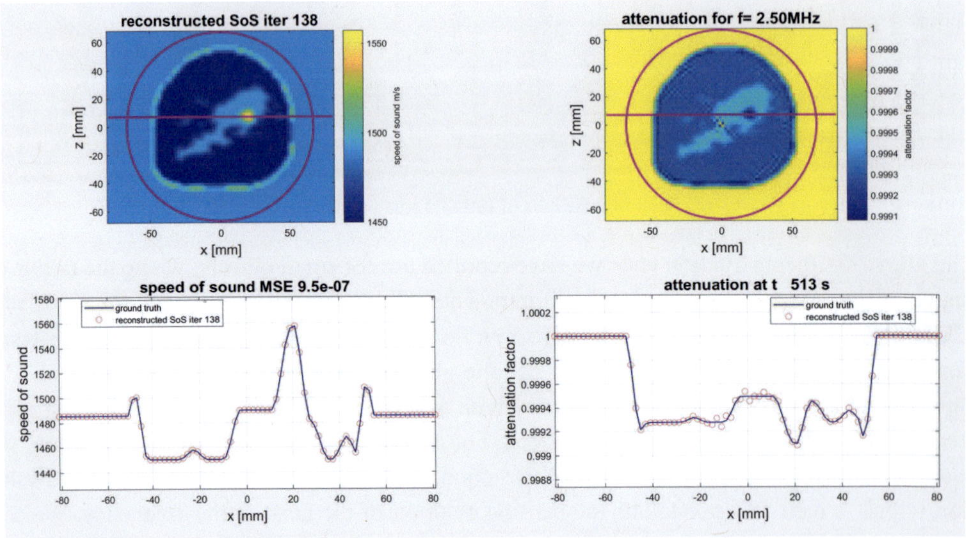

Fig. 3: Visulization of reconstructed speed of sound (blue image) and attenuation (yellow imag) of phantom 3.

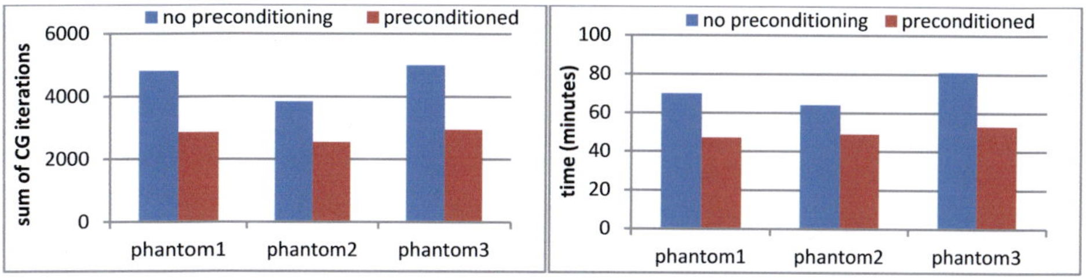

Figure 4: Results of multi-frequency reconstruction with PREQN preconditioning.

4 Conclusions

We use the Gauss-Newton method for USCT image reconstruction by minimizing a nonlinear least-squares problem defined according to measurements data and the forward split-step formulation of the wide-angle parabolic equation (WAPE). The system is linearized in the form of a Jacobian and we choose the conjugate gradient (CG) method to solve the normal equation inside the Gauss-Newton loop, since CG does not need the explicit Jacobian matrix but only matrix-vector products. The commonly used incomplete Cholesky preconditioning for CG can reduce about 70%~85% CG iterations but the computation time for the Jacobian matrix is dominating, and as a result, it fails to reduce the overall computation time significantly. The matrix-free preconditioner via Quasi-Newton update, on the other hand, does not need to form the Jacobian explicitly and saves about 30% of the computation time on average. Reconstruction for large-size problems with high ultrasound frequencies requires starting solutions which are near to the true solutions. We use a multigrid scheme to firstly get a convergent rough reconstruction at lower frequency and then interpolate it for the starting solution with higher frequency. Together with the matrix-free preconditioning, multi-frequency reconstruction gives decent SoS reconstruction for 344×270 parameters at 2.5MHz in reasonable computation time. In future work, more effective problem-dependent preconditioning techniques will be studied for our USCT image reconstruction. Especially for the multigrid reconstruction framework, the non-uniform convergence rates for coarse scale features and fine scale features should be taken into consideration.

Acknowledgements

The research was supported by the Deutsche Forschungsgemeinschaft (DFG) under grants no. HE 3011/37-1 and HO 5565/2-1.

References

[1] H. Gemmeke and N. V. Ruiter, “3D Ultrasound Computer Tomography for medical imaging”, NIM Nucl. Instr. & Meth. In Phys. Res. Vol. Ax, pp. 1057-65, 2007.

[2] J. Greenleaf and R. C. Bahn, "Clinical imaging with transmissive ultrasonic computerized tomography", IEEE Trans. Biomedical Engineering, vol. 4, no. 4, pp. 177-85, Feb., 1981.

[3] A. Fichtner, "Full seismic waveform modeling and inversion", Springer, 2011, pp. 86-123.

[4] L. Althaus, "On acoustic tomography using paraxial approximations", M.S. thesis, Darmstadt University of Technology, Department of Mathematics, Darmstadt, Germany, 2016.

[5] M. D. Feit and J. A. Fleck, "Light propagation in graded-index optical fibers", Appl.Opt. 17(24), 3990-98, Dec., 1978.

[6] H. F. Trotter, "On the product of semi-groups of operators", Proc. Am. Math. Soc., 10, 545-551, 1959.

[7] J. Nocedal and S. Wright, "Numerical Optimization (Second Edition)", Springer-Verlag New York, 2006.

[8] J. R. Shewchuk, "An introduction to the conjugate gradient method without the agonizing pain", 1994.

[9] J. L. Morales and J. Nocedal, "Automatic preconditioning by limited memory quasi-Newton updating", SIAM Journal on Optimization 10.4 (2000): 1079-1096.

[10] J. Nocedal, "Algorithm PREQN: Fortran 77 Subroutines for Preconditioning the Conjugate Gradient Method", (2000).

[11] J. Nocedal, "Updating quasi-Newton matrices with limited storage", Mathematics of computation 35.151 (1980): 773-782.

[12] F. Natterer and F. Wubbeling, "A propagation-backpropagation method for ultrasound tomography", Inverse problems 11.6 (1995): 1225.

[13] P. C. Hansen, "Regularization tools: A Matlab package for analysis and solution of discrete ill-posed problems", Numerical algorithms 46 (2007): 189-194.

[14] Y. Saad and M. H. Schultz, "GMRES: A generalized minimal residual algorithm for solving nonsymmetric linear systems", SIMA J. Sci. Stat. Comput. 7, 856–869 (1986)

[15] J. D. Tebbens and M. Túma, "Efficient preconditioning of sequences of nonsymmetric linear systems", SIAM J. Sci. Comput. 29, 1918–1941 (2007)

[16] W. Xu and T. Coleman, "Efficient (partial) determination of derivative matrices via automatic differentiation", SIAM J. Sci. Comput. 35, A1398–A1416 (2013)

[17] W. Xu, N. Zheng and K. Hayami, "Jacobian-Free Implicit Inner-Iteration Preconditioner for Nonlinear Least Squares Problems", Journal of Scientific Computing 68.3 (2016): 1055-1081.

[18] Y. Saad, "Iterative methods for sparse linear systems", 2nd edn. SIAM, Philadelphia (2003)

[19] K. Morikuni and K. Hayami, "Inner-iteration Krylov subspace methods for least squares problems", SIAM J. Matrix Anal. Appl. 34, 1–22 (2013)

Efficient simulation of ultrasonic waves using an extended spectral element method

C. Boehm, N. Korta Martiartu, M. van Driel, L. Krischer, M. Afanasiev, and A. Fichtner

Department of Earth Sciences, ETH Zurich, Zurich, Switzerland
E-mail: christian.boehm@erdw.ethz.ch

Abstract

We present methods for accurate and computationally efficient simulations of ultrasonic waves in the time domain. Our approach is based on the spectral element method and adaptively changes the computational domain over time. The key idea is to utilize the spatio-temporal localization of the wavefield, and to take advantage of the finite speed at which energy propagates through a medium. By skipping the computation of the wavefield in regions that have no impact on the measurements, we can reduce the computational cost significantly. This is important for a wide range of applications, and particularly useful for waveform inversion, which typically requires a large number of simulations in every iteration. Furthermore, we present tools to accurately mesh the shape of a scanning device for ultrasound breast tomography with conforming unstructured hexahedral meshes. This includes custom-tailored refinement styles as well as strategies to mask out elements based on the opening angle.

Keywords: wave equation, spectral element method, mesh generation

1 Introduction

Waveform inversion for ultrasound computed tomography (USCT) is a promising tool to image the acoustic properties of breast tissue. In recent years, several studies applied waveform tomography to different scanning setups in both 2D and 3D, and simulated wave propagation in both time and frequency domain [11, 17, 19, 22, 23, 25].

Despite the availability and ever-increasing power of high-performance computing architectures, waveform inversion remains computationally challenging. Because of the non-linearity and the absence of an analytic inverse operator, the problem can only be solved iteratively. At its numerical core, waveform inversion requires the recurring simulations of acoustic waves propagating through breast tissue to generate synthetic data, which can be compared to data measurements.

Hence, using efficient simulation methods is crucial to make waveform inversion computationally feasible. In this paper, we present extensions to the spectral element method that are tailored to consecutively simulating multiple scans for ultrasound tomography. The spectral element method is a high-order numerical scheme for accurate time-domain simulations of the wave equation. It was originally introduced by Patera [16] for applications in fluid dynamics and has since then become widely used to model seismic wave propagation from regional to global scale [3, 8, 12, 18, 24].

While finite difference methods usually require rectilinear grids for the discrete system, spectral element methods work with fully unstructured meshes and thus offer a lot of flexibility. In particular, they facilitate (1) to represent the wavefield at arbitrary points in space, (2) to handle complex shapes and geometries, (3) to apply boundary conditions, and (4) to model emitting and receiving transducers accurately.

The rest of the paper is organized as follows. After briefly outlining the key principles of the spectral element method, we show that it is possible to truncate the computational domain without losing accuracy in the simulated waveforms. Furthermore, we outline a strategy to overlap the simulation of multiple scans in time. In addition, we discuss the generation of conforming hexahedral meshes to model the scanning device.

2 Method

2.1 Spectral element discretization

Consider the acoustic wave equation on the spatial domain $\Omega \subset \mathbb{R}^d$ $(d = 2,3)$ and time interval $[0,T]$ given by

$$\beta(\mathbf{x})\partial_t^2\mathbf{u}(\mathbf{x},t) - \nabla \cdot \left(\rho^{-1}(\mathbf{x})\nabla(\mathbf{u})(\mathbf{x},t)\right) = \mathbf{f}(\mathbf{x},t), \quad \text{on } \Omega \times [0,T], \tag{1}$$

with the initial conditions

$$\mathbf{u}(\mathbf{x},0) = 0, \quad \partial_t\mathbf{u}(\mathbf{x},0) = 0, \quad \text{on } \Omega, \tag{2}$$

and homogeneous Neumann-type boundary conditions

$$\nabla\mathbf{u}(\mathbf{x},t) \cdot \vec{\mathbf{n}}(\mathbf{x}) = 0 \quad \text{on } \partial\Omega \times [0,T]. \tag{3}$$

Here, $\mathbf{u}$ denotes the pressure field, $\mathbf{f}$ is an external source generated by an emitting transducer, and $\vec{\mathbf{n}}(\mathbf{x})$ is the outward pointing normal direction. The model is parameterized by the density ρ and the compressibility β, but we could change this easily to different parameters, e.g., by the relation $\beta^{-1} = \rho c^2$, where c denotes the speed of sound. We have omitted attenuation in equation (1), but extensions to visco-acoustic formulations using memory variables are possible [9]. Furthermore, we keep the boundary conditions simple to improve the readability.

Equations (1) - (3) give the so-called *strong form* of the wave equation. This is the starting point of finite difference methods that replace all differential operators appearing in these equations by point-wise approximations defined on a discrete grid. In contrast, finite element methods are based on the *weak form* of the wave equation, which can be obtained by multiplying equations (1) and (3) with test functions $\mathbf{v}$ defined on Ω and integrating over the domain. Applying the Gauss-Green theorem and integration by parts allows us to shift the spatial derivatives onto the test functions and to eliminate the boundary term from the equation. This gives for all $t \in (0,T]$ and all test functions $\mathbf{v}$:

$$\int_\Omega \beta(\mathbf{x})\,\mathbf{v}(\mathbf{x})\,\partial_t^2\mathbf{u}(\mathbf{x},t)\,d\mathbf{x} + \int_\Omega \rho^{-1}(\mathbf{x})\,\nabla\mathbf{v}(\mathbf{x})\cdot\nabla\mathbf{u}(\mathbf{x},t)\,d\mathbf{x} = \int_\Omega \mathbf{v}(\mathbf{x})\,\mathbf{f}(\mathbf{x},t)\,d\mathbf{x}. \tag{4}$$

Detailed reviews of the spectral element method can be found several times in the literature, e.g. in [4, 6, 7, 13]. Here, we briefly summarize the main components. The spatial domain is subdivided into a finite number of elements, where the wavefield is approximated locally by high-order Lagrange polynomials. Hence, the integrals in (4) are replaced by the sum of integrals over all elements, and the majority of the computations are carried out locally on the elements. A key concept of the spectral element method is to use the Gauss-Lobatto-Legendre collocation points for both the interpolation nodes of the Lagrange polynomials and the quadrature rule. This yields two main advantages: (1) the approximation error decays very fast (e.g., exponentially for analytic functions) and hence, fewer grid points per wavelength are required to properly discretize the wave equation. (2) this quadrature rule naturally yields a diagonal mass matrix, which enables the use of explicit time stepping schemes without the need to solve a linear system. Furthermore, all computations can be carried out in a matrix-free fashion. This results in a very low memory consumption and excellent scaling properties.

2.2 Lazy wave propagation

All acquisition geometries of USCT scanning devices have in common, that the transducers cover a relatively small area, e.g., along a ring or the side walls of the scanning device. This means that although the waves propagate through the entire computational domain over the course of the simulation, we actually only require the solution in small subregions towards the beginning and the end of the simulation. In the following, we outline how to exploit this characteristic feature in the design of the spectral element method, and to reduce the computational cost of the simulation. Further details can be found in [2]. The main ingredient is a time-dependent partition of the computational domain into the inactive subdomain $\Omega_i(\tau)$ and the active subdomain $\Omega_a(\tau)$. Here, $\Omega_i(\tau)$ consists of all points $\mathbf{x} \in \Omega$, which are either

(i) outside of the *region of influence* of all emitter locations, or,

(ii) outside the *domain of dependence* of the receiver locations.

In other words, the inactive domain contains all points to which either the travel time from all source locations is greater than τ, and/or the travel time to all receiver locations is greater than $T-\tau$. All remaining points belong to the active subdomain, which we define as $\Omega_a(\tau) = \Omega \setminus \Omega_i(\tau)$.

By construction, we can skip the computations in the inactive domain, because either no energy has been transmitted to it yet, or energy will not be transmitted from here to any point where it can be measured before the end of the simulation. When comparing the resulting wavefield to the solution of the original set of equations (1) – (3), we see that the differential wavefield of the two solutions can be interpreted as solution to a wave equation with a source emitted at the boundary $\partial\Omega_a \cap \partial\Omega_i \subset \Omega_i$ in the interval $[\tau, T]$. By definition of the inactive subdomain, energy emitted by this source will not reach any of the receiver locations before the end of the simulation. Hence, ignoring the inactive subdomain Ω_i in the computations, still gives the exact wavefield at all receiver locations. This concept is called lazy wave propagation [2].

The approach is particularly powerful for simulating multiple consecutive scans with a similar set of receiving transducers. Here, we can stack multiple sources in time and introduce time lags that start the simulation of the subsequent scan as soon as its source location becomes inactive during the previous simulation. In contrast to classical source encoding techniques that superimpose individual wavefields [14, 25], this strategy still accurately computes every individual signal without any artificial interference. Furthermore, mesh initialization and domain decomposition are only required once.

Lazy wave propagation is easy to integrate into conventional implementations of the spectral element method. For each emitter, we need to precompute the time intervals, in which each element will be active during the simulation. Note that approximate travel times between each element and all locations of emitters and receivers are sufficient, as long as they do not underestimate the travel time. For instance, we can work with the Euclidean distance and an upper bound for the speed of sound. If there are multiple sources, we can compute time delays based on the time when the source location gets inactive during the previous simulation. Then, in each time step, the following tasks need to be carried out:

(i) Partition the elements into the active and inactive subdomain based on the precomputed time intervals.

(ii) Set the wavefield to zero in all inactive elements.

(iii) Compute internal and external forces for all active elements.

(iv) Advance the global fields in time and continue with the next time step.

The second step is only necessary in the case of several consecutive sources. It ensures all energy is removed from the inactive subdomain before the new source starts.

Lazy wave propagation applies to both forward and adjoint simulations. In addition to decreasing the computational cost of the simulation, this is also particularly interesting to reduce the memory requirements for buffering the forward wavefield for the adjoint simulation.

2.3 Mesh generation

One of the main advantages of spectral element methods is the ability to accurately represent complex shapes and the geometry of the domain in the mesh. Creating a conforming hexahedral mesh of the scanning device is a non-trivial task though, because the grid must avoid hanging nodes. In addition, we seek to avoid unnecessarily small elements, because this would put a strong restriction on the time step for the numerical wave simulation due to the CFL condition. Although extensions to tetrahedral meshes are possible [5], using hexahedral conforming meshes are key to efficient simulations. This is due to the tensorized structure of the spectral element basis on hexahedra, which can be utilized for highly efficient computations.

Fortunately, the shape of USCT scanning devices is typically topologically similar to a hemisphere or a cylinder. For these shapes it is possible to create hexahedral meshes efficiently by extending the so-called *cubed sphere* method [20]. Starting with a cubed sphere we first mask out all the elements in the upper hemisphere. Then, we compute the radially symmetric distance between the hemisphere and the actual semi-ellipsoidal shape. Finally, we apply this deformation to the mesh by stretching the elements where necessary. This keeps the conforming structure of the mesh and it provides a nearly optimal ratio, when comparing the smallest and largest element sizes. Section 3.2 shows how such meshes can be generated for a USCT scanning device.

3 Numerical Examples

In this section, we show how the spectral element method can be applied efficiently to scanning systems that took part in the SPIE USCT Data Challenge [21]. All examples presented in this section were computed with Salvus [1], a high-performance software package designed to solve large-scale waveform tomography problems. Salvus is a comprehensive collection of packages that cover the complete toolchain of time-domain waveform inversion with modules for numerical wave propagation, meshing, inversion, and workflow management. Our goal with Salvus is to bridge the gap between research and production codes with a design based on C++ and Python wrappers that separate the physical equations from the numerical core. This design together with the use of open-source high-level libraries, such as PETSc and Eigen, ensures that Salvus is both flexible and scalable.

3.1 2D CSIC/UCM USCT

We consider the dataset from the SPIE USCT Data Challenge [21] provided by the Spanish National Research Council (CISC) and the Complutense University of Madrid (UCM).

The setup consists of two plates with 16 transducers each that circumscribe a circular region of interest with a diameter of 20 cm. The transducers of one plate act as emitters and the elements on the other plate record the pressure field. The receiving plate is placed at 11 different positions during the acquisition, which cover a segment of 180 degrees. To generate synthetic waveforms, it is sufficient to consider all positions of the receiving plate at once. This gives a total of 176 receivers per emitting transducer.

Figure 1 shows snapshots of the pressure wavefield using lazy wave propagation. The grey-shaded area depicts the inactive region where we skip the computation of the wavefield. Although the artificial boundary between the active and the inactive domain changes the wave equation, errors do not propagate inside the active subdomain. Over the course of the simulation, only 27 % of the elements are active on average. Although this would ideally save about 73 % of the computational cost, this reduction is hard to achieve in practice if the simulation runs on multiple processors. This is due to the time-dependence of Ω_a, which makes it difficult to achieve a good load balancing without frequent repartitioning of the domain.

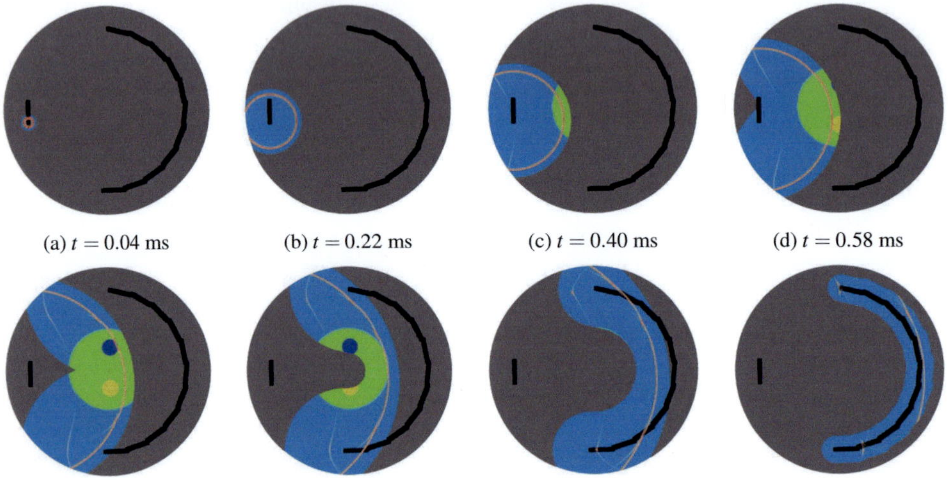

(a) $t = 0.04$ ms (b) $t = 0.22$ ms (c) $t = 0.40$ ms (d) $t = 0.58$ ms

(e) $t = 0.76$ ms (f) $t = 0.94$ ms (g) $t = 1.12$ ms (h) $t = 1.3$ ms

Figure 1: Snapshots of lazy wave propagation. The black dots indicate the transducer locations. The emitting plate is on the left half of the disk and all receiving plates are on the right. The grey-shaded areas indicate the inactive subdomain in which the wavefield is not computed. There are no errors propagating from the artificial boundary into the active subdomain.

However, during the acquisition, each transducer on the emitting plate is activated consecutively and we can overlap the individual simulations in time. We consider a simulation time of

1.4 ms per emitter, which results in a total simulation time of 22.4 ms for all 16 transducers in a conventional spectral element simulation. By overlapping the individual emitters in time, we can start the simulation of the next scan already 0.75 ms after the previous one. Thus, by stacking the sources, we require only 12.65 ms of simulation time in total. This reduces the cost by 43.5 %, and these savings are now independent of the parallel decomposition. In addition to that, we benefit form the inactive regions that still exist for the stacked simulation, and which yield a further reduction of the computational cost. Figure 2 shows snapshots of the stacked simulation. There is no difference to the previous example (Figure 1) during the first 0.75 ms of the simulation, except for the slightly increased size of the active domain, which now considers the region of influence of all emitters. Afterwards, the second emitter is triggered and the method automatically maintains two active regions. We deliberately use imperfect absorbing boundaries along the exterior ring in this example to show that the previous wavefield does indeed not contaminate the active region of the following emitter. Furthermore, the definition of the inactive subdomain guarantees that the signals of the individual sources do not overlap, and so they can easily be extracted from the stacked simulation.

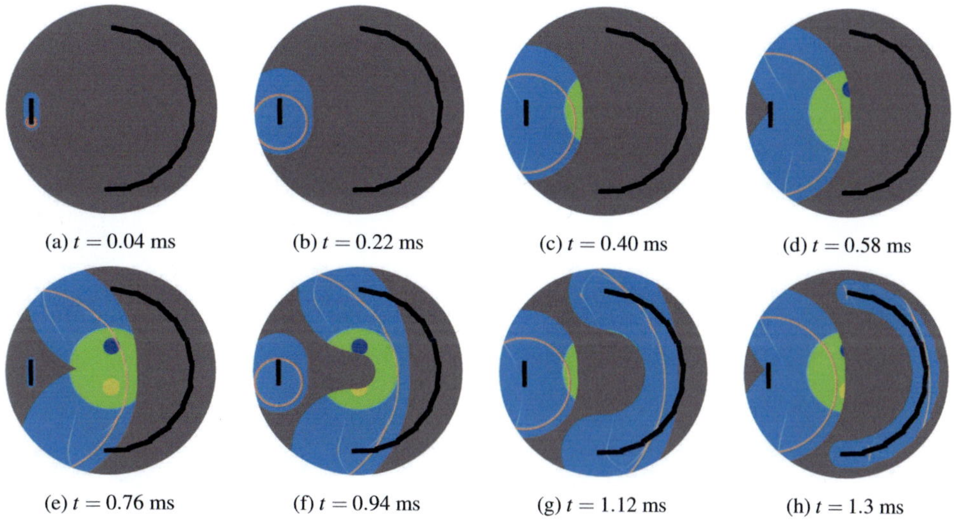

(a) $t = 0.04$ ms (b) $t = 0.22$ ms (c) $t = 0.40$ ms (d) $t = 0.58$ ms

(e) $t = 0.76$ ms (f) $t = 0.94$ ms (g) $t = 1.12$ ms (h) $t = 1.3$ ms

Figure 2: Snapshots of lazy wave propagation with stacked sources. The grey-shaded areas indicate the inactive subdomain. After 0.75 ms the second emitter is triggered, which creates a second active domain.

3.2 3D KIT USCT

In this example, we consider the 3D USCT system developed at the Karlsruhe Institute of Technology [10, 21]. It has a hemi-ellipsoidal 3D aperture, which is 16 cm tall and has a diameter of 26 cm.

Figure 3(a)-(c) show the three steps of the mesh generation process. The ellipsoidal shape requires small deformations of the cubed sphere, where the elements are stretched in vertical direction. The ratio of the largest to the smallest local time steps required by the CFL condition indicates the quality of the mesh. In this example, the minimum value is only 38 % smaller than the largest local time step.

To improve the visibility, Figure 3 shows the mesh for a dominant frequency of only 100 kHz to obtain larger and fewer elements. The total number of elements in the mesh depends, of course, on the highest frequency to be resolved. Here, we use approximately two elements per dominant wavelength and fourth-order polynomials, which results in approximately 9 grid points per wavelength. Figure 3(d) shows a snapshot of a spectral element simulation for a dominant frequency of 300 kHz and a mesh with approximately 520'000 elements. The synthetic breast phantom was created using the OA-Breast Phantom toolbox [15].

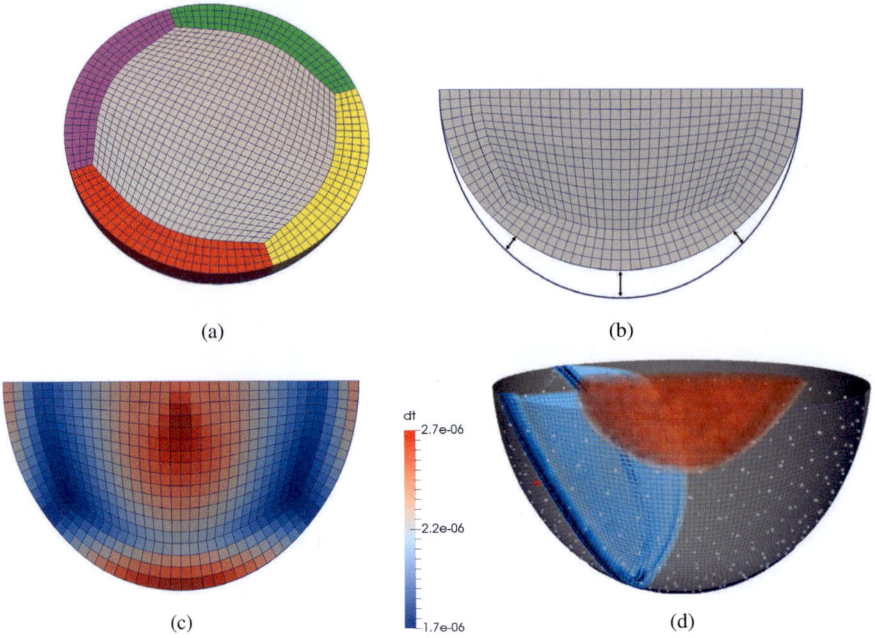

Figure 3: (a) Top view of the cubed hemisphere that consists of a deformed cube in the interior and shells attached to each face of the cube that accurately follow the shape of the sphere. (b) Vertical cut through the cubed sphere before applying the mesh deformation. (c) Vertical cut through the final hemi-ellipsoidal mesh. The colour encodes the time step required by the CFL condition. (d) Snapshot of a spectral element simulation with a synthetic breast phantom.

In addition to the shape of the device, we can also take the transducer characteristics into account when generating the mesh. In particular, we can use the opening angle of the emitter to mask out areas where the amplitude of the pressure field will be negligible. This can easily be done with Salvus with a few lines of Python code. To avoid reflections from the artificially introduced surfaces, we apply absorbing boundary conditions during the simulation. Truncating the domain reduces the number of elements in the mesh, which directly translates into a reduction of the computational cost. Figure 4 shows an example of a truncated mesh, where incorporating the opening angle into the mesh generation reduces the number of elements by almost 50 %.

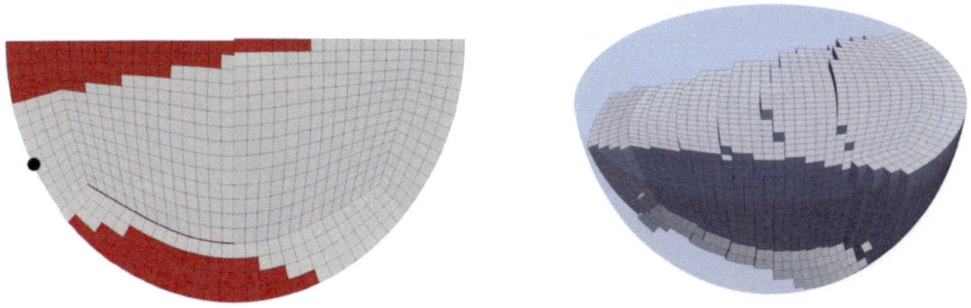

(a) (b)

Figure 4: (a) Vertical cut through the truncated mesh. The black circle indicates the location of the emitter. The red elements were removed from the mesh. (b) Top view of the truncated mesh generated by masking out elements along 4 cutting planes.

4 Conclusions

Applying full-waveform inversion to USCT data remains computationally challenging. Because the recurring simulations of the wave equation vastly dominate the total cost, it is crucial to employ efficient solvers. In this paper, we have presented methods to reduce the cost of waveform simulations without losing accuracy. Our approach is based on the spectral element method and adaptively changes the computational domain over time. By combining lazy wave propagation with conforming hexahedral meshes that are tailored to the acquisition geometry, the computational cost per simulation can be reduced considerably.

Acknowledgments

The authors would like to thank the organizers of the International Workshop on Medical Ultrasound Tomography 2017 for a truly inspiring conference, and for the opportunity to submit this manuscript. Furthermore, we gratefully acknowledge support by the Swiss National Supercomputing Centre (CSCS) under project grant d72.

References

[1] M. Afanasiev, C. Boehm, M. van Driel, L. Krischer, M. Rietmann, D. A. May, M. Knepley, and A. Fichtner. Salvus: A high-performance package for full waveform modelling and inversion from laboratory to global scales. submitted to Geophys. J. Int., 2017.

[2] C. Boehm and A. Fichtner. Lazy wave propagation. submitted to Geophys. J. Int., 2017.

[3] C. Boehm and M. Ulbrich. A semismooth Newton-CG method for constrained parameter identification in seismic tomography. SIAM Journal on Scientific Computing, 37(5):S334–S364, 2015.

[4] E. Chaljub, D. Komatitsch, J.-P. Vilotte, Y. Capdeville, B. Valette, and G. Festa. Spectral-element analysis in seismology. In V. Maupin R. Wu and R. Dmowska, editors, Advances in Wave Propagation in Heterogenous Earth, volume 48 of Advances in Geophysics, pages 365 – 419. Elsevier, 2007.

[5] G. Cohen, P. Joly, J. E. Roberts, and N. Tordjman. Higher Order Triangular Finite Elements with Mass Lumping for the Wave Equation. SIAM Journal on Numerical Analysis, 38(6):2047–2078, 2001.

[6] A. Ferroni, P.F. Antonietti, I. Mazzieri, and A. Quarteroni. Dispersion-dissipation analysis of 3d continuous and discontinuous spectral element methods for the elastodynamics equation. Geophys. J. Int., page ggx384, 2017.

[7] A. Fichtner. Full Seismic Waveform Modelling and Inversion. Springer, Heidelberg., 2010.

[8] A. Fichtner, B. L. N. Kennett, H. Igel, and H.-P. Bunge. Spectral-element simulation and inversion of seismic waves in a spherical section of the Earth. J. Num. An. Ind. Appl. Math., 4:11–22, 2009.

[9] A. Fichtner and M. van Driel. Models and Fréchet kernels for frequency-(in)dependent Q. Geophys. J. Int., 198:1878–1889, 2014.

[10] H. Gemmeke, T. Hopp, M. Zapf, C. Kaiser, and N. V. Ruiter. 3D ultrasound computer tomography: Hardware setup, reconstruction methods and first clinical results. Nuclear Instruments and Methods in Physics Research Section A: Accelerators, Spectrometers, Detectors and Associated Equipment, 873(Supplement C):59 – 65, 2017. Imaging 2016.

[11] A.V. Goncharsky, S. Y. Romanov, and S. Y. Seryozhnikov. A computer simulation study of soft tissue characterization using low-frequancy ultrasonic tomography. Ultrasonics, 67:136–150, 2016.

[12] D. Komatitsch and J. Tromp. Introduction to the spectral element method for three-dimensional seismic wave propagation. Geophys. J. Int., 139:806–822, 1999.

[13] D. Komatitsch, S. Tsuboi, and J. Tromp. The Spectral-Element Method in Seismology, pages 205–227. American Geophysical Union, 2013.

[14] J. R. Krebs, J. E. Anderson, D. Hinkley, R. Neelamani, S. Lee, A. Baumstein, and M.-D. Lacasse. Fast full-wavefield seismic inversion using encoded sources. Geophysics, 74(6):WCC177–WCC188, 2009.

[15] Y. Lou, W. Zhou, T. P. Matthews, C. M. Appleton, and M. A. Anastasio. Generation of anatomically realistic numerical phantoms for photoacoustic and ultrasonic breast imaging. Journal of Biomedical Optics, 22(4):041015–041015, 2017.

[16] A. T. Patera. A spectral element method for fluid dynamics: Laminar flow in a channel expansion. Journal of Computational Physics, 54(3):468 – 488, 1984.

[17] M. Perez-Liva, J. L. Herraiz, J. M. Udías, B. T. Cox, and B. E. Treeby. Full-wave attenuation reconstruction in the time domain for ultrasound computed tomography. In Biomedical Imaging (ISBI), 2016 IEEE 13th International Symposium on, pages 710–713. IEEE, 2016.

[18] D. Peter, D. Komatitsch, Y. Luo, R. Martin, N. Le Goff, E. Casarotti, P. Le Loher, F. Magnoni, Q. Liu, C. Blitz, T. Nissen-Meyer, P. Basini, and J. Tromp. Forward and adjoint simulations of seismic wave propagation on fully unstructured hexahedral meshes. Geophys. J. Int., 186:721–739, 2011.

[19] R. G. Pratt, L. Huang, N. Duric, and P. Littrup. Sound-speed and attenuation imaging of breast tissue using waveform tomography of transmission ultrasound data. Proc. SPIE, 6510:65104S, 2007.

[20] C. Ronchi, R. Iacono, and P.S. Paolucci. The cubed sphere: A new method for the solution of partial differential equations in spherical geometry. Journal of Computational Physics, 124(1):93 – 114, 1996.

[21] N. V. Ruiter, M. Zapf, T. Hopp, H. Gemmeke, and K. W. A. van Dongen. USCT data challenge. Proc. SPIE, 10139:101391N–101391N–8, 2017.

[22] G. Y. Sandhu, C. Li, O. Roy, S. Schmidt, and N. Duric. Frequency domain ultrasound waveform tomography: breast imaging using a ring transducer. Physics in medicine and biology, 60(14):5381, 2015.

[23] G. Y. Sandhu, E. West, C. Li, O. Roy, and N. Duric. 3D frequency-domain ultrasound waveform tomography breast imaging. Proc. SPIE, 10139:1013909–1013909–14, 2017.

[24] C. Tape, Q. Liu, A. Maggi, and J. Tromp. Seismic tomography of the southern California crust based on spectral-element and adjoint methods. Geophys. J. Int., 180(1):433–462, 2010.

[25] K. Wang, T. Matthews, F. Annis, C. Li, N. Duric, and M. Anastasio. Waveform inversion with source encoding for breast sound speed reconstruction in ultrasound computed tomography. IEEE Trans. Ultrason. Ferroelectr. Freq. Contr., 62, 2014.

Medical ultrasound tomography: lessons from exploration geophysics

R. Gerhard Pratt

University of Western Ontario, London ON N6A 5B7, Canada
E-mail: gpratt2@uwo.ca

Abstract

The seismic method is a widely-used geophysical method in the hydrocarbon exploration industry. This has led to the development of powerful imaging tools, in some cases inspired by and akin to those used in medical ultrasound tomography. In both exploration seismology and in medical imaging, the experiment involves the propagation of sound waves over distances of a few tens of wavelengths to a few hundred wavelengths. In both cases the transmitters and receiver design is used to control bandwidth and illumination apertures. However, in exploration seismology i) access to the target is unusually restricted, ii) geological targets are often embedded in strongly scattering material, iii) we cannot ignore 3-D heterogeneity, elastic wave effects including mode conversions, and anisotropic wave propagation, and iv) we must account for the presence of high amplitude dispersive modes associated with the free surface of the Earth.

In seismic exploration, the past decade has seen the emergence of 'Full Waveform Inversion' (FWI) as a remarkably successful innovation. Historically, seismic imaging methods have been most successful when applied to back-scattered (aka reflected) waves. FWI, in contrast, has to date been most successful with transmitted (aka refracted) waves. FWI of reflected data is progressing, but significant problems remain. These include i) handling the significant non-linearity and non-uniquenesses that are inherent in the experiment, and ii) convincing skilled interpreters that FWI yields a new type of image that contributes in significant (but unusual) ways. It is suggested that the field of medical ultrasound tomography shares these problems and that there is much to be learned by cross-fertilization in both fields.

Keywords: Seismic imaging, Full Waveform Inversion, Ultrasound

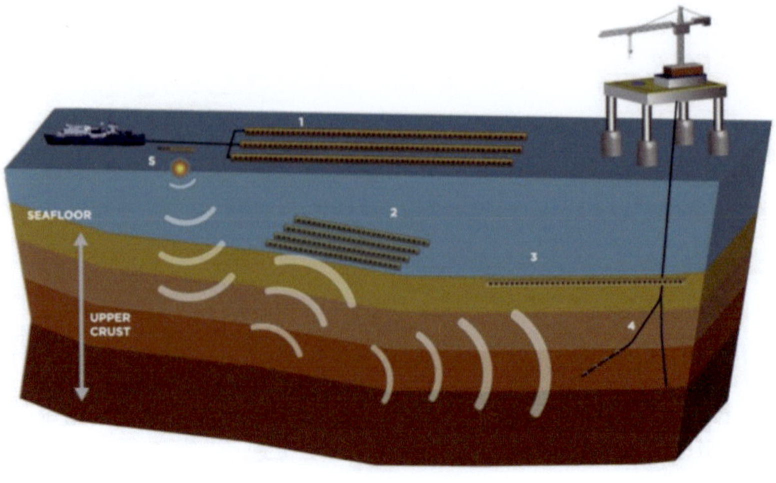

Figure 1: A schematic illustration of marine seismic reflection surveying. Acoustic energy is generated at the source (S), propagates through the seabed into the subsurface, and is reflected (and refracted) back to the surface, where it is recorded using towed hydrophone arrays, or 'streamers' (1). In some cases data might also be recorded using sea-floor arrays (2), buried sea-floor arrays (3), or borehole arrays (4). [4].

1 Introduction

Seismic reflection methods are a critical technology in the world's search for hydrocarbon resources. They are also widely used in a wide variety of other applications, including mineral resource exploration, environmental enginering, geotechnical engineering, and archeological investigations. These methods evolved throughout the 1950's to the present day, enormously aided by the development of the digital computer from the 1960's onward [1]. There are obvious parallels between reflection seismology and medical ultrasound that have been recognized for many years [2, 3]. The seismic reflection method has benefitted from a wide range of innovations since its inception right up to the present day. The purpose of this paper is to share some of the recent innovations in 'Full Waveform Inversion' (FWI) that have received wide spread attention in reflection seismology. It is suggested that some of the lessons learned in the exploration field may be useful in the field of medical ultrasound.

2 Seismic reflection method

In marine environments reflection data are typically acquired from purpose-built vessels (see Figure 1), using air gun arrays that direct energy downwards, and recorded using hydrophones deployed using 'streamers' towed behind the vessel. Streamers can be many kilometers in length, and may contain many hundreds of hydrophone elements. Data volumes are enormous

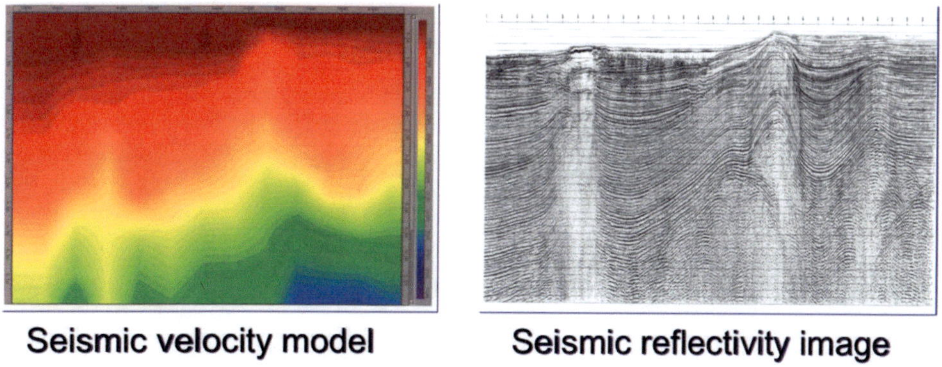

Figure 2: Seismic reflection imaging separates the subsurface representation into a low wavenumber 'velocity model' (left) and a high wavenumber 'reflectivity image' [5].

since seismic 'shots' are typically triggered at intervals of 25 m to 50 m, and data from each shot is recorded in each individual element along the streamers.

Seismic reflection data require extensive processing before the data can be interpreted and used for decision-making in the development of a potential reservoir. In contrast to conventional, B-scan medical ultrasound, seismic sources and receivers are not beam-forming; any beam-forming required is applied at the processing stage. Seismic data processing typically requires many weeks or months before a final product is available, and a team of many processing scientists may be involved. Perhaps the definitive description of the processing workflow is that provided by the well known textbook, 'Seismic Data Processing' [5]. As a crucial step in the processing, the data are regathered into 'Common Midpoint gathers' in which the redundancy of the data acquisition is used to analyze a multiplicity of reflections with a wide aperture from subsurface imaging points. By analyzing the coherency of these reflections an estimate can be made of the subsurface sound-speed (this is referred to in the industry as 'velocity analysis').

Once the sound-speed (velocity) model has been estimated, this smooth, low wavenumber model is then used in a variety of 'seismic migration' methods to form reflectivity images of the subsurface. The two representations of the subsurface (the model, and the image, Figure 2) are derived from distinct aspects of the data: velocity models are informed by the the reflection traveltimes obtained from velocity analysis, and the reflectivity images arise from the reflection waveforms themselves; the two representations contain distinct spectral characteristics (the former contain primarily low wavenumbers, whereas the latter contain primarily high wavenumbers). This is similar to the manner in which sound speed images and reflection images may be computed from the same medical ultrasound scan (Figure 3).

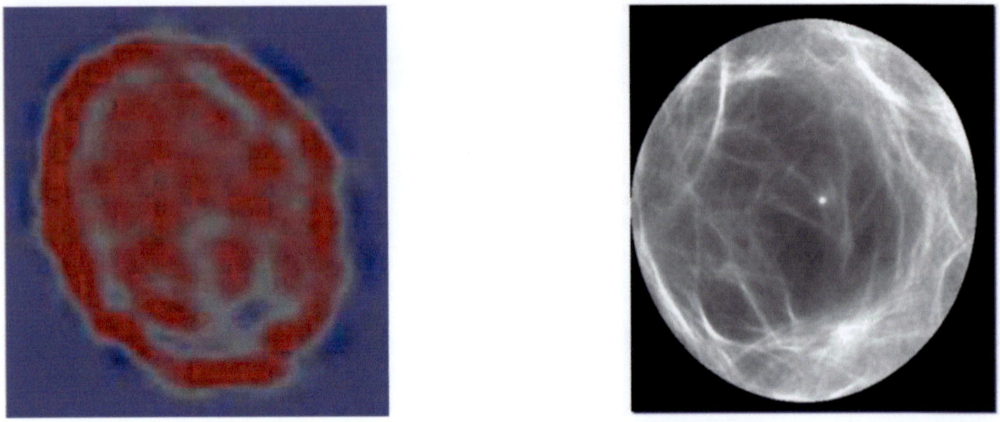

Figure 3: Medical ultrasound tomography can produce multiple modalities, such as the sound-speed (left) and the reflection image (right) (N.Duric, personal communication)

3 Full waveform inversion (FWI)

In the past two decades it has become possible to formally invert seismic waveform data in order to obtain models of the subsurface that are objectively consistent with observed shot gathers. The possibility arises from elegant mathematical results obtained in the 1980's and 1990's [6, 7, 8, 9, 10], from concerted efforts to solve the computational challenges in innovative ways, and from the significant increase in computational power available. Early results with real data were first published in the mid-1990's [11], but for many years the method remained relatively obscure, as the industry viewed the approach as i) too esoteric and unproven, and ii) too computationally intensive for routine use (especially in 3-D).

3.1 Development of FWI – theoretical aspects

FWI has a distinct relationship to 'Diffraction Tomography', a technique developed in the early 1980's in the medical tomography field to overcome the diffraction limitation on ultrasound images [12, 13], and attempts were soon made to apply the method to geophysical settings [14, 15]. Unfortunately Diffraction Tomography was not suitable for application to most real geophysical problems (at least in the original form in which the anomalies were sought in a constant background medium) [1]. Contemporaneously with the emergence of Diffraction Tomography, a series of papers were published [6, 7, 8] that filled the gap by providing a formal inverse method for seismic data that potentially solved the problem of heterogeneous background media. The method later became known as FWI, and it implemented the use of

[1] Recently developments in diffraction tomography [16] claim that this issue can be overcome by treating refraction and diffraction effects in consecutive steps during the imaging.

iterative methods to handle the inherent non-linearity of the wave equation (with respect to the velocity parameter). The methodology was first developed for time-domain problems, but in keeping with Diffraction Tomography, our group [8, 10] developed the method in the frequency domain, in which case the forward problem can be cast as the matrix problem

$$\mathbf{S}(\omega, \mathbf{p})\, \mathbf{u}(\omega) = \mathbf{f}(\omega), \tag{1}$$

where $\mathbf{S}$ is the 'differencing matrix' that captures the finite approximation to the Helmholtz operator (i.e., the acoustic wave operator $\nabla^2 + \omega^2/c^2$), $\mathbf{u}$ is a vector containing the acoustic wavefield solution, and $\mathbf{f}$ is the (mostly zero-valued) vector of source terms. All terms depend on ω, the frequency of the experiment, and the differencing matrix depends on $\mathbf{p}$, the parameter vector (representing the full distribution of acoustic velocities with each cell). We solve this matrix equation to generate simulated (synthetic) data for a given velocity model.

The inverse problem is to find a distribution of model parameters, $\mathbf{p}$ (i.e., velocities) that predict the observed data. Introducing a data residuals vector $\delta\mathbf{d}(\omega)$ representing the differences between the frequency domain predicted and observed data, we define a misfit functional

$$E(\mathbf{p}) = \frac{1}{2}\delta\mathbf{d}^T\mathbf{d}, \tag{2}$$

for which the gradient (steepest ascent direction)

$$(\nabla_p E)_i = \frac{\partial}{\partial p_i} E(\mathbf{p}) = \mathscr{R}\left\{\mathbf{u}^T \left[\frac{\partial \mathbf{S}}{\partial p_i}\right] \mathbf{v}\right\} \tag{3}$$

[10], where a new, 'backpropagated' wavefield $\mathbf{v}$ is introduced satisfying

$$\mathbf{S}\,\mathbf{v} = \delta\mathbf{d}^* \tag{4}$$

(i.e., the conjugated data residuals are used as source terms to backpropagate the wavefield). This shows that the gradient calculation is the result of a classic double-focussing operation in which the forward propagated wavefield $\mathbf{u}$ is correlated with the backpropagated wavefield $\mathbf{v}$ at each imaging point. This double-focussing is equivalent to acoustic holography [17], and is also equivalent to a single pass of seismic migration [6, 10].

In order to proceed to a model update we require the computation of a step length α, chosen to optimally update the model in the negative gradient (steepest descent) direction, following which we may then iterate the method using

$$\mathbf{p}^{(k+1)} = \mathbf{p}^{(k)} - \alpha\nabla_p E^{(k)}. \tag{5}$$

Following convergence for the current frequency, ω (or block of frequencies) we may move on to the next imaging frequency to improve the reconstruction. In total each iteration requires that at minimum 3 forward models be solved per frequency, per iteration, and per source location (the forward model, the backpropagation model, and at least one further model to estimate the step length).

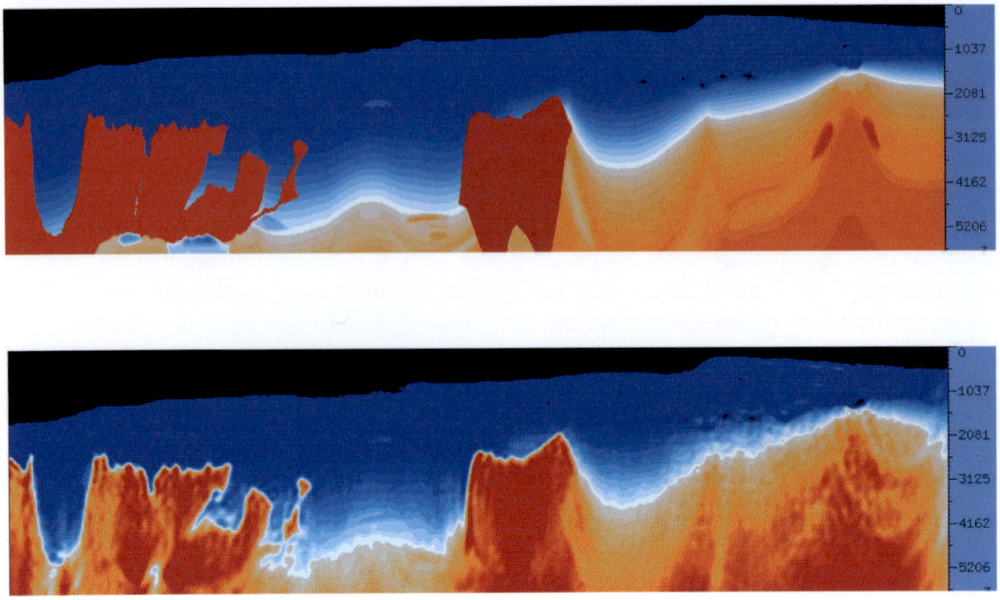

Figure 4: Bottom: An FWI result produced by the author and members of his research group in a blind test in 2004, compared with the (then unknown) true model (top) (F. Billette, personal communication).

3.2 Development of FWI – applications

While the elements of FWI were in place in the mid 1980's, it was at least a decade before enough was understood (and enough compute power was available) to enable real data results to be obtained [11]. A key moment in seismic FWI took place in 2004 when a blind test organized by BP [18] provided an opportunity to showcase the potential of FWI in a controlled setting. The image in Figure 4 was presented at that workshop by our group, and it proved highly influential. Within a few years FWI research groups had been formed by many of the major Oil & Gas exploration companies and service companies, and a significant body of literature subsequently emerged. FWI is now considered to have allowed many producers to realize significant economic uplift. Nevertheless research into FWI continues in order to improve the convergence characteristics of the optimization, to efficiently handle the massive computational burden, and to extend the method to more general physics (i.e. to properly handle the properties of a subsurface which is 3-D, elastic, attenuating and anisotropic)[19, 20].

4 Application of FWI to Medical Ultrasound Data

The scaling comparison illustrated in Table 1 provides motivation for applying methods from Exploration Seismics to Medical Ultrasound data.

It may be seen that at 1 MHz the medical ultrasound system shares the same number of wavelengths with those encountered in long-offset seismic exploration data (at 25 MHz, for maximally distal source-receiver pairs). Thus the numerical grids used for 2-D FWI in Exploration Seismics are appropriate for 2-D reconstructions of these ultrasound data.

Kinematic scaling		Exploration Geophysics		Medical Ultrasound	
		Low frequency	High frequency	Low frequency	High frequency
Propagation distance	L	16 km	16 km	15 cm	15 cm
Frequencies	f	2.5 Hz	25 Hz	1 MHz	3 MHz
Sound speed	c	4000 m/s	4000 m/s	1500 m/s	1500 m/s
Wavelength	$\lambda = c/f$	1.6 km	0.16 km	.15 cm	0.05 cm
Fresnel zone size	$\sqrt{L\lambda}$	4.9 km	1.5 km	1.9 cm	11.2 cm
Number of wavelengths	$N_\lambda = L/\lambda$	10	100	100	300

Table 1: A comparison of kinematic scaling parameters in both Exploration Seismology and in Medical Ultrasound. The first two columns represent the low and high frequency cases for exploration, with approximately 10 wavelengths from source to receiver for the lowest frequencies, and 100 wavelengths for the highest frequencies. For medical ultrasound, even at 1 MHz we already have 100 wavelengths of propagation. The parameters for Medical Ultrasound are taken from the Computed Ultrasound Risk Evaluation (CURE) system [21], comprising a 20 cm diameter solid-state ultrasound ring array with 256 active, non-beamforming transducers.

It is understood in FWI that the achievable spatial resolution is of the order of $\lambda/4$. A comparison of the scaling parameters in Table 1 indicates that 1 MHz ultrasound data may yield a resolution of $\lambda/4 \approx 0.4$ mm. This spatial resolution is already competitive with X-ray CT resolutions. Although Table 1 indicates that using higher frequencies of, say, 3 MHz could push the resolution limit to perhaps 0.1 mm, there are difficulties in using higher frequencies for FWI: First, as we increase the frequency (and decrease the wavelength) the total number of wavelengths, N_λ in the transmission path grows significantly larger than 100. The larger N_λ, the greater the computational cost, and also the greater the risk of non-convergence in FWI due to 'cycle-skip' non-linearity [22]. Second, the increased number of wavelengths at higher frequencies also implies an increase in total attenuation. In seismic exploration it is common to express attenuation through the seismic 'Q-factor', a dimensionless parameter the inverse of which measures the energy loss per cycle in a propagating wave. The conversion from Seismic Q to the attenuation factor used in medical ultrasound is provided in Appendix A. Seismic Q is approximately frequency-independent, so that when measured in dB the attenuation varies approximately linearly with both propagation distance and frequency. As may be seen on Table 2, attenuation losses in human tissue are more significant than in the sedimentary rocks encountered in exploration seismics. At 1 MHz we expect to experience approximately 14 dB of total attenuation, whereas at 3 MHz this triples to 41 dB. This creates a signal detection issue, all the more important for FWI which relies on the fidelity of the waveform data.

Dynamic scaling		Exploration Geophysics		Medical Ultrasound	
		Low frequency	High frequency	Low frequency	High frequency
Propagation distance	L	16 km	16 km	15 cm	15 cm
Frequencies	f	2.5 Hz	25 Hz	1 MHz	3 MHz
Sound speed	c	4000 m/s	4000 m/s	1500 m/s	1500 m/s
Number of wavelengths	$N_\lambda = L/\lambda$	10	100	100	300
Seismic Q	Q	500	500	200	200
Attenuation factor α	$\frac{20}{\ln 10}(\pi/cQ)$	0.14 dB/cm/MHz	0.14 dB/cm/MHz	0.91 dB/cm/MHz	0.91 dB/cm/MHz
Total attenuation		0.55 dB	5.5 dB	14 dB	41 dB

Table 2: A comparison of dynamic scaling parameters in both Exploration Seismology and in Medical Ultrasound. As in Table 1, the first two columns represent the low and high frequency case for exploration, and the second two columns represent the low and high frequency case for medical ultrasound.

In 2007 the author and several collaborators from the medical ultrasound community published a study [23] in which FWI was applied to data from the CURE system. The results of the sound-speed (time-of-flight) reconstruction is shown in the middle panel of Figure 5, and the FWI sound-speed reconstruction is shown in the right-hand panel. The improvement in the resolution of the reconstruction in the FWI image is evident: the smallest simulated breast masses are not visible on the time-of-flight reconstruction, whereas the FWI reconstruction shows all simulated masses, as well as the details of the skin and subcutaneous fat layers. In the original paper the method was also successfully applied to in-vivo breast scanning data.

Although FWI has proven in many exploration case studies to be of great utility, this has not led to full scale replacement of seismic migration as an imaging technique. Migration is a well understood method for obtaining high-resolution reflectivity images, and seismic interpreters continue to rely on the migration/reflectivity images for decision-making purposes. There are several reasons for this: First, FWI appears to be limited to cases where $N_\lambda \lesssim 100$; higher frequency results are both computationally very expensive (especially in 3-D), and are at greater risk of cycle-skipping non-linearity problems. Second, FWI is limited in depth, due to the difficulty in penetrating the subsurface with transmission (refraction) energy to reservoir depths when the streamer length is limited. Nevertheless, even if higher resolution FWI images were available at reservoir depths, interpreters are not familiar or comfortable with the high-resolution velocity images, and prefer to use tried-and-tested reflectivity images. Even though these images may suffer from limitations and artifacts, these too are well understood and interpreters are familiar with these.

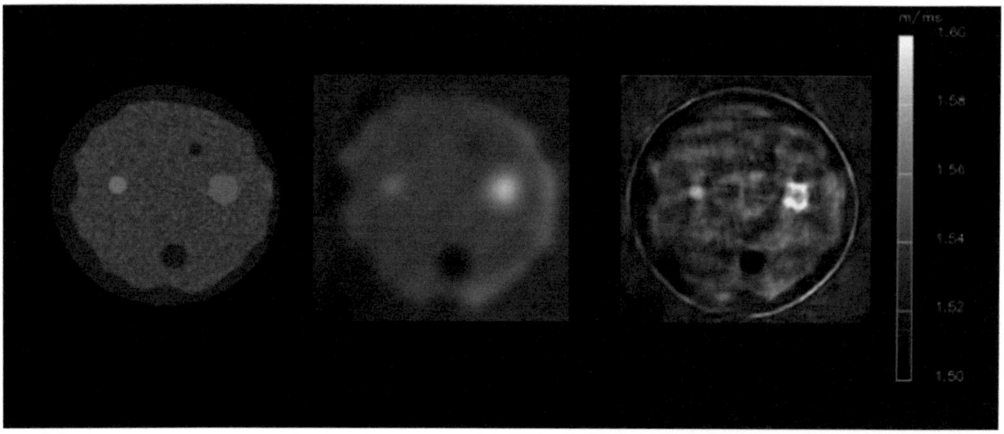

Figure 5: Left: An X-ray CRT reconstruction of a breast phantom. Middle: The sound-speed reconstruction of the breast phantom using CURE ultrasound data. Right: An FWI reconstruction of the phantom using 1 MHz data frequencies.

The reluctance of interpreters to accept FWI as a primary tool for decision-making appears to have a direct parallel in medical ultrasound, where radiologists are trained in the use of backscattering (B-scan) images and may be equally reluctant to use FWI sound-speed images for decision-making diagnoses. As a result, we have pursued 'Reverse Time Migration' (RTM) with medical ultrasound data. Compared to traditional B-mode techniques, RTM uses a much more accurate propagation model to re-focus the forward and backpropagated wavefields. Recently we published the application of RTM to the same breast phantom used above [24]. Figure 6 shows the result of that application; the images are much more consistent with those expected from B-scan imaging, and therefore more amenable to diagnostic purposes.

5 Conclusions

Exploration seismics is a parallel technology to medical ultrasound. The seismic method is well established and relies extensively on the imaging methods of seismic migration to produce high-resolution reflectivity images. In recent years, Full Waveform Inversion, or FWI has attracted great interest due to the potential for creating more informative images of the subsurface, using formal inverse methods. FWI works well with transmission data (i.e., seismic refractions), but FWI for back-scattered data (i.e., seismic reflections) remains challenging due to convergence issues; non-linearity in seismic FWI is especially challenging in presence of strong heterogeneity. Recent mathematical advances show some promise in this regard [25].

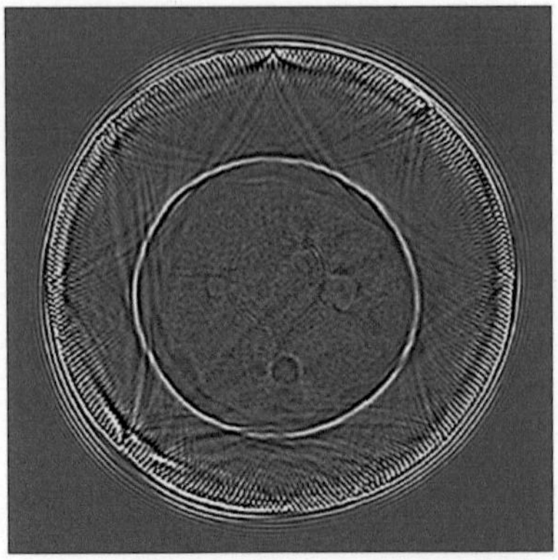

Figure 6: Filtered RTM reconstructions of the breast phantom. A Laplacian filter is used to remove low wavenumber artifacts related to the presence of direct arrivals in the data. The migration was performed using a sound-speed model using time-of-flight tomography [24].

The advent of FWI presents new challenges for users and decision makers (i.e., seismic interpreters, and medical radiologists): the method yields a new type of image that responds to sound-speed variations rather than reflectivity. The contributions of FWI images are significant but unusual, and making effective use of this technology may require a paradigm shift in interpretative science.

6 Acknowledgements

The author thanks Neb Duric, Olivier Roy and Cuiping Li of Delphinus Medical Technologies Inc. for many fascinating and fruitful discussions, and for several collaborations involving medical ultrasound data. I also wish to thank Mohammed Akbar Zuberi for his contributions in computing the image shown in Figure 6.

References

[1] Bill Dragoset. A historical reflection on reflections. *The Leading Edge*, 24(s1):s46–s70, 2005.

[2] A Witten. Geophysical Diffraction Tomography: Theory, Implementation and Results. *Oak Ridge National Laboratory*, Report No., 1992.

[3] J F Greenleaf. Computerized tomography with ultrasound. *Proc. Inst. Electr. Electron. Eng*, 71(9):330–337, 1983.

[4] International Association of Oil and Gas Producers (OGP) and the International Association of Geophysical Contractoors (IAGC). An overview of marine seismic operations. *Report No. 448*, 2011.

[5] Ozdogan. Yilmaz, Stephen M. Doherty, Ozdogan. Yilmaz, and Society of Exploration Geophysicists. *Seismic data analysis : processing, inversion, and interpretation of seismic data.* Society of Exploration Geophysicists, 2001.

[6] Patrick Lailly. The seismic inverse problem as a sequence of before stack migrations. In *Conference on Inverse Scattering: Theory and Application. Edited by J B Bednar, R Redner, E Robinson and A Weglein*, pages 206–220. SIAM Philadelphia, 1983.

[7] Albert Tarantola. Inversion of seismic reflection data in the acoustic approximation. *Geophysics*, 49(8):1259–1266, 1984.

[8] R Gerhard Pratt and M H Worthington. Inverse Theory Applied To Multi-Source Cross-Hole Tomography- Part 1: Acoustic Wave-Equation Method. *Geophysical Prospecting*, 38(3):287–310, 1990.

[9] R Gerhard Pratt and M H Worthington. Inverse theory applied to multi-source cross-hole tomography.. Part 2: Elastic wave-equation method. *Geophysical Prospecting*, 38(3):311–329, 1990.

[10] R. Gerhard Pratt, Changsoo Shin, and Hicks. Gauss-Newton and full Newton methods in frequency-space seismic waveform inversion. *Geophysical Journal International*, 133(2):341–362, 1998.

[11] Zhong-Min M Song, Paul R Williamson, and R Gerhard Pratt. Frequency-domain acoustic wave modeling and inversion of cross-hole data: Part II – Inversion method, synthetic experiments and real data results. *Geophysics*, 60(3):796–809, 1995.

[12] A J Devaney. A filtered backpropagation algorithm for diffraction tomography. *Ultrasonic Imaging*, 4:336–350, 1982.

[13] M Kaveh, M Soumekh, and J F Greenleaf. Signal processing for diffraction tomography. *IEEE Trans. on Sonics and Ultrasonics*, SU-31:230–238, 1984.

[14] AJ J Devaney. Geophysical diffraction tomography. *Inst. Electr. Electron. Eng*, GE-22(1):3–13, 1984.

[15] R G Pratt and M H Worthington. The application of diffraction tomography to cross-hole seismic data. *Geophysics, 53*, 10:1284–1294, 1988.

[16] P. Huthwaite and F. Simonetti. High-resolution imaging without iteration: a fast and robust method for breast ultrasound tomography. *The Journal of the Acoustical Society of America*, 130(3):1721–1734, sep 2011.

[17] RS Wu and MN N Toksöz. Diffraction tomography and multisource holography applied to seismic imaging. *Geophysics*, 52(I):11–25, 1987.

[18] F J Billette. The 2004 BP Velocity Benchmark. *EAGE 67th Conference & Exhibition Madrid, Spain, 13 - 16 June 2005, Paper B035*, (June):13–16, 2005.

[19] L. Sirgue, O.I. Barkved, J. Dellinger, J. Etgen, U. Albertin, and J.H. Kommedal. Thematic Set: Full waveform inversion: the next leap forward in imaging at Valhall. *First Break*, 28(1728):65–70, 2010.

[20] Michael Warner, Andrew Ratcliffe, Tenice Nangoo, and Joanna Morgan. Anisotropic 3D full-waveform inversion. *Geophysics*, 78(2), 2013.

[21] N Duric, P Littrup, A Babkin, D Chambers, S Azevedo, K Arkady, R Pevzner, M Tokarev, E Holsapple, O Rama, and R Duncan. Development of ultrasound tomography for breast imaging: Technical assessment. *Med. Phys.*, 32(5):1375–1386, 2005.

[22] R G Pratt. Waveform tomography - Successes, cautionary tales, and future directions. *EAGE Conference & Exhibition - Rome, Italy, 9 - 12 June 2008*, (June):9–12, 2008.

[23] R. Gerhard Pratt, Lianjie Huang, Neb Duric, and Peter Littrup. Sound-speed and attenuation imaging of breast tissue using waveform tomography of transmission ultrasound data. *Medical Imaging 2007: Physics of Medical Imaging*, 6510:1–12, 2007.

[24] O. Roy, M. A. H. Zuberi, R. G. Pratt, and N. Duric. Ultrasound breast imaging using frequency domain reverse time migration. *Medical Imaging 2016: Ultrasonic Imaging and Tomography, edited by Neb Duric, Brecht Heyde, Proc. of SPIE*, 9790:97900B, 2016.

[25] Michael Warner and Lluís Guasch. Adaptive waveform inversion: Theory. *GEOPHYSICS*, 81(6):R429–R445, nov 2016.

[26] K Aki and P G Richards. *Quantitative seismology, theory and methods*. W. H. Freeman and Co, 1980.

Appendix A. Conversion from Seismic Q to attenuation

Seismic Q is a dimensionless parameter defined by

$$\frac{1}{Q} \equiv -\frac{\Delta E}{2\pi E} \approx -\frac{1}{\pi}\frac{\Delta A}{A}, \tag{6}$$

(for $Q \gg 1$), where E and A are the peak strain energy and the peak amplitude, and $-\Delta E$ and $-\Delta A$ are the energy and amplitude losses per cycle, [26]. The loss in amplitude measured in Decibels over one cycle is therefore

$$20\log_{10}\left(\frac{A-\Delta A}{A}\right) = 20\log_{10}\left(1-\frac{\Delta A}{A}\right) \tag{7}$$

$$= 20\log_{10}\left(1+\frac{\pi}{Q}\right) \tag{8}$$

$$\approx \frac{20}{\ln 10}\left(\frac{\pi}{Q}\right) \tag{9}$$

(again, for $Q \gg 1$), and given the wavelength $\lambda = c/f$, the loss per distance per frequency is thus

$$\alpha = \frac{20}{\ln 10}\left(\frac{\pi}{cQ}\right). \tag{10}$$

Non-linear Ultrasonic Computed Tomography (USCT) for soft and hard tissue imaging

P. Lasaygues, J. Rouyer, S. Mensah, E. Franceschini, G. Rabau, R. Guillermin, S. Bernard, V. Monteiller, D. Komatitsch

Aix Marseille Univ, CNRS, Centrale Marseille, LMA, Marseille, France
E-mail: lasaygues@lma.cnrs-mrs.fr

Abstract

Ultrasonic Computed Tomography (USCT) is an imaging technique that has proven effective for soft-tissue characterization. The classical tomography procedures are adapted to broadband data acquired in scattering configurations under Born approximation for homogeneous media and far-field conditions, while the heterogeneous objects are probed by spherical waves in near-field conditions. An elliptical Fourier transform theory is then derived to solve the near-field inverse problem in case of harmonic ellipsoidal waves. More recently, the use of USCT has been envisaged for bone imaging. In this field, the large variations of impedance distribution (high impedance contrast) require that the modelling of wave propagation be integrated into the reconstruction scheme. In that case, iterative inversion schemes are proposed. These various reconstruction procedures are validated against experiments and numerical simulations.

Keywords: Ultrasonic Computed Tomography, Inverse Born Approximation, Iterative Approximation, Full Waveform Imaging, Breast, Bones

1 Introduction

This paper presents the theoretical framework that enables to find specific responses, on the one hand, to the problem of soft tissue imaging (typically breast cancer detection) and, on the other hand, to the problem of bone characterization (typically osteoporosis, bone infection and cancer detection). The difficulties raised are somewhat different as in soft tissues the very small fluctuations to be quantified suffer from their very low values. This poor echogenic index generally induces low detection probability, for instance in the case of large diffuse masses. In addition, invasive lesions that must not be overlooked, may be of millimetric size. In bone imaging, the difficulties arise from the very high echogenic index of the bone that strongly alters the propagation of the ultrasonic waves. Solutions consist in optimally assessing these non-linear effects in an iterative approach aiming at local linearization. In this paper, we describe a Ultrasonic Computed Tomography (USCT) method based on the use of the first-order inverse Born approximation (IBA) method, applied to the case of a homogeneous and constant background. The unknown object function, which is assumed to be weakly heterogeneous, is linearly related to the field measured via a spatial Fourier transform. The inverse problem is based on the filtered back-projection algorithm. However, such approaches are limited for breast inspection, in which the probe is either in contact with the skin or located within a near-field distance when using a coupling device (water bag or water tank). In this case, an extension of the method is proposed via a tool called Elliptical Fourier transform [1]–[3]. Nevertheless, the first-order Born USCT has some limitations when dealing with highly-contrasted scatterers. When the problem can be reduced to the study of a fluid-like cavity buried in an elastic cylinder surrounded by water, an extension of the IBA method can be proposed, taking into account physical phenomena such as wave refraction [4]. The first approach is purely experimental and consists in performing reflection and transmission measurements, using an iterative correction procedure, which compensates for refraction effects arising at the boundary between bone and the surrounding tissues. The main limitation of the method is the heavy experimental costs involved (multiple iterative experiments). We have then suggested a numerical non-linear inversion algorithm, in which the minimization procedure between the full recorded and simulated data is performed using a Polak-Ribière conjugate-gradient method mainly developed in non-destructive testing domain, or an efficient quasi-Newton technique mainly developed in seismology (related to the full waveform inversion method). An overview of the performances and the limitations of these tomography methods applied to breast and bone imaging problems are presented and discussed.

2 USCT Formulation

2.1 Physical background

Ultrasonic Computed Tomography (USCT) applied to soft tissues has been studied in several publications [5]–[8], and the use of powerful computers makes it possible nowadays to introduce more complex algorithms [1], [9]. Numerous experimental devices have been developed [10]–[12].

Let A be the operator that describes the acoustic propagation or the scattering phenomena in the heterogeneous medium of interest (including boundary and/or Sommerfeld conditions). Let S be the acoustic sources, which are assumed to be known. The variable φ denotes the resulting acoustic field, and satisfies the equation:

$$A\varphi = S \tag{1}$$

Let us assume the medium to be composed of a known domain (the reference medium as the background) resulting in an operator A_0, and an unknown domain (the object) resulting in an operator A' such as:

$$A = A_0 + A' \tag{2}$$

Assuming that φ_0 , the solution of the unperturbed problem, is known:

$$A_0\varphi_0 = S \tag{3}$$

Let φ' be the difference between φ and φ_0, that is the field perturbation induced by the perturbation by the object of the reference medium. Therefore φ' is the solution of

$$A_0\,\varphi' = -A'(\varphi_0 + \varphi') \tag{4}$$

If the Green function G_0 of the unperturbed problem is given by $G_0 = -A_0^{-1}$, the Eq.4 can be written:

$$\varphi' = G_0\,A'(\varphi_0 + \varphi') \tag{5}$$

The latter equation is the Lippmann-Schwinger non-linear equation, and a solution can be found by using a perturbation scheme, based on successive linear approximations. The "Born series" is one of these schemes introducing different development orders. Within the first-order Born approximation, the field perturbation φ' is neglected in every internal point of the scatterer. The solution φ_1' can be written:

$$\varphi_1' = G_0\,A'\,\varphi_0 \tag{6}$$

In the frequency range (> 3 MHz) of USCT of weakly heterogeneous soft tissues, in first approximation the reference medium is considered to be constant, leading to an Inverse Born Approximation (IBA) method with a constant background. The final objective is to obtain suitable images from scattered measurements $(\varphi')^m$, where the subscript *m* stands for measurements. Rotating the transducers around the object and transmitting broadband pulses at each angular position can be handled using the same approach as in *X*-ray tomography. This provides a slice-by-slice spectral coverage of the object spectrum (*2-D*-spatial Fourier transform, F_{2D}):

$$A' = (F_{2D}^{-1})\,(\varphi')^m \tag{7}$$

where $\left(F_{2D}^{-1}\right)$ denotes the inverse two-dimensional spatial Fourier transform. The first reconstruction method was then performed using a classical algorithm of the summation of filtered back-projections [1], [13], [14]. This IBA formulation assumes a far-field propagation hypothesis, but often the object to be inspected is excited in a near-field region by a spherical wave (harmonic ellipsoidal waves). The functions of domain decomposition then have as spatial support an ellipse whose foci are the position of the transducers. This decomposition has been called the Elliptic Fourier Transform [2].

The expression of the diffracted field φ' depends on the transfer function of the medium, the wave number k, and the diffraction angle. Depending on the fluid or elastic configuration, the transfer function, denoted $H(\theta, \omega)$, can be written:

- for fluid modeling

$$H(\theta, \omega) = k_0^2[\hat{\gamma}_\chi + \hat{\gamma}_\rho cos\theta](\vec{K}) = -k_0^2[\hat{\gamma}_Z(1 - cos\theta) + \hat{\gamma}_c(1 + cos\theta)](\vec{K}) \quad (8)$$

$$\gamma_\chi = \frac{\chi - \chi_0}{\chi_0} ; \gamma_\rho = \frac{\rho - \rho_0}{\rho} ; \gamma_Z = log\left(\frac{Z}{Z_0}\right) ; \gamma_c = \frac{c^2 - c_0^2}{c^2} ; \quad (9)$$

- for elastic modeling

$$H(\theta, \omega) = -k_0^2[\hat{\gamma}_\lambda - \hat{\gamma}_\mu cos\theta + 2\hat{\gamma}_\rho cos\theta](\vec{K}) ; \quad (10)$$

$$\gamma_\lambda = \frac{\lambda}{\lambda_0 + 2\mu_0} , \gamma_\mu = \frac{\mu}{\lambda_0 + 2\mu_0} ; \quad (11)$$

$$\vec{K} = k(\vec{n}_0 - \vec{n}) ; cos\theta = \vec{n}_0 . \vec{n} ; \quad (12)$$

with χ is the compressibility, ρ is the density, Z is the impedance, c is the compressional speed of sound, and λ, μ, are the Lamé coefficients. $\hat{\gamma}$ stands for the 2D elliptical Fourier transform of the parameter γ. The subscript "*0*" represents the parameters related to the background medium. $\vec{n}_0$ and $\vec{n}$ are the normal vectors in the incidence direction and in the observed direction (θ is the diffraction angle). These equations involve the acoustic parameters offering distinct directivity patterns that can be separated according to spatial scanning performed: transmission ($\theta = 0°$), reflection ($\theta = 180°$) and diffraction ($\forall\theta$).

2.2 From soft to hard tissue modeling

With hard biological tissues, such as bones, having larger acoustic impedances than those of the surrounding medium, the weak scattering assumption is no longer realistic. Indeed, the path of the transmitted wave changes from its initial course because of refraction. This results in the propagation of more complex waves, such as those occurring in elastic volumes (compressional and shear waves). The weak scattering hypothesis is therefore not realistic.

Provided some assumptions, the application of USCT can be extended to bone imaging. If the object to be imaged can be modeled by a set of concentric isotropic homogeneous noncircular fluid-like media representing the homogenized surrounding tissues, bone and marrow, only compressional waves are taken into account. Using low frequency transducers (< 3 MHz), the wavelength of the compressional wave (propagating at velocities ranging between 2000 and 4000 $m.s^{-1}$) in the cortical bone is typically greater than 1 mm, which remains much larger than the typical size of bone microstructures. Therefore, the cortical shell of the bone can be intrinsically seen as a weakly heterogeneous medium, and ultrasonic wave propagation will be minimally disturbed. Thus, the Born approximation is satisfied in this area. The IBA method with a variable background can be used; the background being the set consisting of the homogeneous solid cylinder and the homogeneous fluid surrounding medium. The solution φ_1' can be then written:

$$\varphi_1' = G_p \, A' \, \varphi_b \tag{13}$$

where G_p is the suitable Green function of the variable background. φ_b and A_b are respectively the corresponding field and the corresponding operator such as:

$$A_b \varphi_b = S \text{ and } A_b G_b = I \tag{14}$$

where I is the identity operator. The strategy can be applied iteratively:

$$\varphi_n' = G_b^{n-1} \, A_n' \varphi_b^{n-1} \tag{15}$$

where G_b^n is the inhomogeneous Green function of the variable background adapted for every iteration step n. This non-linear inversion scheme is called Compound USCT, and the reconstruction algorithm is therefore the same as the previous classical one. The solutions are iteratively determined using Eq. 7. Experimentally, this approach was adapted to bone sample considered as a tube-like sample. The refraction effects are cancelled using a specific set-up in order to impose straight ray propagation inside the shell of the tube/bone [4]. Despite limitations due to heavy data processing requirements and complex acoustic signals resulting from multiple physical effects involved (various paths into the shell, roughness of the water/bone interfaces etc…), this approach gives images that are quantitatively related to the compressional wave velocities in a cross-section of a cortical shell, and the error remains within reasonable limits (about 7%).

A second non-linear inversion method was investigated. In this case, the medium is modeled without any *a priori* knowledge by performing a simple geometrical discretization of the object. The algorithm involves successive linearizations of the Lippmann-Schwinger representation. The initial guess in the iterative process is provided by the first-order Born approximation. If the solution is known with the order (n-1), the n-order solution A_n' will satisfy:

$$[(\varphi')^m - \varphi_{n-1}'] = G_b^{n-1} \, [A_n' - A_{n-1}'] \varphi_b^{n-1} \tag{16}$$

At each iteration, the algorithm numerically solves a forward diffraction problem in order to calculate the appropriate inhomogeneous Green function G_b^{n-1} and the internal field φ_b^{n-1}. Contrary to what occurs with the Compound USCT, this method requires only one series of experimental data, and involves the inversion of a huge, full and complex matrix. The matrix inversion procedure is the key point in this method. A mean-square solution can be calculated using a conjugate-gradient method associated with a regularization procedure. Our first approach is iterative, and the inversion procedure is carried out frequency by frequency from the sinogram in the frequency domain. The stability of the algorithm is improved using a Tikhonov regularization process. The minimization of the cost function (the difference between recorded and simulated waveforms) is computed using the Polak-Ribière conjugate gradient process. The detail of the algorithm is presented in [15], [16] for a numerical and experimental academic targets, and in [17] for a real lamb shoulder bone. To make use of the broadband frequency content of the impulse signal used, the idea is to begin with the low frequencies, which carry overall information, and to gradually inject the high frequencies to simultaneously improve both the qualitative aspects (the resolution) and the quantitative aspects (the characterization). However, this technique is computationally time consuming. The second proposed method consists in resorting to the more advanced Full Waveform Inversion (FWI) techniques that are at the forefront in the field of geophysics [18], [19]. The term "full" refers to the use of the full-time series. The aim is to simultaneously reconstruct the compression and shear waves in the bone without considering that the tissue density is spatially constant as in the previous method. Indeed, full waveform inversion is an imaging method that is based on full numerical modeling of wave propagation in the medium. The gradient of the cost function is obtained as the convolution product of the forward field with an adjoint field obtained by calculating the propagation of the time-reversed residuals. In this iterative process, some artifacts can alter the quality of the reconstruction. In order to reduce these artifacts and ensure a coherent reconstruction of the parameters, different pre-conditioning or regularization techniques can be proposed. The minimization of the cost function that we use is based on the quasi-Newton technique called Limited-memory Broyden-Fletcher-Goldfarb-Shanno (L-BFGS) [20], which is far more efficient in terms of convergence than conjugate-gradient techniques. The details of the algorithm are presented in [21].

3 Results

The feasibility of these different algorithms was tested on data obtained using mechanical and electronical ultrasonic scanners, allowing diffraction-, reflection- and/or transmission-mode measurements.

3.1 Breast phantom imaging

The breast training phantom CIRS™ Model 052A mimics the ultrasonic and anatomic characteristics of tissues found in an average patient. The soft tissue mimicking phantom made of

Zerdine™ contains cystic and solid masses which appear respectively dark and bright on B-mode (ultrasound sonography) and USCT images. B-mode images were made using a clinical ultrasound device, Esaote™ AU5, with a 7-MHz linear probe. Near-field USCT images were made using the 1024-element electronical and mechanical scanner developed by our laboratory and presented in detail in [22]. Figure 1 shows, in the center, the USCT map of the analyzed phantom containing 5 dark masses and one bright mass. The two images on the side represent the B-mode images made of the areas of the phantom identified by the white rectangles. Differences arise because the scanner performs an entire 2D circular scan (Ø = 30 cm, 720 reflection measurements) around the breast phantom whereas a unique position of the probe (one incident direction) is considered with the B-mode system.

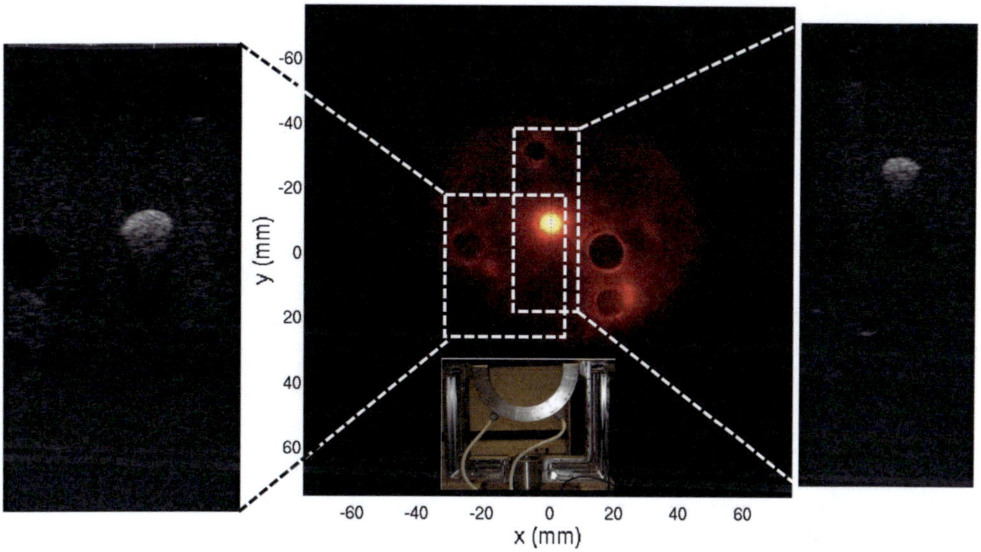

Figure 1: Imaging of the CIRS™ breast phantom. At the center, the USCT image (using the 1024-element scanner built by our laboratory), and on the sides, two B-mode images (using 7-MHz Esaote™ AU5 scanner) of the areas marked by the white rectangles. The inlaid picture shows the semi-circular 1024-element array used. Details can be found in [23]

3.2 Bone qualitative imaging

The USCT device, in this application, is a circular antenna having an internal radius of 150 mm and equipped with 8 fixed 1-MHz transducers distributed over a 360 ° angle ($\Delta\theta_{fixed} = 45°$) [24]. The validity of USCT was tested on artificial and fresh bone sample. As fresh sample, in-vitro experiments were conducted on a fibula from a 10-year old child, containing water in the inner cavity. The mean cross-section of the bone was 17 ± 2 mm and that of the inner cavity was 6 ± 2 mm. Figure 2 shows the USCT map (255 x 255 pixels) of the fibula. On the image, the outer and inner boundaries (i.e. the marrow area) were defined from image processing using an active contour method (Snake algorithm). If the outer contour is well defined, the resolution for the inner boundary is poor. The active contour method corrects its calculation by successive apodisations. This results in a smoothing of the boundary, which does not represent the actual bone area.

A human bone mimicking phantom (Sawbones™, tibia-fibula) was also studied. The cavity diameter of the tibia is 12.5mm. The fibula mimicking phantom had no inner cavity. The distance between bones was ~8 mm [24]. The USCT images of objects were compared with X-ray computed tomography (X-ray CT) images obtained at the same cross-section levels, with an X-ray CT device (Mediso™, Hungary) (Figure 2).

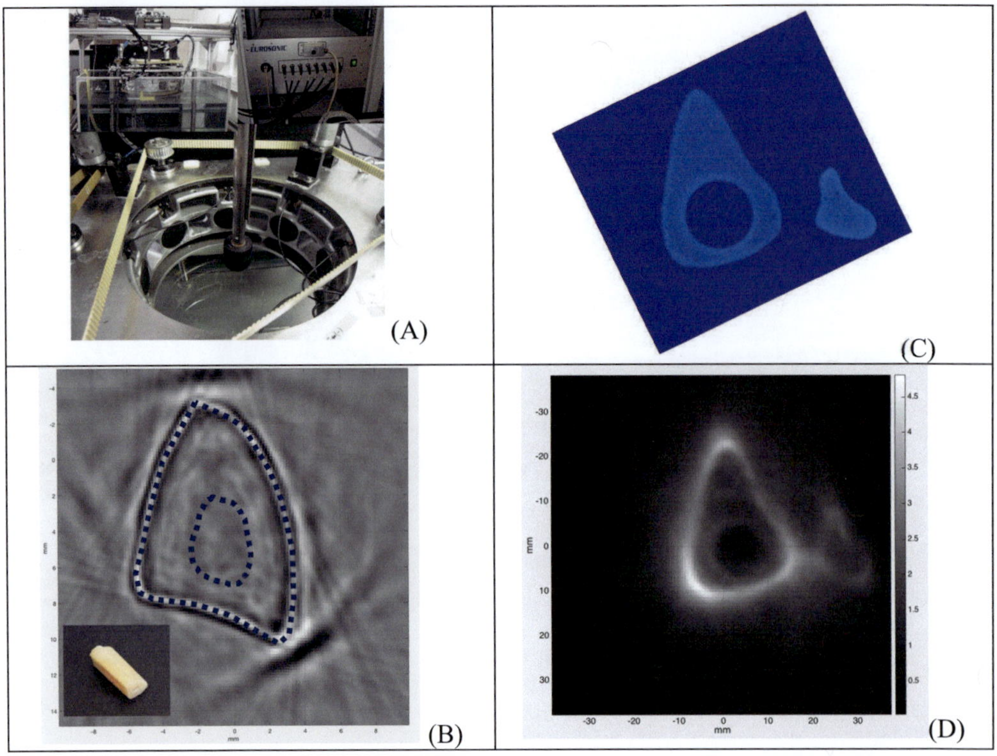

Figure 2: (A) Circular antenna with an internal radius of 150 mm, 8 fixed 1-MHz transducers (Imasonic™), and a multiplexer electronic setup (8x8 channels, 12 bits, sampling frequency of 20 MHz) (Mistras-Eurosonic™) (B) The USCT-image of a child fibula. The inlaid picture shows the fresh bone sample. In dotted lines, the outer and inner boundaries are plotted using a Snake algorithm. (C) X-ray CT, and (D) USCT of a Sawbones™ composite bone-mimicking phantom. Details can be found in [24].

3.3 Bone quantitative imaging

The third results are obtained based on the non-linear schemes and quantitative USCT of bones. The first non-linear method (frequency-hopping method) was performed with a fresh and cleaned lamb shoulder bone, immersed in a water tank. Data acquisition was performed using a mechanical scanner, with one 500 kHz-transducer (Imasonic^{TM}) as a transmitter, and one hydrophone (Reson^{TM}) as a receiver. The usable bandwidth ranges from approximately 150 kHz to 750 kHz. The received signals were digitized (14 bits, 20 MHz) using a data acquisition sheet (Spectrum Mi4031). The sector scanned was 360 degrees with both transmitter and receiver, with an angular increment of 10 degrees (36 x 36 signals). The compressional wave and shear wave velocity in bone were respectively 2700 (± 200) m/s and 1250 (± 200) m/s (1476 m/s for the speed of sound in the water tank). Iterations were performed by gradually increasing the working frequency with four frequencies chosen within the useful bandwidth: 150 kHz, 250 kHz, 500 kHz and 750 kHz. Regarding the quantitative aspects, the compressional wave velocity was reconstructed with a relative error of about 30% [17].

For the full waveform inversion method, the results are purely numerical. No experimental results were obtained yet, but that will be the focus of future work. Figure 3 shows the main quantitative (compressional wave velocity and density) reconstruction obtained with a numerical phantom. The phantom has a realistic geometry of a tibia/fibula paired bone, surrounded by a water-like medium. The incident signal is a Ricker (second derivative of a Gaussian) 200 kHz-wavelet, and the virtual array has 8 sources and 128 receivers, with 9 cm of radius [21].

4 Conclusions and future work

Ultrasonic Computed Tomography (USCT) appears as an alternative imaging tool capable of revealing the internal structure of soft tissues (mammography), delineating the shape of bones (cortical thickness), and even providing the possibility of parametric estimation (the sound speed and density map). In this work, the scope of USCT methods was extended from low impedance contrasted media such as soft tissues (the classical domain of USCT) to more contrasted domains such as cortical bone structures using non-linear and correction schemes. The wave field and associated Green function of the reference background medium were determined iteratively at the various steps. In future work, we plan to investigate various ways of improving these methods. Work is in progress, for instance, on the matrix inversion procedure involved in the FWI method and particularly on the regularization process, which is a very important aspect of the inversion scheme, especially in the case of high-contrast targets. Optimization, signal and image processing studies on how to handle the heavy experimental data are also ongoing (wavelet analysis, blind deconvolution, segmentation, Cramer-Rao bounds) [24]–[26].

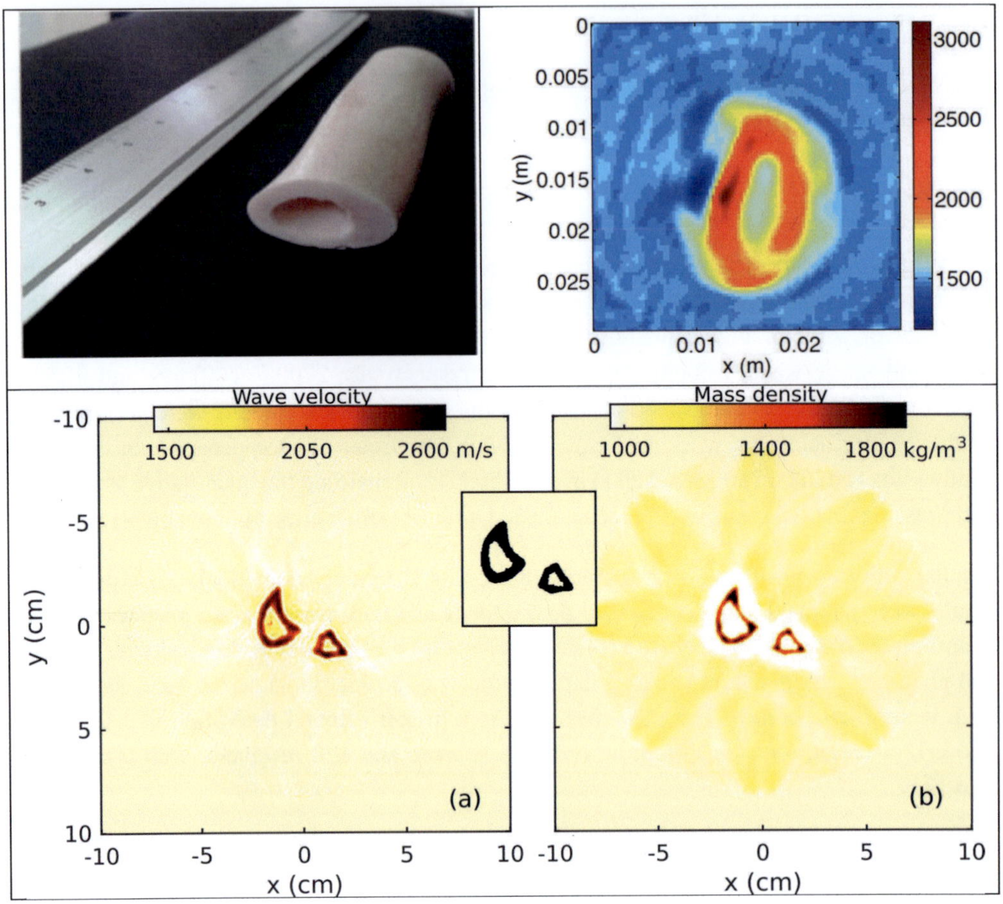

Figure 3: (Top) Experimental quantitative USCT of a lamb shoulder bone using non-linear frequency-hopping method. Images and details can be found in [17]. (Bottom) Numerical quantitative USCT of a tibia/fibula paired bone using non-linear full waveform inversion method. Images and details can be found in [21].

Acknowledgements

The authors are grateful to Eric Debieu and Vincent Long at the Laboratory of Mechanics and Acoustics, (LMA) for their help in setting up experiments. The authors are grateful for medical assistance from Dr Philippe Petit and Dr Jean-Luc Jouve at the "*Timone*" Children's Hospital (APHM). The *X*-ray CT were performed by Laure Balasse and Samantha Fernandez at the European Center for Research in Medical Imaging (CERIMED), Marseille.

References

[1] S. Mensah and J.-P. Lefebvre, "Enhanced compressibility tomography," *IEEE Trans. Ultrason. Ferroelectr. Freq. Control*, vol. 44, no. 6, pp. 1245–1252, Nov. 1997.

[2] S. Mensah and R. Ferriere, "Near-Field Diffraction Tomography," *Ultrason. Imaging*, vol. 24, no. 1, pp. 13–24, Jan. 2002.

[3] S. Mensah and R. Ferriere, "Diffraction tomography: a geometrical distortion free procedure," *Ultrasonics*, vol. 42, no. 1–9, pp. 677–682, Apr. 2004.

[4] P. Lasaygues, E. Ouedraogo, J.-P. Lefebvre, M. Gindre, M. Talmant, and P. Laugier, "Progress towards in vitro quantitative imaging of human femur using compound quantitative ultrasonic tomography," *Phys. Med. Biol.*, vol. 50, no. 11, pp. 2633–2649, Jun. 2005.

[5] J. F. Greenleaf and R. C. Bahn, "Clinical Imaging with Transmissive Ultrasonic Computerized Tomography," *IEEE Trans. Biomed. Eng.*, vol. BME-28, no. 2, pp. 177–185, Feb. 1981.

[6] M. P. André *et al.*, "A New Consideration of Diffraction Computed Tomography for Breast Imaging: Studies in Phantoms and Patients," in *Acoustical Imaging*, J. P. Jones, Ed. Boston, MA: Springer US, 1995, pp. 379–390.

[7] N. V. Ruiter, T. O. Müller, R. Stotzka, and H. Gemmeke, "Evaluation of Different Approaches for Transmission Tomography in Ultrasound Computer Tomography," in *Bildverarbeitung für die Medizin 2005*, H.-P. Meinzer, H. Handels, A. Horsch, and T. Tolxdorff, Eds. Berlin/Heidelberg: Springer-Verlag, 2005, pp. 430–434.

[8] N. Duric *et al.*, "Detection of breast cancer with ultrasound tomography: First results with the Computed Ultrasound Risk Evaluation (CURE) prototype: Detection of breast cancer with ultrasound tomography," *Med. Phys.*, vol. 34, no. 2, pp. 773–785, Jan. 2007.

[9] E. Franceschini, S. Mensah, L. Le Marrec, and P. Lasaygues, "An optimization method for quantitative impedance tomography," *IEEE Trans. Ultrason. Ferroelectr. Freq. Control*, vol. 54, no. 8, pp. 1578–1588, Aug. 2007.

[10] M. P. André, H. S. Janée, P. J. Martin, G. P. Otto, B. A. Spivey, and D. A. Palmer, "High-speed data acquisition in a diffraction tomography system employing large-scale toroidal arrays," *Int. J. Imaging Syst. Technol.*, vol. 8, no. 1, pp. 137–147, 1997.

[11] R. C. Waag and R. J. Fedewa, "A ring transducer system for medical ultrasound research," *IEEE Trans. Ultrason. Ferroelectr. Freq. Control*, vol. 53, no. 10, pp. 1707–1718, Oct. 2006.

[12] J. Rouyer, P. Lasaygues, and S. Mensah, "Novel Ultrasound Tomograph for Anatomical Inspection," in *Acoustical Imaging*, vol. 31, A. Nowicki, J. Litniewski, and T. Kujawska, Eds. Dordrecht: Springer Netherlands, 2012, pp. 3–10.

[13] J.-P. Lefebvre, "Progress in linear inverse scattering imaging : NDE application of Ultrasonic Reflection Tomography," in *Inverse Problem in Engineering Mechanics*, Rotterdam/Brookfield: A.A.Balkema, 1994, pp. 371–375.

[14] J. P. Lefebvre, P. Lasaygues, S. Mensah, S. Delamare, and A. Wirgin, "Born Ultrasonic Tomography: Some Limits and Improvements," in *Acoustical Imaging*, vol. 25, M. Halliwell and P. N. T. Wells, Eds. Boston: Kluwer Academic Publishers, 2002, pp. 79–86.

[15] P. Lasaygues, R. Guillermin, and J.-P. Lefebvre, "Distorted Born diffraction tomography applied to inverting ultrasonic field scattered by noncircular infinite elastic tube," *Ultrason. Imaging*, vol. 28, no. 4, pp. 211–229, Oct. 2006.

[16] R. Guillermin, P. Lasaygues, G. Rabau, and J.-P. Lefebvre, "Quantitative non-linear ultrasonic imaging of targets with significant acoustic impedance contrast—An experimental study," *J. Acoust. Soc. Am.*, vol. 134, no. 2, p. 1001, 2013.

[17] R. Guillermin, P. Lasaygues, and G. Rabau, "Quantitative Ultrasonic Imaging of Bones," in *The 22nd International Congress on Sound and Vibration*, Florence, Italy, 2015, pp. 1–6.

[18] J. Tromp, D. Komatitsch, and Q. Liu, "Spectral-Element and Adjoint Methods in Seismology," *Communications in Computational Physics*, pp. 1–32, 2008.

[19] V. Monteiller, S. Chevrot, D. Komatitsch, and Y. Wang, "Three-dimensional full waveform inversion of short-period teleseismic wavefields based upon the SEM-DSM hybrid method," *Geophys. J. Int.*, vol. 202, no. 2, pp. 811–827, May 2015.

[20] J. Nocedal and S. J. Wright, *Numerical optimization*. New York: Springer, 2006.

[21] S. Bernard, V. Monteiller, D. Komatitsch, and P. Lasaygues, "Ultrasonic computed tomography based on full-waveform inversion for bone quantitative imaging," *Phys. Med. Biol.*, Jul. 2017.

[22] J. Rouyer, S. Mensah, E. Franceschini, P. Lasaygues, and J.-P. Lefebvre, "Conformal ultrasound imaging system for anatomical breast inspection," *IEEE Trans. Ultrason. Ferroelectr. Freq. Control*, vol. 59, no. 7, pp. 1457–1469, Jul. 2012.

[23] J. Rouyer, S. Mensah, C. Vasseur, and P. Lasaygues, "The benefits of compression methods in acoustic coherence tomography," *Ultrason. Imaging*, vol. 37, no. 3, pp. 205–223, Jul. 2015.

[24] P. Lasaygues *et al.*, "Contrast resolution enhancement of Ultrasonic Computed Tomography using a wavelet-based method – Preliminary results in bone imaging," in *Proceedings of the Int. Workshop on Medical Ultrasound Tomography*, Speyer, Germany, 2017.

[25] M. L. Diong, A. Roueff, P. Lasaygues, and A. Litman, "Precision analysis based on Cramer–Rao bound for 2D acoustics and electromagnetic inverse scattering," *Inverse Probl.*, vol. 31, no. 7, p. 075003, Jul. 2015.

[26] M. L. Diong, A. Roueff, P. Lasaygues, and A. Litman, "Impact of the Born approximation on the estimation error in 2D inverse scattering," *Inverse Probl.*, vol. 32, no. 6, p. 065006, Jun. 2016.

Real-Time Ultrasound Transmission Tomography based on Bézier Curves

Mailyn Perez-Liva[1,2], José M. Udías[1], Jorge Camacho[3] and Joaquín L. Herraiz[1]

[1] *Grupo de Física Nuclear and UPARCOS, Univ. Complutense de Madrid, CEI Moncloa, Spain;*
[2] *Centre de RechercheCardiovasculaire. Hôpital Européen Georges Pompidou, Paris, France*
E-mail: mailyn.perez-liva@inserm.fr
[3] *Spanish National Research Council (CSIC), Madrid, Spain*

Abstract

Refraction-corrected ray-tracing methods in Ultrasound Transmission Tomography (USTT) are able to reconstruct the acoustic properties of tissues with good accuracy when using medium to high frequencies (>3 MHz). However, these methods, are generally time-consuming in comparison with reconstructions based on straight lines, which provide on the other hand, very low-quality images. In this work, we propose an on-the-flight reconstruction method that exploits the computing capabilities of current GPUs. The method uses Bezier polynomials to asses the geodesic path joining a pair of ultrasound detectors for a given sound speed map. The outcome of the proposed algorithm demonstrates that Bezier curves can be an effective and accurate method to compute bent-rays for fast USTT reconstruction. Besides, the method is faster than typical acquisition times in USTT, so it can be considered a step towards real-time reconstructions suited for clinical practice.

Keywords: USTT, USCT, refraction-corrected ray-tracing, Bezier polynomials

1 Introduction

Ultrasound Transmission Tomography is a promising technique that provides quantitative images of the speed of sound and acoustic attenuation of tissues under study. To reconstruct these acoustic parameters of tissue, it is necessary to employ an appropriate model for wave propagation that finds the right balance between computational efficiency and physical accuracy to describe the processes taking place in breast tissue. To achieve that, it is needed to analyze which are the dominant physical processes that take place in the medium explored, in this case breast tissues. Zhu and Steinberg [1] showed for both *in vivo* and numerical phantoms, that refraction is the most important process, while scattering is a secondary process dominating the distortion of the ultrasound wave front. This supports the adoption of bent-rays methods in USTT, as it has been demonstrated that they are able to reproduce well refraction effects up to 20%, which is larger than the changes in sound speed inside the breast (typically <8% [2,3]).

When using relatively high frequencies (>3 MHz), refraction-corrected ray-tracing methods can reconstruct the mentioned acoustic properties of tissue with high image quality. However, most of these methods are based on the numerical solution of the eikonal equation, which provides the time at which the wavefront will arrive at any given point of the domain, with the posterior use of algorithms to extract the geodesic path. This procedure increases the computational cost of these algorithms in comparison with straight-rays methods, therefore precluding real-time applicability. On the other hand, straight-rays methods fail around structures with large sound speed variations, because they ignore refraction, which makes them not suitable to obtain high-quality images of breast tissue.

In order to develop refraction-corrected ray-tracing USTT in a computationally efficient manner and being able to perform on-the-flight reconstructions, in this work we propose a fast and straightforward ray-linking method that exploits the large computational capabilities of current GPUs in parallelized problems. The proposed method avoids solving the eikonal equation and the gradient methods commonly employed to obtain optimal paths between detectors. In our method, each thread of the GPU evaluates the travel-time along a smooth curve chosen out of a family of restricted Bezier curves, connecting emitters and receivers. The curve with the shortest travel-time (geodesic curve) is the one used for the reconstruction [4].

2 Materials and methods

2.1 Ray-linking problems with Bezier polynomials

There are multiple methods to join two points with optimal curves. One possible approach is the use of Bézier polynomials. According to Bézier's method, a given curve can be obtained from a polygon [5]. If the curve is created as a polynomial of degree n, the polygon will have (n+1) vertices. We will define these vertices with the vector P. The initial and final points of this vector, P_0 and P_N, will represent the extremes of the curve. The Bézier curve defined this way will always pass through the extreme points, but not neccessarily through the remaining vertices of the polygon. Most common Bézier curves used are based on n=1 to 3. With n=1 the Bezier curve are straight lines linking two given points, for n=2 the Bézier curve is a quadratic polynomial, and so on.

A quadratic Bézier curve, given by the function B(t) and determined by the vertices: P_0, P_1 and P_2 is given by the following parametric expression:

$$B(t) = (1-t)^2 P_0 + 2t(1-t)P_1 + t^2 P_2, \quad t \in [0,1]. \tag{1}$$

If P_1 is shifted in both x and y directions, many curves can be obtained. P_1 choice will determine the characteristics of the Bézier curve. The parameter t provides points to sample the Bézier function and therefore, $B(t)$ will contain the set of points that belongs to the Bézier curve.

Given a family of paths that connects two points obtained with Bézier polynomials, the optimal path among them can be calculated by for a given sound speed map and selecting the curve that provides the lowest TOF. The strategy we propose to use the quadratic Bézier curves (n=2) for bent-ray tracing is schematically represented in Fig. 1. The points P_0 and P_2 correspond to the coordinates of emitter and receiver, respectively. The total set of points P_1 that defines different curves can be obtained by providing a range of shifts in directions parallel and perpendicular ($N_\perp$ and $N_\parallel$) to the straight line that links the detectors. Once the center point is found, if a shift in each direction is given ($d_\perp$ and $d_\parallel$), it is straightforward to move the point P_1 in the grid.

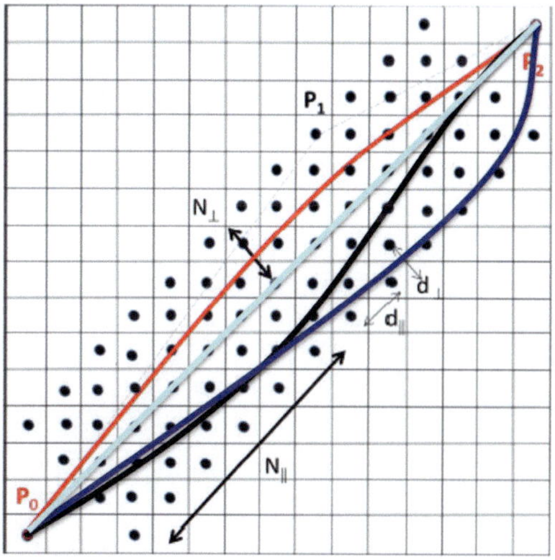

Figure 1: Bent-ray tracing with quadratic Bézier polynomial curves

We can numerically evaluate the time-of-flight (TOF) for each given path subdividing it into small segments and then computing the sum of the product of their lengths dl_i and the inverse of the speed (from the SS map) in that segment:

$$TOF = \sum_{i=0}^{N} \left(\frac{1}{c_i}\right) dl_i \qquad (2)$$

In equation (1) c_i is the SS at the pixel determined by the parameter i, being N the number of points used to evaluate the Bézier curve, and dl_i is the distance between two contiguous points of the curve.

We used CUDA to implement the method, as the different evaluations of the Bézier curves for different points P_1 can be done in parallel using GPUs, speeding up the calculations considerably. In the method proposed, the curvature of the path can be controlled by changing the range of the shift in the parallel and perpendicular direction of P_1.

For the seek of comparison with a reference method, we analyzed the output curves provided by our method against the ones provided by an implementation of the Fast Marching Method (FMM), which solves numerically the eikonal equation. All the details of the implementation of FMM used can be found in reference [6]. In Fig. 2, we represented the differences of simulated paths obtained with the classical FMM method and the proposed Bézier-based method, for a water-breast tissue interface (1480 m/s and 1550 m/s respectively).

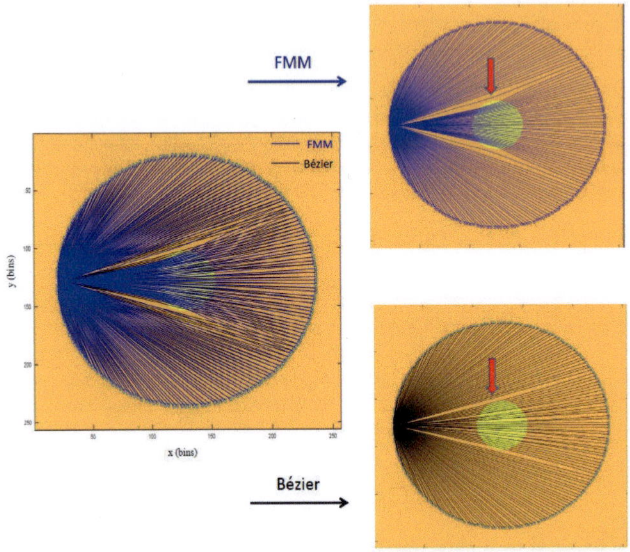

Figure 2: Comparison between the estimations with FMM and Bézier trajectories. Around the simulated object, FMM bend the paths even when rays travel along a homogeneous medium. Bézier ray tracing can be adjusted to overcome that issue

Due to the higher SS value of breast tissue, some of the rays around the interface will bendtheir trajectories. In our case, when using FMM, some rays around the inclusion, that only travel in water, appear bent, which is clearly not correct (those rays are indicated by red arrows in the right panel of Fig. 2). However, we can adjust the parameters of the Bézier-based method ($N_{\perp}$ and $N_{\parallel}$) to avoid this problem and still retain the right behavior in the regions close to the inclusion. It is important to note that other implementations of FMM exists, but they need higher-order interpolations to achieve good enough accuracy, which requires much longer computational time.

Once the method to simulate the wave propagation is determined, any general method to solve the optimization problem can be formulated, as for example, the Maximum Likelihood - Expectation Maximization (ML-EM), whose updating expression is given by:

$$\xi_j^{(n+1)} = \frac{\xi_j^{(n)}}{\sum_{i=1}^{M} A_{i,j}} \sum_{i=1}^{M} A_{i,j} \frac{p_i}{\sum_{k=1}^{N} A_{i,k}\, \xi_k^{(n)}} \tag{3}$$

where $\xi_j^{(n+1)}$ is either the sound speed or the absorption coefficient value in the pixel j for the next iteration based on the value $\xi_j^{(n)}$ at the current iteration. $A_{i,j}$ represents the sensitivity coefficients or the path followed by the wave and p_i is the parameter used to characterize the measured pressure field at the receiver location and with which we can reconstruct the acoustic parameter of interest.

2.2 Ray tracing for sound speed reconstructions

The reconstruction of SS maps using geometrical acoustics is done from TOF values. The algorithms used to obtain SS maps are based on the following system of equations:

$$TOF_i^{sim} = \sum_{j=1}^{n} A_{i,j} S_j \ , \qquad i = 1{:}M \tag{4}$$

Where j represents the scanned pixel, i identifies the receiving transducer, S_j is the slowness at pixel j and the coefficients $A_{i,j}$, are the sensitivity kernel elements that relate the data with the pixels involved in the wave propagation. These coefficients represent the discrete version of the ray in the image grid. TOF_i^{sim} is the simulated TOF value estimated at detector i.

With the previous equation, an estimate of the TOF value with a given model of the slowness can be obtained. This value will differ in an amount δT from the measured data TOF_i^{exp}, which can be use to formulate the inverse problem for the reconstruction:

$$\delta T_i = TOF_i^{exp} - TOF_i^{sim} \tag{5}$$

2.3 The amplitude-decay method for attenuation reconstructions

When an acoustic wave propagates through a medium, it will experience a loss of amplitude due to geometrical spreading and by the absorption and scattering characteristics of the medium of propagation given by:

$$A = A_0 e^{-\alpha(f)x} \tag{6}$$

Where A and A_0 are the final and initial amplitudes of the wave once it has a distance x in a given medium, with an attenuation that present a certain dependence with the frequency of the wave as $\alpha(f)$.

The amplitude-decay method assumes [8]:

- A linear dependence on the frequency in the attenuation coefficient:

$$\alpha(f) = \alpha_0 f \tag{7}$$

- The attenuation in water is neglected.
- The energy is assumed to be concentrated at the central frequency of the signal.

Using the former assumptions and measurements in water, a way to avoid calculating the geometrical spreading of the wave is obtained. A simple expression to formulate the inversion problem for the attenuation reconstruction can be given as

$$\sum_{j=1}^{n} A_{i,j} \alpha_{0_j} = \frac{1}{f_c} \ln\left(\frac{A_{water}}{A_{phantom}}\right) \tag{8}$$

Where, as before, j represents the scanned pixel, i identifies the receiving transducer, α_{0_j} is the absorption coefficient at the pixel j and the coefficients $A_{i,j}$ will relate the data with the pixels connected with the ray that represents the energy propagation of the wave. A_{water} is the amplitude of the signal at the i receiver when there is only water in the field of view (FOV) and $A_{phantom}$ is the amplitude at the same position as before but with the phantom located in the FOV.

2.4 *In-vitro* real data experiments

To evaluate the performance of the algorithm proposed, we used experimental data acquired with the Multimodal Ultrasound for Breast Imaging (MUBI) system. The MUBI scanner is a USCT prototype (see Fig. 3(a)) [7] comprising two coplanar medical 128-element linear arrays of transducers, with a central frequency of 3.2 MHz and a 50% bandwidth (Prosonic, Korea). Array probes and breast phantoms are arranged inside a water tank to ensure good acoustic coupling. The arrays can be moved independently of each other using stepper motors with high mechanical precision (0.1°) to cover several locations around the breast phantom. The radius of rotation is variable between 45 mm and 100. A SITAU 112 (Dasel, Spain) 128 channel ultrasonic equipment is used, with parallel acquisition, beam steering and dynamic depth focusing capabilities. The data measured is transferred through a USB interface to a computer for data post-processing.

To acquire transmission data, one of the arrays acts as emitter and the other one as receiver (as it is indicated in Fig. 3 (a)). For each emitting position, the location of the receiver is shifted several times in order to cover a variable area describing a fan-beam. This process is performed sequentially changing the orientation of the fan-beam until the whole field of view is scanned. Fan-beams are taken at regular angular intervals. Total acquisition time with this prototype is around 10 minutes per coronal plane. Most of the time is spent in arrays motion.

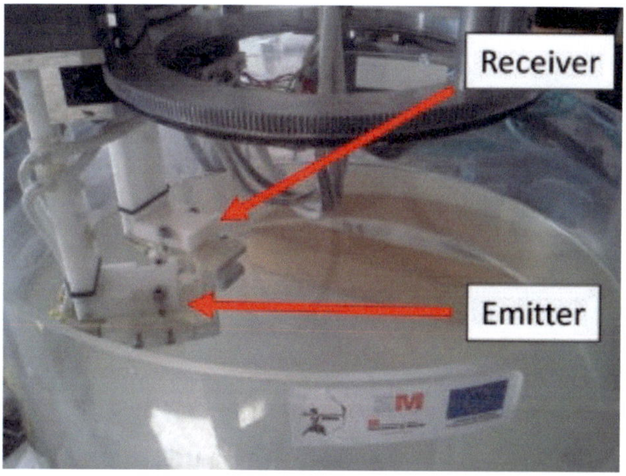

Figure 3: Experimental arrangement of the MUBI scanner with rotating fan-beams. A variable number of fan-beams can be used in this setup to scan the whole field of view [7].

The data acquired with the MUBI system consisted on a tissue-mimicking phantom whose main characteristics can be seen in Fig. 4 and Table I. Two holes were performed inside the phantom. The first one was filled with water once the phantom was located inside the water tank and in the second one we mixed different concentrations of alcohol and graphite, resulting in a region with small differences in terms of SS with respect to the background of the phantom, but increased attenuation. Due to the axial symmetry of the phantom only a central slice was acquired.

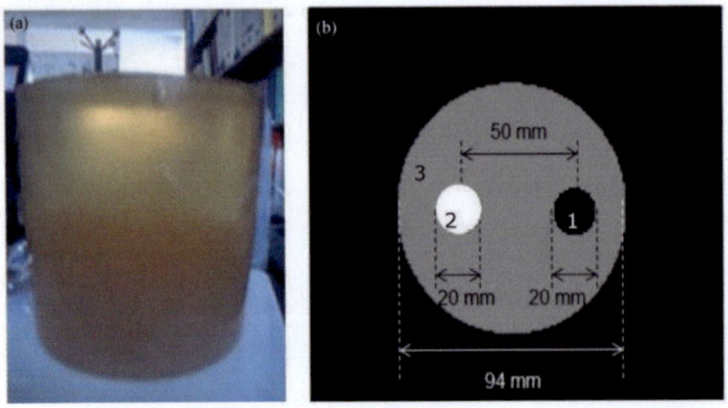

Figure 4: *In-vitro* tissue mimicking phantom created for USTT reconstructions. (a). lateral view of the phantom. (b). depicsts a scheme of the top view of this phantom.

Region	**Water (ml)**	**Gelatin (ml)**	**Graphite (ml)**	**Formaldehyde (ml)**	**Ethanol (ml)**
Background	800.0	63.0	78.4	2.4	64.2
Cyst	400.0	61.0	58.8	1.2	16.0

Table 1: *In-vitro* tissue mimicking phantom composition for measurements in the MUBI scanner.

To reconstruct this phantom, we used the proposed Bézier-based reconstruction method and also, a simple analytic straight-rays method based on filtered back-projection (FBP) for comparison. To obtain the TOF and amplitude values of the signals acquired, we used cross-correlation and envelope-based methods respectively [4]. To provide a reference for our reconstructions, for all the USTT acquisitions performed in the MUBI scanner, a high-resolution reflectivity acquisition of the same tomogram was also obtained. The reflectivity reconstructions are based on the Full Angle SpatialCompound (FASC) technique [7].

3 Results and Discussion

Fig. 5 shows the SS and AA reconstructions of the phantom under study with analytic and Bézier iterative methods. The reconstruction time per slice was ~0.23 seconds for both FBP-SS and FBP-AA (top and bottom left panels of Fig. 5 respectively) as the same angular and radial sampling is used for both reconstructions. The reconstructions using Bézier took ~10 seconds/slice for the SS and using the pre-calculated Bézier bent-rays from the SS reconstruction, the AA maps can be obtained in 2 seconds/slice.

The information obtained from both reconstruction algorithms is similar. Nevertheless, FBP reconstructions tend to miss-estimate the actual size of the structures inside the phantom, as they do not take into account refraction. Due to the considerable changes of SS in this phantom, refraction is an important phenomenon in order to obtain accurate reconstructions.

The proposed Bézier-based reconstruction method requires an amount of time similar to the one required for acquiring and processing USTT data, so it can be considered a real-time reconstruction method suited for clinical practice, while providing SS and AA images with good enough quality.

One advantage of the proposed method is that it can be easily extended to 3D-Data, for scanners such as the USCT developed at KIT [8]. In this kind of systems, the amount of recorded data is very large, and approximated reconstruction methods can be very useful to obtain images in a reasonable amount of time. Furthermore, the proposed method can be used to provide the initial estimated image for full wave-inversion (FWI) methods [9]. These methods are known to provide better image quality than ray-tracing ones, but they require to start the iterative process with an initial image that is close enough to the actual one to avoid convergence problems. For that reason, starting a FWI algorithm with an image obtained with a ray-tracing method such as the one proposed here, with refraction effects corrected, can reduce possible artifacts and improve its convergence.

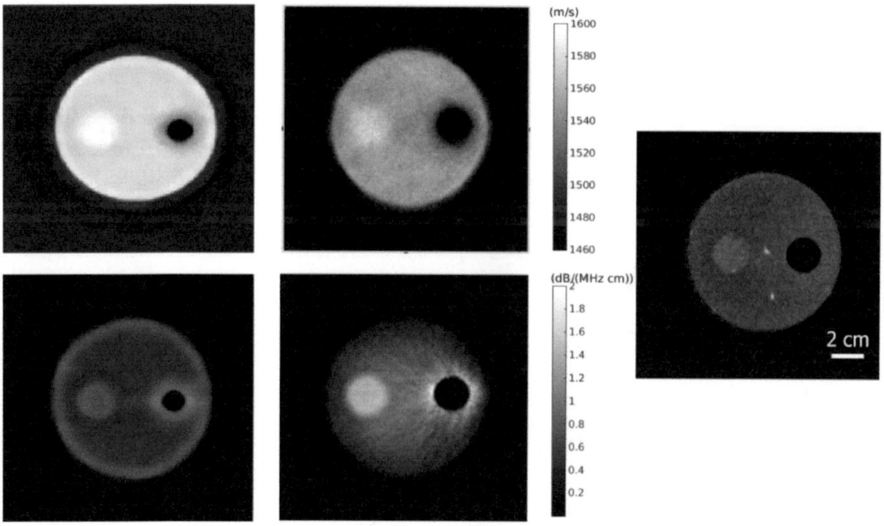

Figure 5: Sound speed (SS) and Acoustic attenuation (AA) reconstruction for the tissue-mimicking phantom. Left panel shows FBP reconstructions of the phantom, central panel Bézier-based bent rays reconstructions and right panel the reflectivity reconstruction as reference. At the top are SS reconstructions and at the bottom AA ones. FBP reconstructions miss-estimate the actual dimensions of the structures in the phantom.

References

[1] Q. Zhu and B. D. Steinberg: Wavefront amplitude distribution in the female breast. The Journalof the Acoustical Society of America, 96(1) (1994) 1–9.

[2] A. H. Andersen: A ray tracing approach to restoration and resolution enhancement inexperimental ultrasound tomography. Ultrasonic imaging, 12(4) (1990) 268–291.

[3] S. Li, M. Jackowski, D. P. Dione, T. Varslot, L. H. Staib, and K. Mueller: Refraction corrected transmission ultrasound computed tomography for application in breast imaging. Medical physics, 37(5) (2010) 2233–2246.

[4] M. Pérez-Liva: PhD Thesis University Complutense of Madrid (2017).

[5] A. R. Forrest: Interactive interpolation and approximation by bézier polynomials. The Computer Journal, 15(1) (1972) 71–79.

[6] M. Pérez-Liva, J. Herraiz, N. González-Salido, L. Medina-Valdés, J. Camacho, C. Fritch, and J. Udías: Ultrasound computed tomography for quantitative breast imaging. IEEE Global Medical Engineering Physics Exchanges/Pan American Health Care Exchanges (GMEPE/PAHCE), (2016) 1–6.

[7] J. Camacho, L. Medina, J. F. Cruza, J. M. Moreno, and C. Fritsch: Multimodal ultrasonic imagingfor breast cancer detection. Archives of Acoustics, 37(3) (2012) 253–260.

[8] Ruiter, N.V., Zapf, M., et al.: "First Results of a Clinical Study with 3D Ultrasound Computer Tomography," Proc. IEEE Internat. Ultrasonics Symp., (2013).

[9] M. Pérez-Liva, J. L. Herraiz, and J. M. UdíasE. MillerB. T. Cox and B. E. Treeby, Time domain reconstruction of sound speed and attenuation in ultrasound computed tomography using full wave inversion. The Journal of the Acoustical Society of America 141, 1595 (2017);

3D imaging of the breast using full-waveform inversion

Oscar Calderon Agudo[1], Lluis Guasch[1], Peter Huthwaite[2], and Michael Warner[1]

[1]*Imperial College London, Department of Earth Science and Engineering, London, United Kingdom*
E-mail: oc14@imperial.ac.uk
[2]*Imperial College London, Department of Mechanical Engineering, London, United Kingdom*

Abstract

Full-waveform inversion (FWI) is an iterative method that produces high-quality quantitative models by minimising the misfit between observed and modelled data. Its application to medical imaging is still in its infancy, especially when FWI is applied to datasets and models in 3D. Here we implement a robust, efficient and reliable 3D FWI algorithm to invert a synthetic 3D ultrasound dataset obtained from a realistic phantom of the breast and we study the impact of having low-frequency data as well as neglecting absorption, density and 3D effects. We then apply our FWI algorithm to a 2D *in vivo* dataset with no information other than the recorded data, the total number of transducers and their nominal position. Our results suggest that 3D data acquisition as well as 3D data FWI and low-frequencies are essential to produce high fidelity models with enough quality to improve breast cancer diagnostics with ultrasound.

Keywords: 3D full-waveform inversion, 3D acquisition, low-frequency ultrasound

1 Introduction

Breast cancer is the most common type of cancer amongst women worldwide and the second with the highest mortality rate [1]. Advances in imaging techniques are key to improve its early detection and diagnosis in order to reduce its mortality rate. Due to its low cost, mammography is generally the preferred technique for standard routine screenings. It is based on the projection of X-rays through the breast and the assumption that the cancer mass is denser than the surrounding tissue. This imaging technique has helped reduce the number of breast cancer deaths considerably, but it has some disadvantages: it uses ionising radiation that is harmful for the patient, it has a low sensitivity when applied to dense breasts, it does not provide quantitative images of different tissue properties and it can lead to false-positive diagnostics when trying to detect breast cancer early [2].

Recently, ultrasound tomography has emerged as a safe alternative imaging method for breast cancer diagnosis that does not rely on ionising radtiation and which can provide images of speed of sound in tissue, sound attenuation and tissue density, amongst others. Typically, ultrasound tomography algorithms are based on ray theory, which limits their spatial resolution to the first Fresnel zone [3]. On the other hand, full-waveform inversion (FWI) honour the physics of finite-frequency wave propagation and is able to image variations of acoustic properties at sub-wavelength scales, which is significantly better than the resolution power of ray-based approaches [4].

Despite the computational burden of FWI algorithms, three-dimensional (anisotropic) FWI is nowadays standard practice in the oil industry [4]. In breast imaging, 2D FWI has been previously applied to *in vivo* ultrasound datasets [5], but the application of 3D FWI to these datasets has not yet been demonstrated in *in vivo* 3D data, partly due to the lack of adequate data-acquisition systems.

In this paper we demonstrate the potential of 3D FWI for imaging the breast and we show its feasibility on a realistic 3D breast phantom. We then analyse the benefits of having low-frequency data (below 0.5 MHz) for FWI and we investigate the impact of neglecting density, absorption and 3D effects. In the last section of this manuscript we apply our algorithm to a 2D *in vivo* ultrasound dataset having very little prior information of the acquisition system, and obtain a high-resolution model of the breast. We finally discuss briefly how the results could be improved, especially in terms of the acquisition strategy.

2 Methodology

The theoretical framework of FWI is well established. Here we present the basic formulation in order to understand its application to the medical imaging problem. The goal of FWI is to find a model $\mathbf{m}$ that minimises the misfit between the observed data, $\mathbf{d_{obs}}$, and the modelled data $\mathbf{d}(\mathbf{m})$. In other words, this is equivalent to minimising the least-squares norm:

$$f(\mathbf{m}) = \frac{1}{2}||\mathbf{d_{obs}} - \mathbf{d}(\mathbf{m})||_2^2 \tag{1}$$

with respect to the model parameter vector $\mathbf{m}$. This requires solving the forward problem $\mathbf{G}(\mathbf{m}) = \mathbf{d}(\mathbf{m})$, where $\mathbf{G}$ is an operator that decribes how to calculate the data from the model parameters - in practice, $\mathbf{G}$ is the implementation of the (acoustic) wave equation. The optimisation problem in equation (1) is non-linear because the wave equation does not have a linear relation between model parameters and pressure. In FWI we seek a local minimum of the functional described in equation (1), $\mathbf{m_0}$, such that the updated model after one iteration is the starting model plus a model perturbation, $\mathbf{m} = \mathbf{m_0} + \delta\mathbf{m}$. After linearising the problem by assuming that a small model perturbation introduces a small perturbation in the difference between observed and modelled data, the perturbation can be expressed as:

$$\delta \mathbf{m} = -\mathbf{H}^{-1} \frac{\partial \mathbf{f}}{\partial \mathbf{m}} \tag{2}$$

Where **H** is the Hessian operator, which contains all the second-order differentials of the misfit function, and $\partial f / \partial \mathbf{m}$ is the gradient. Due to the large dimensions of the Hessian, only an approximate magnitude of the diagonal elements is retained. To compute the gradient, we perform forward wavefield propagations from each source as well as backward propagations of the residual between observed and modelled data for each receiver and cross-correlate the two at each time-step for every cell in the model.

The computational cost of FWI is larger than that of ray-based methods because it requires full wave equation propagations but it leads to models with significantly higher resolution. Our parallel algorithm is able to perform 3D time-domain FWI with or without absorption by solving the visco-acoustic wave equation using a fourth-order in time and sixth-order in space finite-difference (FD) time-stepping algorithm. To optimize its performance, the accuracy of the FD stencil in 3D is tenth-order in space. The code is parallelised across distributed and shared memory systems, and it is optimised to minimise memory and CPU footprint, which makes it suitable for large 3D problems. In the next section we demonstrate the feasibility of 3D FWI to image a numerical breast phantom with our FWI implementation and we apply our algorithm to a 2D *in vivo* dataset. Further details of our algorithms can be found in [4].

3 Results

In this section we show the result of applying our FWI algorithm to two ultrasound datasets: 1) a 3D dataset from a realistic numerical breast phantom and 2) a 2D *in vivo* breast dataset. For the first dataset we study the impact of low-frequency content in the ultrasound, absorption, density and 3D effects. We then discuss the workflow used to obtain a model of speed of sound for the second dataset, which requires minimal user interaction, and we review the importance of low frequencies and the consequences of ignoring 3D effects in *in vivo* data inversions.

3.1 3D breast phantom

The first ultrasound dataset is generated from the 3D breast phantom in Figure 1, which simulates the human breast [6]. We design velocity, density and absorption models based on typical measured values, and these are respectively shown in Figures 1a, 1b and 1c. The bulk of the model is formed by a glandular region and is represented by a random medium, which is surrounded by an irregular subcutaneous fat layer and an outer thin skin layer. Several spherical inclusions have been added inside the glandular region to simulate cancer and fat masses. The dimensions of the discretised model are $95 \times 431 \times 431$ in cells, with a grid spacing of 0.29 mm that ensures there is no dispersion of P-waves beyond the maximum inverted frequency.

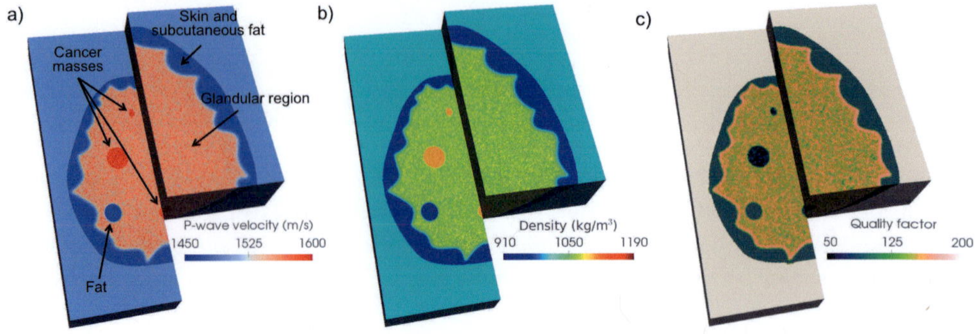

Figure 1: 3D numerical phantom of the breast with realistic a) P-wave velocity, b) density and c) absorption models.

We now perform several tests by generating ultrasound data with or without absorption, with fixed or variable density and with a 2D or 3D data acquisition geometry and we analyse the results of inverting these data using our FWI code. First, we generate synthetic ultrasound data for the 3D breast phantom in Figure 1a and fixed values of density and absorption, equal to the values for water (density of $1000 kg/m^3$ and $Q = 10^3$). The data is generated using 350 sources equally distributed across 3 rings and a three-cycle toneburst source wavelet with a center frequency of $750 kHz$ and a time sampling of $0.11 \mu s$ is used to generate $120 \mu s$ of data. The ultrasound signal is then recorded at 1280 receivers distributed across 5 rings with 256 receivers in each ring. The source and receiver rings have a diameter of $12 cm$, their center is at the center of a coronal view of the breast and the distance between rings is constant - but different for source and receiver rings so that these are uniformly distributed in the vertical direction. Figure 2 shows the results of applying 3D FWI on the data up to a frequency of $1.4 MHz$ by using different starting models and starting frequencies for the inversion. To reduce the computation time, 35 out of 350 sources are used at each iteration and these are different for each iteration so that all sources are used in each iteration block.

Pairs of coronal and sagital views for two particular slices are shown in Figure 2 for each model, respectively. The true model for these two views is shown in Figures 2a and 2b, in which the dotted lines indicate the position at which the slices for the complementary view are taken. Figures 2c and 2d show the simplest starting model used for the inversions, which only contains water. This is used to invert the data starting at a frequency of $700 kHz$ and the results are shown in Figures 2e and 2f. The recovered model differs significantly from the true model such that only the skin and outer region of the subcutaneous fat are recovered well, whereas anything inside the glandular region is distorted. This behaviour commonly appears when the starting model is not good enough or/and when there is a lack of low frequencies so that the modelled data is delayed by more than half a cycle with respect to the observed data, leading to what is known as cycle skipping. To test this hypothesis, we design a better starting model by smoothing the true model with a three-dimensional Gaussian filter, which is shown in Figures 2g and 2h, and we run FWI again with this starting model and the same starting frequency. Figures 2i and 2j show the resulting recovered model. In this case, the modelled data for the first iterations is not delayed by more than half a cycle with respect to the observed

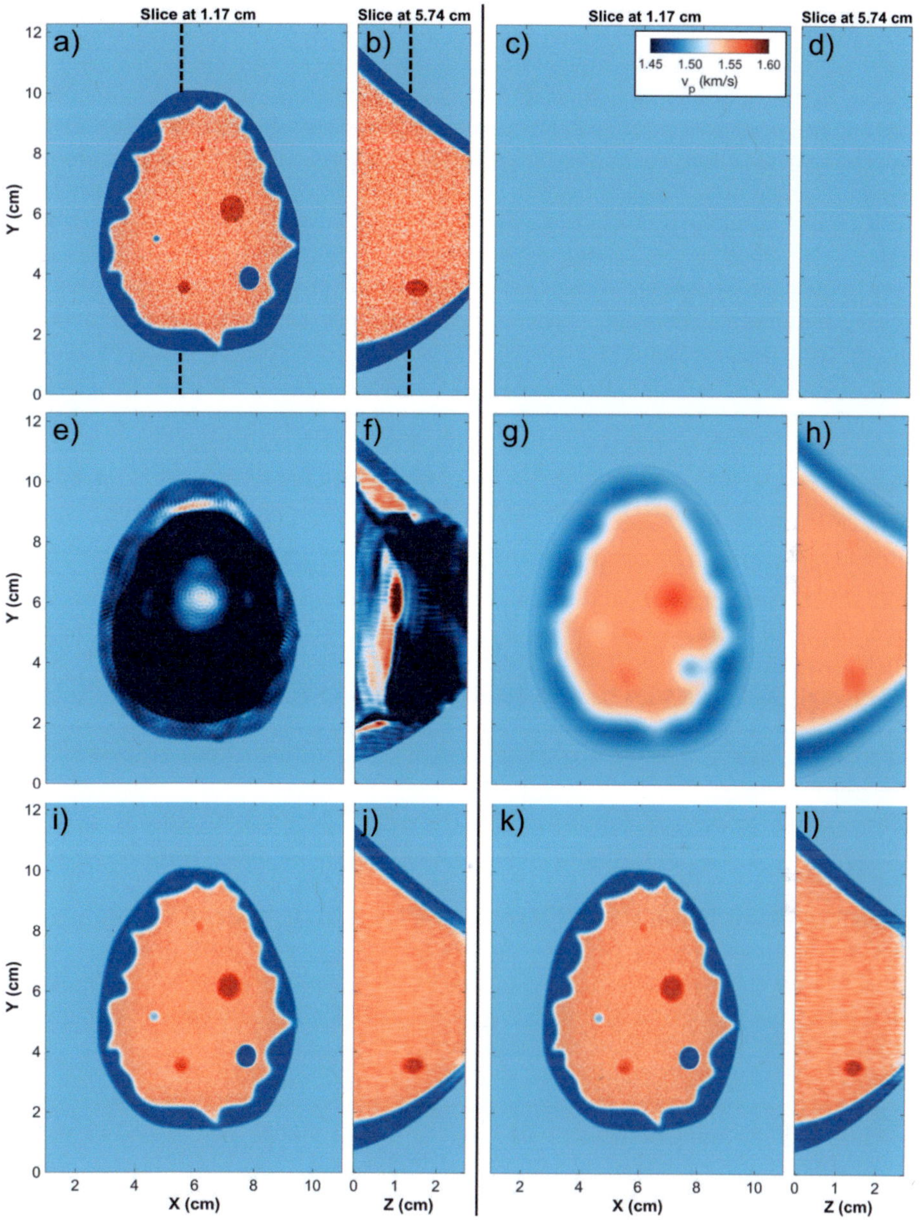

Figure 2: Pairs of coronal and sagital views of speed of sound for the true model (a and b, respectively), a water starting model (c and d), the recovered model starting from water and at $f_{min} = 700\,kHz$ (e and f), a smooth starting model (g and h) and the recovered models starting from the smooth model and at $f_{min} = 700\,kHz$ (i and j) and starting from water and at $f_{min} = 300\,kHz$ (k and l). All inversions are in 3D, the maximum inverted frequency is $1.4\,MHz$ and density and absorption are fixed during modelling and inversion.

data and FWI successfully recovers an accurate velocity model of the breast. The recovered model is more resolved than the starting model and the different spherical masses inside the glandular region as well as the irregular boundaries of the subcutaneous fat layer are well recovered. However, obtaining a good starting model sometimes requires the intervention of the user and is not the best practice to have a well-conditioned inversion problem. Instead, the presence of low frequencies can overcome this issue directly from the data without requiring any other algorithm or user's intervention. This is shown in Figures 2k and 2l, in which FWI has been applied using the water starting model in Figures 2c and 2d and starting the inversion at $300kHz$. We observe that, unlike the result in Figures 2e and 2f, starting the inversion at lower frequencies is enough to recover a very accurate model of the breast, provided low frequencies are present in the data. The resolution of the recovered model is only limited by the maximum frequency at which the inversion is performed - increasing the frequency increases the computation cost - and the limited number of transducers. In terms of computation run time for these tests, it takes approximately 21 hours when running the code in parallel accross 36 nodes. Although several strategies could be implemented to reduce the compute time, these results already suggest that high resolution 3D models of the breast can nowadays be obtained by performing 3D FWI, which require minimal user intervention.

Next, we investigate the effects of neglecting density and absorption on the recovered models after 3D FWI. We first repeat the previous tests by modelling data with fixed density and absorption - equal to those of water - but we now run FWI up to $1MHz$ to reduce the compute cost. We start the inversion at $300kHz$ by using a water starting model and we keep density and absorption fixed, which leads to the result shown in Figures 3a and 3b. We then generate observed data by using the visco-acoustic wave equation with the density and absorption models in Figures 1b and 1c, and we perform acoustic FWI of the new observed data by ignoring density and absorption effects, i.e. by keeping them constant and equal to those of water. The boundaries of the recovered model as well as the spherical inclusions are well recovered, as shown in Figures 3c and 3d. Nevertheless, ignoring absorption and density leads to a recovered model that is generally slower and not as accurate as when we do not have these effects in the modelling. This is in part because absorption delays and attenuates the wavefield and also because the dynamics of the wavefield is not correct due to an incorrect density. Overall, we conclude that the consequences of ignoring density and absorption effects for a typical breast during FWI are not significant, although this may differ for denser breasts. For the rest of this manuscript, density and absorption are therefore ignored.

In the last test on this section we investigate the impact of neglecting 3D effects and performing 2D FWI. In order to compare 2D and 3D inversions, we generate data with a single circular array of transducers that contains 50 emitters and 256 receivers and which has its center at the center of a coronal view and is at $z \approx 1.66cm$. Figure 4 shows the data generated for a single emitter as a function of time for each transducer in the array when we consider a 2D model of the breast at the same location as the array (left picture) and when we model data using the full 3D model (right picture). We observe there are differences in the reflected part of the signal (black arrow) and also in the transmitted part (black circle), which is due to off-plane effects when we consider the full 3D model. For these tests, a three-cycle toneburst source wavelet with a centre frequency of $500kHz$ has been used to avoid numerical dispersion introduced by using different modelling codes in 2D and 3D with different stability conditions.

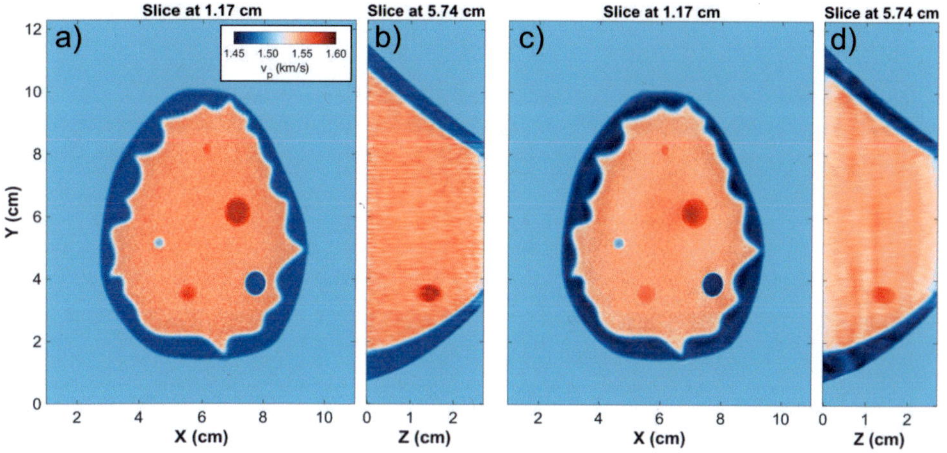

Figure 3: Pairs of coronal and sagital views of speed of sound for the recovered models in which density and absorption are fixed during the inversion and the modelling (a and b) and in which they are variable during the modelling but fixed during the inversion (c and d). All inversions are in 3D at $f_{min} = 300\,kHz$ and the maximum inverted frequency is $1\,MHz$.

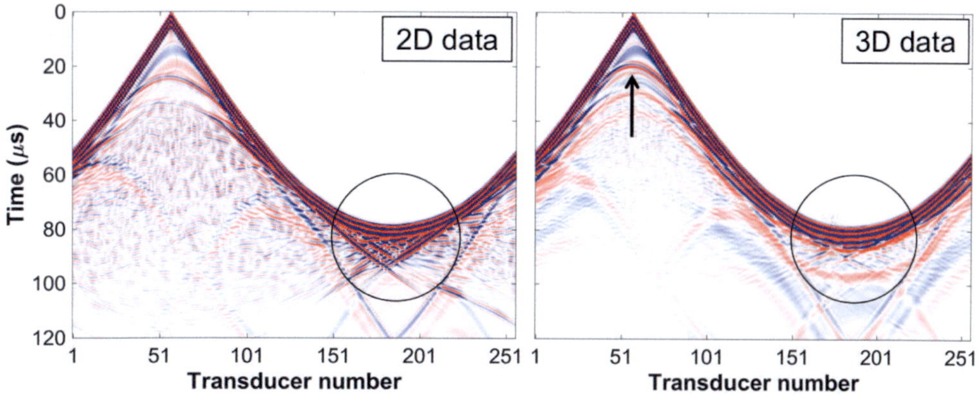

Figure 4: Modelled data for a source in a 2D circular array around a 2D section of the breast phantom (left) and around the 3D breast phantom (right).

The 3D data generated with a single transducer ring is now inverted using both a 2D and 3D water starting models, and 2D and 3D FWI are respectively performed starting at a frequency of $150\,kHz$ up to $1\,MHz$. The resulting recovered models as well as the true model corresponding to the same coronal slice in which the ring of transducers is located are shown in Figure 5.

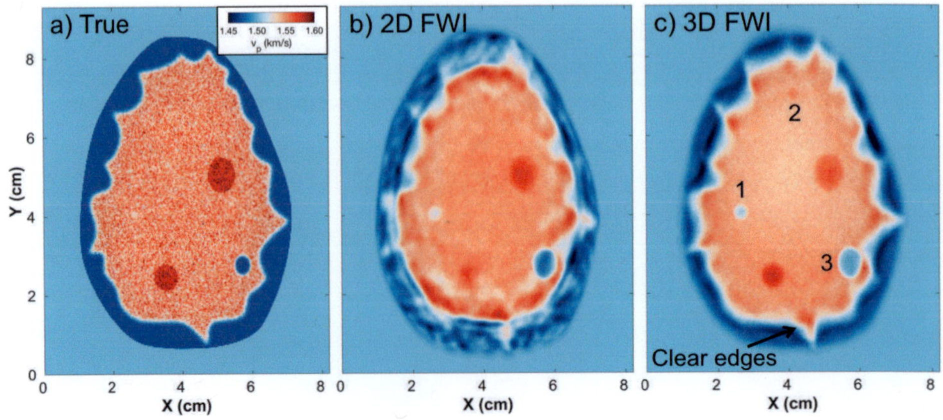

Figure 5: Coronal views of a) the true model and the recovered models after b) 2D FWI and c) 3D FWI of the 3D data acquired with a single circular array of 50 transducers around the 3D breast phantom. All inversions are at $f_{min} = 150\,kHz$ and a maximum frequency of $1\,MHz$.

From these results we conclude the following: 1) 2D FWI of 3D data leads to a less accurate model than that obtained with 3D FWI and 2) 3D FWI of data acquired with a single acquisition ring leads to off-plane effects in the recovered model. The first observation is made by comparing Figures 5b and 5c and noting that the edges of the breast as well as the spherical inclusions are better defined in Figure 5c than those in Figure 5b. On the other hand, the second remark is made by comparing Figures 5a and 5c and observing that the spherical inclusions in Figure 5c denoted by 1 and 2 are not present in the true model and that the spherical inclusion denoted by 3 is larger than the same inclusion in the true model. Additionally, the edges of the breast skin and subcutaneous fat are also distorted and are slightly larger when compared to those in the true model. These are consequence of waves travelling through planes slightly above or below the current plane, which could be minimised by using focused transducers. Another way to separate off-plane effects is to acquire data in three dimensions by, for instance, using several acquisition rings, and performing 3D FWI as demonstrated in Figure 2 (e.g. compare size of the spherical inclusions or the irregular shape of the subcutaneous fat in the true model in Figures 2a and 2b with those for the recovered model in Figures 2k and 2l).

In summary, the previous tests suggest that high resolution models of a typical density breast can be obtained with no prior information by using FWI if density and absorption are ignored, low-frequency transducers are used and data is acquired and inverted in three dimensions.

3.2 2D *in vivo* data

In this section we perform 2D FWI of an *in vivo* dataset acquired with the CURE (Computed Ultrasound Risk Evaluation) system at the Karmanos Cancer Institute (Wayne State University). This system is formed by a single ring of transducers of $20\,cm$ in diameter with a total of 256 transducers that can act both as sources and receivers. We have no other information regarding the exact location of the transducers or a water shot to calibrate their location, the temperature of the water bath - that determines the velocity of sound in water - or the source wavelet. We apply 2D FWI on this dataset rather than 3D FWI to reduce the computation cost and minimise any external intervention, although 3D FWI would be possible.

First, we do some minimal data processing and interpolate the data so that the time sampling is $0.04\,\mu s$, which allows us to invert the data up to $1.75\,MHz$ without having numerical dispersion given that the grid spacing is $0.15\,mm$. We then remove data generated by a malfunctioning source, which reduces the total number of working sources to 255, and we band-pass filter the data to reduce the noise at frequencies below $200\,kHz$ and beyond $1.75\,MHz$. Figure 6a shows the band-pass filtered data for a working source as a function of time for all transducers. We observe that this data contains strong coherent noise at early times, which is present in the gathers for all the sources and which will negatively affect FWI as it will try to match modelled data to the observed data. To minimise this, we discard data arriving before $30\,\mu s$ during the inversion and we also discard data arriving later than $180\,\mu s$ to further reduce the computation time. But before inverting the data, we need a source wavelet accurate at low frequencies, as well as the location of the transducers. Typically, this is obtained by calibrating the system using a water shot, i.e. an acquisition without any target. As the data we have has been acquired *in vivo* with a target, we can only use the first arrivals present in the data corresponding to the water wave in those regions in which it does not cross with reflections or transmissions. These reduces the amount of traces for calibration from 256 to 50 and it does not allow us to obtain a source wavelet variation with aperture angle but an average wavelet. We calibrate the location of the transducers by using the method suggested by [7] and we extract the source wavelet based on the picked first arrivals on the observed data and the same arrivals for data modelled with an arbitrary source band-pass filtered as the observed data and assuming a constant background of just water [4]. Figures 6b and 6c show the extracted source wavelet and its spectrum, respectively.

We now perform 2D FWI of the minimally pre-processed data by ignoring density and absorption effects. For all the inversions, the starting and recovered models have a dimension of 1464×1464 in cells and we run FWI by using 85 sources per iteration, and the results are shown in Figure 7. The average run time is of 23 hours across 11 nodes.

Figure 7a shows the recovered model obtained by starting the inversion at a frequency of $500\,kHz$ and using a water starting model. Due to the lack of low-frequency data, FWI does not recover a good reconstruction of the breast and it is difficult to identify any feature that, for instance, may allow a radiologist identify the presence of a tumour. Thus, we first obtain a better starting model by using bent-ray tomography [8], which produces the smooth and homogeneous recovered model in Figure 7b. In the latter we can identify the presence of a high-velocity region (red elipse) that might be a tumour, but the recovered model does not have many details and no other features can be distinguished. We then apply FWI again with the latter as a starting model and with a minimum frequency of $800\,kHz$, leading to the recovered model in Figure 7c. In this test we see a clear improvement in terms of details: the structure of the high-velocity mass is changed, the breast skin and the edge of the subcutaneous fat are better defined and some features can be observed inside the breast that were not visible in the bent-ray tomography result. Nevertheless, we also observe the presence of some artefacts that are caused by cycle-skipping, such as the discontinous skin layer on the left-hand-side or a slow velocity semi-circular layer in the middle of the breast that cuts through other features. To overcome cycle-skipping we finally apply FWI using the bent-ray tomography result as a starting model but we now start the inversion at $500\,kHz$, resulting in the recovered model is shown in Figure 7d. From this model we observe that lowering the minimum frequency used in the inversion helps overcome cycle-skipping provided there is data at these frequencies, and results in a detailed model of velocities with coherent structures inside the breast and very well defined breast boundaries. The high degree of detail in the recovered model in Figure 7d is such that some features that may be blood vessels, milk ducts or lymphatic vessels can be observed - see for instance the region from $x = 6\,cm$ to $x = 12\,cm$ and from $y = 8\,cm$ to $y = 15\,cm$.

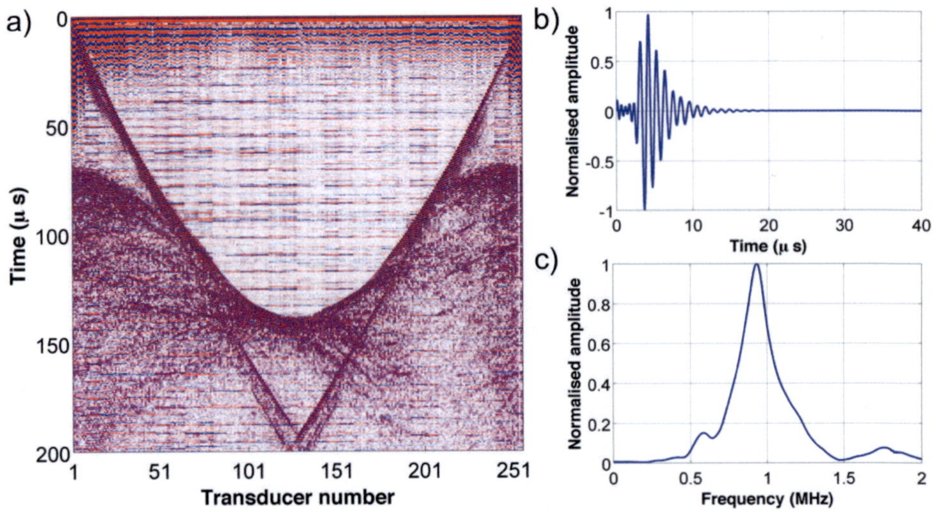

Figure 6: From left to right and top to bottom, a) band-pass filtered raw data for a single source for the 2D *in vivo* data, b) the corresponding extracted wavelet in time and c) its frequency spectrum. The extracted source has a centre frequency near $900\,kHz$.

Nevertheless, we expect a more accurate FWI recovered model when a calibration with a water shot and source extraction in the laboratory are available. Additionally, the structures observed in Figure 7d may not all be from the same plane, and 3D acquisition as well as 3D FWI would be necessary to separate them and determine the volume of the high velocity mass. If 3D acquisition is not available, off-plane effects could be separated to a certain extent by 3D FWI, especially if the radiation pattern of the sources is not strongly de-focused - unlike a point source -, but we recommend 3D data acquisition as well as 3D FWI for a more accurate recovery of breast velocity models.

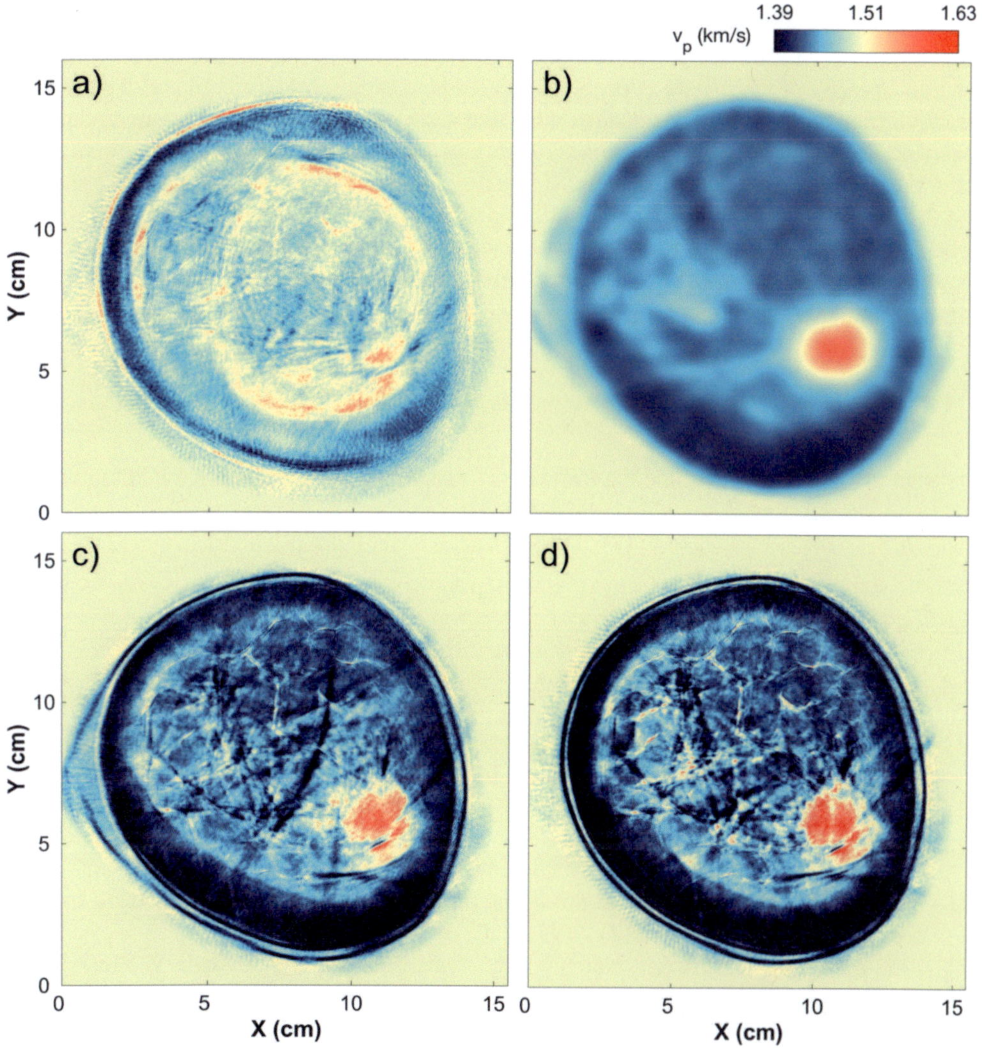

Figure 7: Recovered models of speed of sound obtained from the 2D *in vivo* data after using a) FWI at $f_{min} = 500 kHz$ and a constant water starting model, b) bent-ray tomography and FWI with the time-of-flight model as a starting model at c) $f_{min} = 800 kHz$ and d) at $f_{min} = 500 kHz$. The maximum frequency for all FWI tests is $1.75 MHz$.

4 Conclusions

The application of full-waveform inversion for breast imaging is still in an early stage, especially for 3D datasets. Here we have implemented a robust, reliable and efficient 3D algorithm to invert 3D ultrasound data from a realistic phantom of the breast. Our results show that 3D

FWI leads to more accurate recovered models of the breast than those obtained with 2D FWI and that 3D data aquistion is required in order to separate off-plane effects. We also demonstrate that the use of low-frequency ultrasound transducers – a few hundreds of kHz – mitigates the non-linearity of the inversion problem and leads to high-fidelity models with minimal interaction from the user. The results also show that neglecting absorption and density during the inversion does not have a strong impact for standard density breasts, although it leads to less accurate and slower recovered models of speed of sound. Finally, the successful application to a 2D *in vivo* dataset with little prior information confirms that low-frequency ultrasound or good starting models – e.g. from bent-ray tomography – and 3D data acquisition are required for an accurate reconstruction of the speed of sound in the breast.

Acknowledgements

We want to thank Neb Duric and the Karmanos Cancer Institute for sharing the 2D *in vivo* data and giving us permission to publish the results.

References

[1] J. Ferlay, I. Soerjomataram, R. Dikshit, S. Eser, C. Mathers, M. Rebelo, D. M. Parkin, D. Forman, F. Bray: Cancer incidence and mortaility worldwide: Sources, methods and major patterns in GLOBOCAN 2012. International Journal of Cancer, 136(5), (2015), E359-E386.

[2] S. H. Heywang-Köbrunner, A. Hacker, S. Sedlacek: Advantages and disadvantages of mammography screening. Breast Care, 6(3), (2011), 199-207.

[3] P. R. Williamson: A guide to the limits of resolution imposed by scattering in ray tomography. Geophysics, 56(2), (1991), 202-207.

[4] M. Warner, A. Ratcliffe, T. Nangoo, J. Morgan, A. Umpleby, N. Shah, V. Vinje, I. Stekl, L. Guasch, C. Win, G. Conroy, A. Bertrand: Anisotropic 3D full-waveform inversion. Geophysics, 78(2), (2013), R59-R80.

[5] R. G. Pratt, L. Huang, N. Duric, P. Littrup: Sound-speed and attenuation imaging of breast tissue using waveform tomography of transmission and ultrasound data. SPIE Proceedings, 6510, (2007), 1-12.

[6] P. E. Huthwaite: Quantitative imaging with mechanical waves. Imperial College London, (2012), 1-192.

[7] O. Roy, I. Jovanovic, N. Duric, L. Poulo, M. Vetterli: Robust array calibration using time delays with application to ultrasound tomography. SPIE Proceedings, 7968, (2011), 1-11.

[8] S. Li, M. Jackowski, D. Dione, T. Varslot, L. Staib, K. Mueller: Refraction corrected transmission ultrasound computed tomography for application in breast imaging. Medical Physics, 37, (2010), 2233-2246.

Ultrasound Computed Tomography: Historically Guided Musings

James F. Greenleaf

Mayo Clinic College of Medicine
Rochester, Minnesota, USA

Abstract

Computed Tomography with ultrasound waves, in both through transmission and reflection geometries, has been investigated for over 40 years. In that time investigators have concentrated on the complex interactions of ultrasonic waves with the tissue of the human female breast in an effort to delineate malignant from benign lesions. Over the years the relentless improvement of both electronics and computer power has allowed the inverse solution of more and more complex mathematical models of wave propagation through complex tissue such as the breast. However, the need for complete three-dimensional acquisition of scattering waves from the tissue continues to be a difficult technological problem. In addition to the technical challenges are the challenges of finding where in the flow diagram of breast disease patients traversing the health care system to place ultrasound breast tomography to provide the most effective contribution to the efficacy and efficiency of breast disease detection, diagnosis, and treatment. Meanwhile, other modalities are developing that provide very stiff competition to the field of computed ultrasound tomography of the breast. This paper provides some results and ruminations from the past and some comments about the future.

Keywords: Computed tomography, Breast, Transmission, Reflection

1 Introduction

The earliest and currently most widely used mode of ultrasound for obtaining clinical images is the echo or backscatter mode [1]-[5]. Although the tissue characteristics responsible for generating the backscattering signals as the ultrasound wave passes through biological tissues are not well understood, the resulting qualitative images are widely used for noninvasively diagnosing a variety of diseases with relatively inexpensive equipment [5]. The early clinical ultrasound B-mode scanners obtained tomograms (slice images) of distributions of reflectivity within the tissue without the need for computerized analysis such as required by X-ray or MR computer-assisted tomography (CAT) scanning equipment. This fortuitous circumstance of obtaining tomograms without the need for computational analysis propelled the backscatter B-scan mode of ultrasonic imaging into the forefront of clinical diagnostic instrumentation at a very early stage [2]

Quantitative images (i.e., in which the numerical value of each pixel represents a basic physical property of tissue such as speed) were obtained using computerized transmission ultrasonic tomography in the eighth decade of the last century [6]-[11]. Our group was apparently the first to describe ultrasound transmission tomography [8], Glover et al. [11] were probably the first to apply the newly developed techniques of ultrasonic transmission tomography to patients in vivo. Carson et al.[12] also have imaged soft tissue in patients. McDonnell et al. are using ultrasonic transmission tomography to study ultrasonic mechanisms of attenuation in the infarcted myocardium [13].

Transmission ultrasound tomography currently requires a geometry in which ultrasound can be transmitted from a plurality of directions covering 360^0 around the organ under examination. Approximately 15 percent of American women will develop carcinoma of the breast and many more will develop other diseases which must be distinguished from carcinoma [14].

For these reasons, the breast has been the principal organ to which transmission tomography ultrasound has been applied [7]- M. O'Donnell, J. W. Mimbs, B. E. Sobel, and J. B. Miller, "Ultrasonic attenuation in the normal and ischemic myocardium," in Proc. Nat. Bureau Standards 2ndInt. Symp. Ultrasonic Tissue Characterization, Gaithersburg, MD, June 13-15, 1977, p. 63.] [17].The geometry required by the ultrasound CAT obtained with the patient lying prone with a breast suspended in a tank of water while transducers are scanned around the breast in some fashion to complete the required set of data.

The relationship between the incoming ultrasound wave and the scattered exit wave has been known for several decades [18].

2 Methods

The straight line integral relationships between the real part of tissue refractive index NR (ultrasonic speed) and measured transit time T for ultrasonic pulses traveling through tissue, and the relationship between the imaginary part of refractive index NI (attenuation coefficient) and the log of the amplitude A of the received pulse have been derived elsewhere [10] and are;

$$T(\bar{b}) - T(\bar{a}) = \int_{\bar{a}}^{\bar{b}} N_R \, ds$$

and

$$\log \frac{A(\bar{b})}{A(\bar{a})} = -\int_{\bar{a}}^{\bar{b}} N_I \, ds.$$

The position of the transmitter is at a while b is the position of the receiver and ds is taken along a straight line between a and b in the direction k of the impinging wave. The derivation these equations require that variations in refractive index N to be small to eliminate second-order terms propagation [10]. More accurate models of the transmission tomography problem in tissues which take into account the curved nature of the ultrasound rays were developed by Mueller and Kaveh [17] and Stenger and Johnson [19].

3 Results

As early as 1977 we used reconstructions of distributions of acoustic speed to correct compound B-scans for aberrations due to inhomogeneous refractive indexes [14] and also applied ultrasonic tomography to diagnosing breast cancer [16]. Around that time Mueller et al. [17] and Duck et al. [18] described quantitative tomography methods for the backscattered mode as well. Transmission ultrasound tomography currently requires a geometry in which ultrasound can be transmitted from a plurality of directions covering 360^0 around the organ under examination.

The purpose of this paper is to describe some of the results of early investigators in the field who used very simple ultrasound speed and attenuation tomograms in a set of patients that were scheduled for a biopsy.

Figure 1 illustrates bilateral ultrasound tomograms obtained in the early 70's that indicate a scirrhous carcinoma in the right breast with no such indication in the left breast. The speed and attenuation in the lesion of this fatty breast are high. It was known then that malignant lesions could have either low or high attenuation but normally had a high speed of sound.

Striking visual localization of solid lesions can be produced by the joint colored display of velocity and attenuation. In such displays the solid lesion appears as a localized region of relatively high velocity which in young patients is surrounded by highly attenuating parenchyma and in older patients is either rimmed by a relatively highly attenuating boundary or is congruent with a region of relatively high attenuation (Fig. 2).

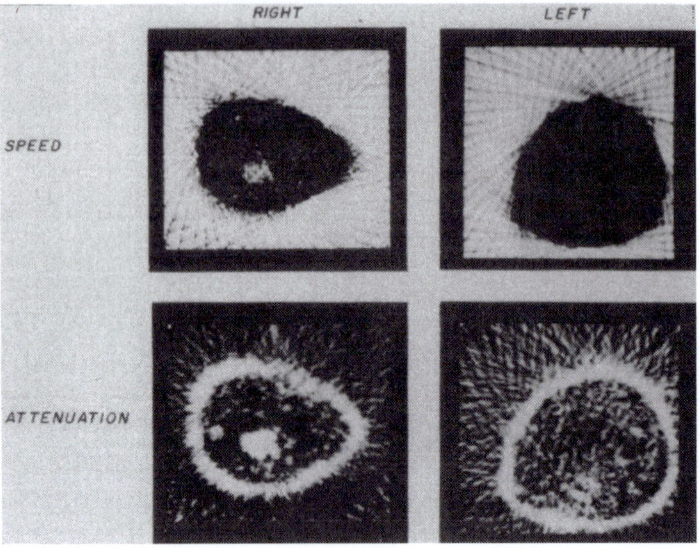

Figure 1: Reconstructions of attenuation and speed in the coronal plane of a 68-year-old woman showing scirrhous carcinoma having high attenuation relative to atrophic background tissue and high acoustic speed. Contralateral breast shows no high-speed region.

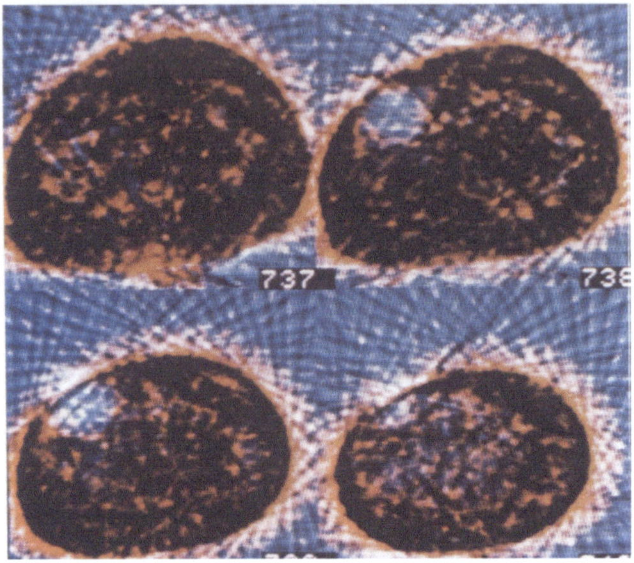

Figure 2: Ultrasonic speed (blue) and attenuation (red) are synergistically displayed by superimposing two images in separate colors. The exact relationship of speed and attenuation images can be seen and aids in evaluation the border and internal characteristics of the lesions.

From these early examples of ultrasound computed tomography, the field has been developed to a point where clinical trials are being conducted with scanners that are nearly ready for commercial application. However, the future may have some revolutionary changes in store as has the past.

4 Future

Ultrasonic computed tomography has improved over the past 5 decades because of the relentless advances in computer power. Most of the methods of solving the wave equation have been known but the forward/back functional minimization methods required massive compute power, which now is possible. Data acquisition remains a problem because the required geometry for a complete inversion of the wave equation requires 360 degrees of scattering information. Because this remains an unsolved problem, at least in clinically relevant times, there needs to be a breakthrough in approaches to the problem. But this author feels there is help on the way.

In the immediate future, there will be a disruptive change in the field of ultrasonics caused by advanced artificial intelligence. Methods similar to those used to master the game of GO will impact the field of clinical ultrasound [21][22]. Already methods of AI have been used to improve the impulse response of ultrasound systems [23]. Whether such AI systems will impact reconstruction algorithms for transmission and reflection computed tomography is yet to be determined but it seems that the probability of such an impact is not zero.

Another area of impact will be in the field of diagnosis from the images produced by the ultrasound transmission tomography systems. Already many projects are focusing on the application of AI methods to image evaluation. Whether this method will be applied to the data or to the images is unknown. One thing is certain, compute power is improving relentlessly along with AI efficacy and the two together will be a powerful tool in the healthcare arena.

References

[1] J. J. Wild and J. M. Reid, "Echographic visualization of lesions of the lining of the intact human breast," Cancer Res., vol. 14, pp. 277- 283, 1954.

[2] D. White and E. A. Lyons, Ultrasound in Medicine, vol. 4. New York: Plenum, 1978.

[3] Y. Kikuchi, R. Uchida, K. Tanaka, and T. Wagai, "Early cancer diagnosis through ultrasonic," J. Acoust. Soc. Amer., vol. 29, pp. 824-833, 1957.

[4] J. Jellins, G. Kossoff, T. S. Reeve, and B. H. Barraclough, "Ultrasonic grey scale visualization of breast disease," Ultrasonics Med. Biol., vol. 1, pp. 393-404, 1975.

[5] P. N. T. Wells, BiomedicalUltrasonics. New York: Academic, 1977.

[6] J. F. Greenleaf, S. A. Johnson, R. C. Bahn, B. Rajagopalan, and S. Kenue, "Introduction to computed ultrasound tomography," in Computer Aided Tomography and ultrasonics in Medicine, IFIP, J. Raviv, J. F. Greenleaf, and G. T. Herman, Eds. Amsterdam, The Netherlands: North-Holland, 1979, pp. 125-136.

[7] J. F. Greenleaf, "Computerized transmission tomography," in Methods of Experimental Physics-Ultrasound, P. D. Edmonds, Ed. New York: Academic, 1979.

[8] J. F. Greenleaf, S. A. Johnson, S. L. Lee, G. T. Herman, and E. H. Wood, "Algebraic reconstruction of spatial distributions of acoustic absorption with tissues from their two-dimensional acoustic projections," in Acoustical Holography, vol. 5, P.S. Green, Ed. New York: Plenum, 1974, pp. 591-603.

[9] J. F. Greenleaf, S. A. Johnson, W. F. Samayoa, and F. A. Duck, "Algebraic reconstruction of spatial distributions of acoustic velocities in tissue from their time-of-flight profiles," in Acoustical Holography, vol. 6, N. Booth, Ed. New York: Plenum, 1975, pp. 71-90.

[10] J. F. Greenleaf, S. A. Johnson, and A. H. Lent, "Measurement of spatial distribution of refractive index in tissues by ultrasonic computer assisted tomography," Ultrasound Med. Biol., vol. 3, pp. 327-339, 1978.

[11] G. H. Glover, "Characterization of in vivo breast tissue by ultrasonic time of flight computed tomography," in Proc. Nat. Bureau Standards 2nd Int. Symp. Ultrasonic Tissue Characterization, Gaithersburg, MD, June 13-15, 1977, p. 221.

[12] P. Carson, T. V. Oughton, W. R. Hendee, and A. S. Ahuja, "Imaging soft tissue through bone with ultrasound transmission tomography by reconstruction," Med. Phys., vol. 4, no. 4, pp. 302-309, 1977.

[13] M. O'Donnell, J. W. Mimbs, B. E. Sobel, and J. B. Miller, "Ultrasonic attenuation in the normal and ischemic myocardium," in Proc. Nat. Bureau Standards 2ndInt. Symp. Ultrasonic Tissue Characterization, Gaithersburg, MD, June 13-15, 1977, p. 63.

[14] 0. H. Beahrs, S. Shapiro, C. Smart, and R. W. McDivitt, "Supplemental and concluding report of a working group to review BCDDP," J. Nat. Cancer Inst., vol. 62, no. 3, pp. 699-709, 1979.

[15] J. F. Greenleaf, S. A. Johnson, W. F. Samayoa, and C. R. Hansen, "Refractive index by reconstruction: use to improve compound B-scan resolution," in Acoustical Holography, vol. 7, L. Kessler, Ed. New York: Plenum, 1977, pp. 263-273.

[16] J. F. Greenleaf, S. K. Kenue, B. Rajagopalan, R. C. Bahn, and S. A. Johnson, "Breast imaging by ultrasonic computer-assisted tomography," in Acoustical Imaging, vol. 8, A. F. Metherell, Ed. New York: Plenum, 1978, pp. 599-614.

[17] R. K. Mueller, M. Kaveh, and G. Wade, "Acoustical reconstructive tomography and applications to ultrasonics," Proc. IEEE, vol. 67, pp. 567-586, Apr. 1979.

[18] L. M. Brekhorvskikh, Waves in Layered Media. New York: Academic, 1960, p. 171.

[19] F. Stenger and S. A. Johnson, "Ultrasonic transmission tomography based on the inversion of the Helmholtz wave equation for plane and spherical wave insonification," Appl. Math. Notes, vol. 4, pp. 102-127, Nov. 1979.

[20] F. A. Duck and C. R. Hill, "Acoustic attenuation reconstruction from backscattered ultrasound," in ComputerAided Tomography and ultrasonics in Medicine, IFIP, J. Raviv, J. F. Greenleaf, and G. T. Herman, Eds. Amsterdam, The Netherlands: North-Holland 1979, pp. 137-150.

[21] Google AI algorithm masters ancient game of Go, Elizabeth Gibney, 27 January 2016 Nature 529: number 7587.

[22] Perez Carlos E., https://medium.com/intuitionmachine/the-strange-loop-in-alphago-zeros-self-play-6e3274fcdd9f

[23] A. Luchies, B Byram, Deep neural networks for ultrasound beamforming, Proceedings of the Ultrasonics Symposium, 2017 http://ieeexplore.ieee.org/document/8092159/

A Multi-Modal Ultrasound Breast Imaging System

J. Camacho[1], J. F. Cruza[1], N. González-Salido[1], C. Fritsch[1], M. Pérez-Liva[2], J.L. Herraiz[2], J.M. Udías[2]

[1] *Ultrasound Systems and Technology Group, Spanish National Research Council (GSTU-CISC), Madrid, Spain*
E-mail: j.camachot@csic.es
[2] *Grupo de Física Nuclear, Universidad Complutense de Madrid (GFN-UCM), Madrid, Spain*

Abstract

This work presents a description of the Multi-Modal Ultrasound Breast Imaging System (MUBI) and our first results obtained with tissue-mimicking phantoms. MUBI is a joint development of the Spanish National Research Council (CISC) and the University Complutense of Madrid (UCM), and it is intended to be a flexible platform for multi-modal ultrasound imaging research, mainly oriented to breast diagnosis. Up to now, four imaging techniques have been implemented in this system: phased-array, phase coherence imaging, acoustic radiation force imaging (these three with full-angle spatial compounding), and ultrasound tomography. A brief introduction to each method is given along with preliminary experimental results.

Keywords: Breast Imaging, USTT, Bézier curves, Phase-coherence imaging.

1 Introduction

While the standard technique for breast cancer screening is X-ray mammography, ultrasound (US) breast imaging is currently considered a complementary procedure useful for further assessment of suspicious findings. US does not use ionizing radiation, provides high-contrast real-time images, allow a cleaner distinction between fluid-filled cysts and solid masses, and it is a pain-free technique [1]. Furthermore, mammographically dense breast tissue produces a high level of false negatives in mamography [2], while ultrasound imaging is not affected by that condition [3]. Nevertheless, there are several reasons why US is not the first choice in screening programs: ultrasonic diagnosis depends on the technician skills, the scanning time is relatively long and imaging and registering the whole breast by a hand-held technique is challenging [4]. As most of these limitations arise from its hand-held nature, automated breast ultrasound scanners have been proposed as an alternative. Several configurations have been proposed, such as a plane transducer arrangement (usually in a ring configuration) that generate coronal slice images [5-8] and moves in the axial direction to collect volumetric data, and a three-dimensional distribution of transducers that generate a 3D image directly [9]. In the first case, the reconstruction problem is simpler (2D imaging), while the resolution in the axial direction is limited by the elevation focusing of the transducers. In the second case the reconstruction problem must be solved in 3D (more computing demanding), but with the advantage of obtaining the same resolution in all directions.

The approach followed for the configuration of MUBI system is the ring configuration. A ring of 16 phased-array transducers of 128 elements each is used to obtain coronal-plane images while moving it in the axial direction for volumetric acquisition. The center frequency is f = 3.2 MHz and the distance between elements is d = 0.22 mm ($\approx \lambda/2$ in water), and the ring opening is 220 mm (Figure 1.a). A multiplexing electronics is embedded in the ring housing, allowing emitting and receiving with each single array (pulse-echo) or with any pair of them (through-transmission). This way, both reflectivity and ultrasound tomography (UST) datasets can be acquired.

The electronics have been in-house developed, based on a 128 channel full-parallel phased-array system, with real-time emission and reception beamforming capabilities (dynamic-depth focusing in reception) as well as full parallel channel acquisition for UST datasets. Different from other approaches, beamforming in emission allows implementing full-angle spatial compounding of B-Mode images and acoustic radiation force impulse elastography. While the final ring system is still under construction, a proof of concept with two moving arrays in a water tank was built for the algorithms development and system validation (Figure 1.b). Two pairs of 3.2 MHz and 5 MHz arrays were attached to independent arms moved by stepper motors, which allows simulating the full ring. A SITAU-112 (Dasel SL) phased-array system was used for emission and reception.

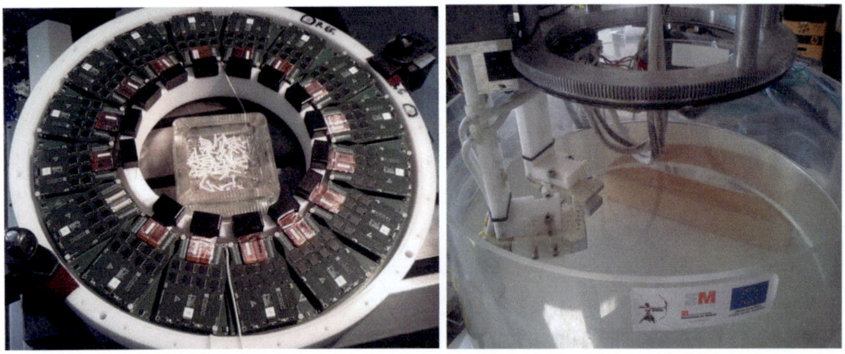

Figure 1: (left) Ring transducer of the MUBI system (right) proof of concept with moving arrays.

In the following sections the first results obtained with the MUBU prototype (Figure 1.b) are presented, showing the implementation of the following imaging techniques: Full angle spatial compound (FASC) of reflectivity images, Phase coherence imaging, full angle spatial compound of ARFI images (FASC-ARFI) and ultrasound tomography images of speed of sound and attenuation.

2 Full angle spatial compound of reflectivity images

Spatial compounding of reflectivity images improves contrast-to-noise ratio by reducing the speckle variability, and hence, generating a more homogeneous image [10-11]. Furthermore, artifacts like shadows and reverberations are attenuated by averaging images acquired from different positions. In the MUBI system the Full Angle Spatial Compound (FASC) method was implemented, where 16 sector-scan images (each one acquired with a different array) are scan converted to a rectangular grid and averaged to obtain a compounded image (Figure 2). In [12] the expected resolution and the point spread function isotropy of this approach were analyzed by simulation and experimentally, concluding that the FASC resolution can be considered homogenous and isotropic in the region of interest, and is about 50% worse than the axial resolution of each B-Scan.

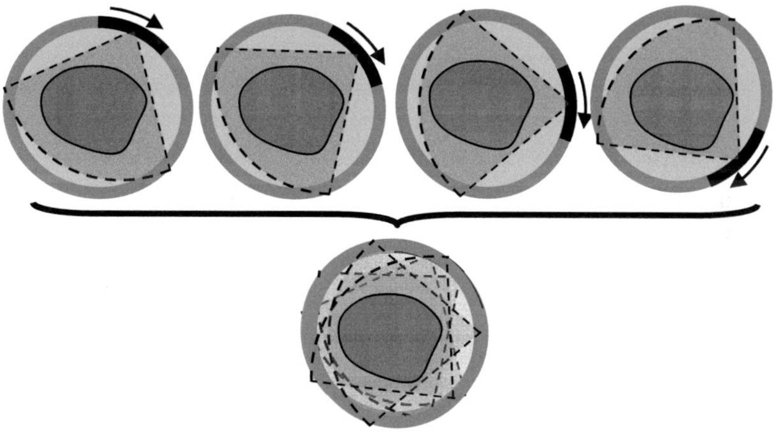

Figure 2: Schematic representation of the Full Angle Spatial Compound process of B-Mode reflectivity images.

One of the main issues for image compounding is the speed of sound variation during propagation of the wave. If the velocity map were previously computed from the USTT dataset, it could be used to correct the beam trajectory and the samples distance for each B-Scan line before scan conversion, completely eliminating the refraction effect. Nevertheless, the higher speed-of-sound mismatch is expected at the water-tissue interface, which can be reasonably corrected without a detailed knowledge of the speed-of-sound distribution inside the breast. In [13] a method for correcting the water-tissue refraction on FASC was proposed, based on estimating the contour of the breast from the B-Scan images and bending each ray at the breast entry point according to the Snell's law, for an assumed constant speed-of-sound. Then, scan conversion to a rectangular grid is performed by bilinear interpolation of each pair of consecutive refracted B-Scan lines, and the compounded image is obtained by averaging. This process is iteratively repeated, modifying each time the average speed of sound to get the maximum image sharpness [14].

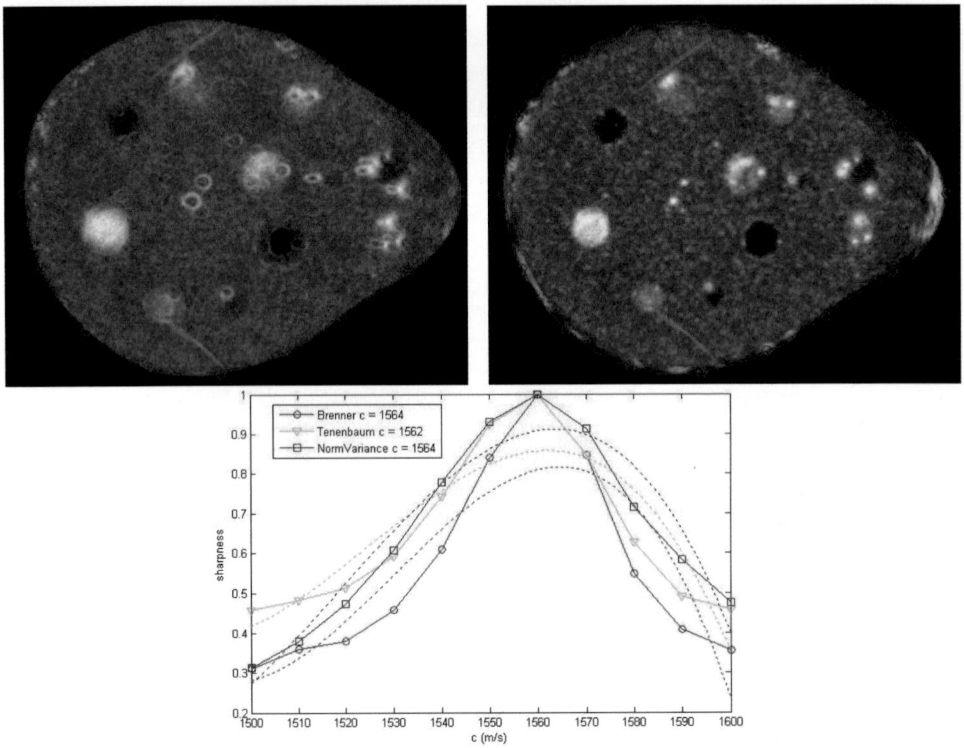

Figure 3: Compounded image of a phantom (top-left) before and (top-right) after refraction correction at the water-tissue interface. (bottom) Global Sharpness value of the compounded image for three different metrics (Brenner, Tenenbaum and Normalized Variance) versus the average speed of sound into the phantom.

Figure 3 top-left shows the FASC image of a breast phantom (Blue Phantom, EEUU) without refraction correction, where the general blurring effect and the artifacts generated by the speed of sound errors are evident. The red dots show the water-tissue interface points automatically detected from the center line of each B-Scan, and the red trace shows the interpolated interface used to correct the beam trajectories. Figure 3 top-right shows the image obtained after applying the proposed method, which clearly shows all the phantom structures with good resolution and contrast. Figure 3 bottom shows the image global sharpness value for three different metrics: Brenner, Tenenbaum and Normalized Variance. With all of them, the maximum sharpness is given for c = 1560 m/s, which is the optimum speed of sound average value for this phantom.

3 Phase Coherence Imaging

Phase Coherence Imaging (PCI) has been proposed to improve the resolution and contrast of ultrasound images [15]. It performs an adaptive beamforming by weighting the beamformer output by a coherence factor (PCF), obtained from the instantaneous phase dispersion along the aperture data. Assuming strict dynamic depth focusing, when all signals come from a reflector at the focus, their instantaneous phases will be equal, coherence factor will be unity and the echo signal will be kept in the output image. On the other hand, if the reflector is not at focus, the phase dispersion increases and the coherence factor becomes lower and reduces the indication amplitude in the output image. This way, resolution and contrast are simultaneously improved, as well as artifacts like grating lobes and reverberations are reduced.

Another property of PCI is reducing grain noise in coarse grained materials (like austenitic steel, titanium alloys, etc.) while keeping the indications of real flaws, even if they have low reflectivity with regard to the noise level [16], which is being exploited for non-destructive-testing. Our hypothesis is that a micro-calcification (or a cluster of them) will increase the phase coherence value with regard to the surrounding tissue, which could be used to enhance their presence in the image, a possible application in the medical field.

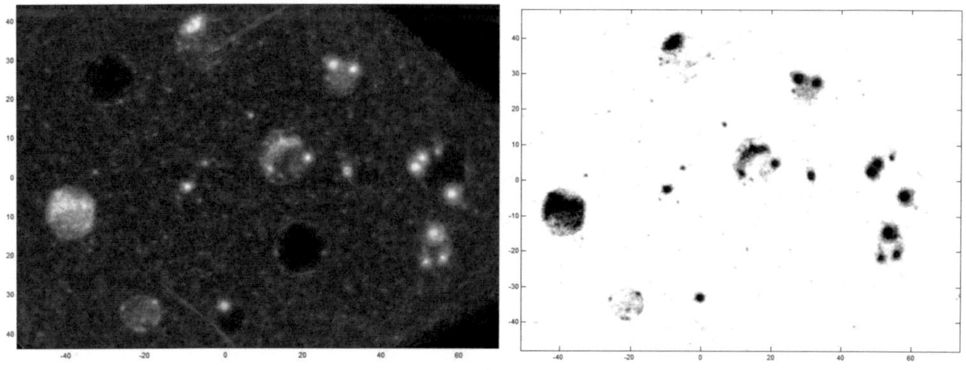

Figure 4: (left) Original FASC image of the phantom and (right) after applying the phase coherence processing. Both images with 50 dB dynamic range and inverted grayscale palette in (right).

Figure 4 left shows a detail of the center region of the phantom, where several bright spots can be observed. They correspond with small air bubbles and material inhomogeneities, which could resemble the echoes generated by micro-calcifications (small point-like reflectors). Figure 4 right shows the image after phase coherence processing, with the same dynamic range and an inverted grayscale palette. While most of the background texture is eliminated by PCF the point-like indications remain, because of their higher phase coherence value with regard to the surrounding tissue. This would help to enhance microcalcifications visibility, a hypothesis that is being verified by manufacturing phantoms with size and concentration controlled calcium carbonate grains.

Despite the MUBI system uses arrays with a pitch below λ/2, it is usually difficult to reach this figure when building large ring or ellipsoid array transducers. For larger pitch arrays grating lobes appear, generating artifacts that could hide the presence of weak reflectors. Figure 5 left shows the image of a set of nylon wires obtained with a 5 MHz, 128 elements and 1.7λ pitch array in water obtained by the total focusing method (TFM), where the grating lobes are clearly visible and partially hide the indications of the leftmost column of wires. Figure 5 right shows the image after applying the phase coherence processing, where the grating lobes artifacts are eliminated (up to 80 dB dynamic range), while the weak indications of the nylon wires are clearly visible.

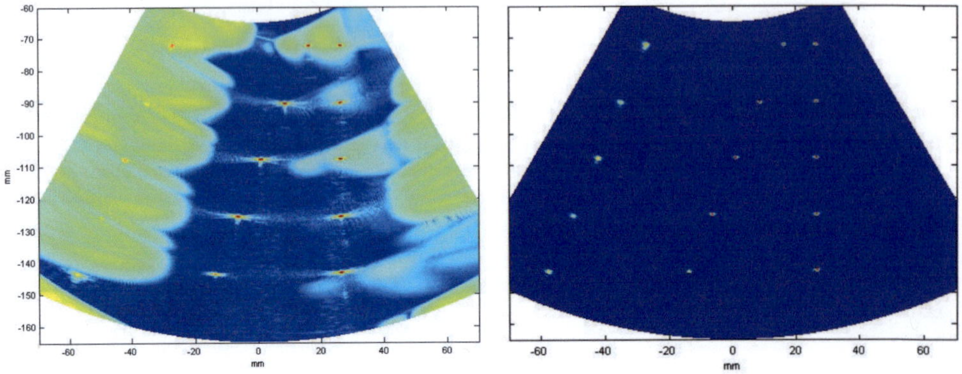

Figure 5: (left) Image of a set of cooper and nylon wires in water obtained by TFM with a 1.7λ pitch array and (right) after phase coherence processing. Dynamic range is 80 dB in both images.

4 Acoustic Radiation Force Impulse imaging

It is generally accepted that lesion stiffness is highly related with tumor malignancy [17] and hence, generating a stiffness map of the tissue (elastography) would be of great value in automated breast imaging systems. The most extended ultrasound technique for this task is quasi-static elastography, where the imaging transducer is used to slightly compress the tissue by hand, producing a deformation measured by cross-correlation of A-Scans before and after compression. For the same applied stress. soft tissue shows higher deformation than hard tissue, which allows creating a color map of the tissue stiffness. Because the applied force is not known, the map is qualitative, showing relative stiffness differences between regions but no a quantitative value of the elastic modulus.

Because the breast is not in contact with the transducer in the MUBI system, the quasi-static approach cannot be followed. Instead, we implemented the acoustic radiation force impulse (ARFI) imaging method [18], based on remotely displacing the tissue by emitting a highly focused (low #F) and long duration burst with the same array used for imaging (pushing pulse). The pushing pulse produces tissue displacements in the focus neighborhood that can be measured by cross-correlation of pre and post compression A-Scans, and a qualitative stiffness map can be generated.

One of the main limitations of ARFI is that the region of measurable displacements is restricted by the focus length, usually short for satisfying the low #F requirement. Hence, for imaging large regions like the breast cross-section, several pushing beams have to be emitted at different focal depths and steering angles, increasing the acquisition time. Furthermore, because the tissue displacement depends on the acoustic intensity and tissue attenuation, both changing with depth and angle, some procedure for normalizing the displacement images is required. In [19] we proposed a procedure to normalize and combine partial ARFI images, based on the system focal configuration, transducer characteristics and global tissue parameters found by ultrasonic measurements. Different from other approaches, the measured displacements are not used for normalization, and it is not required that the operator selects a homogeneous elasticity region as reference.

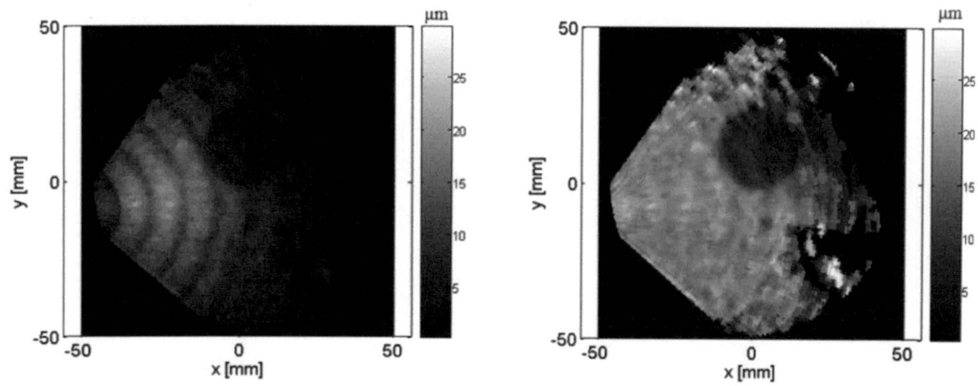

Figure 6: (left) Raw multi-focus ARFI image of a gelatin phantom and (right) after normalization proposed in [19]

Figure 6 left shows the raw ARFI image obtained with the MUBI system for the elasticity phantom described in [20], based on different concentrations of gelatin and graphite for generating a softer background with a hard inclusion of 25 mm diameter. Several bands can be observed because of the non-constant acoustic intensity within each focus region, along with an angular decay in displacements due to the angular array sensitivity, and some fading effect with depth due to tissue attenuation. All these effects are automatically corrected by the proposed algorithm, producing a homogeneous background level and a better delimited hard inclusion (Figure 6 right). Nevertheless, the noise increases in the region far away from the array, because tissue displacements are near the detection limit at large depths.

The spatial diversity of the ring transducer configuration can be exploited to improve the quality of ARFI images. In [20] we performed, for the first time, full angle spatial compounding of ARFI images, showing a significant improvement in contrast-to-noise ratio (CNR) and signal-to-noise ratio (SNR) with regard to conventional single-angle images. Figure 7 left shows the FASC-ARFI image of the phantom used in Figure 6, with an improvement of 3.5 times in CNR with regard to each single-angle image (Figure 6 right). Figure 7 right shows the reflectivity FASC image, where the hard inclusion can be distinguished by its edge but not by speckle differences in both regions. On the other hand, the FASC-ARFI (Figure 7 left) image shows the inclusion with its correct size and with a large contrast with regard to the background, which matches the large stiffness difference of both regions.

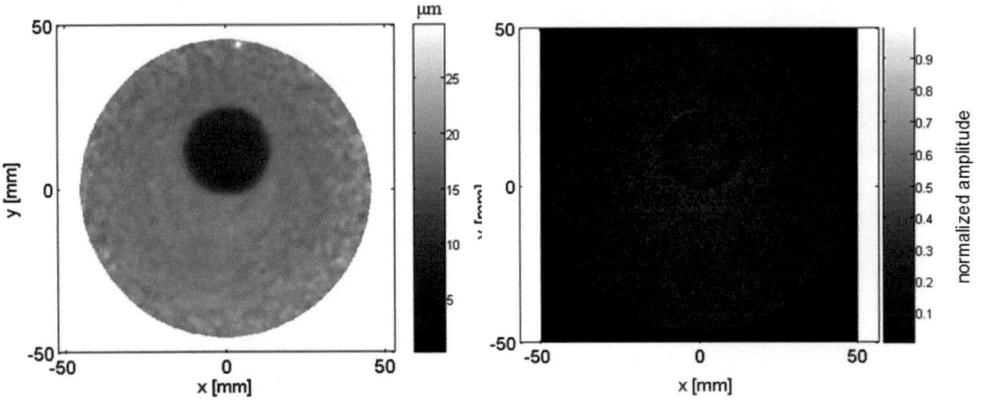

Figure 7: (left) FASC-ARFI image of a gelatin phantom with a 25 mm diameter hard inclusion (right) FASC reflectivity image of the same phantom.

5 Ultrasound Transmission Tomography (USTT)

Using the MUBI scanner in transmission mode we can reconstruct the acoustic properties of the tissues in the field-of-view: their speed-of-sound (SS), and their acoustic attenuation (AA) coefficient (in dB/mm/MHz).

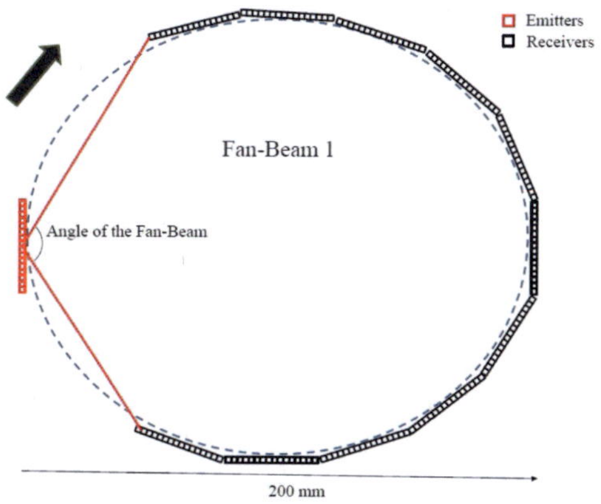

Figure 8: MUBI scanner configuration using the maximum transducer separation of 200 mm.

The acquisition scheme for USTT follows the fan-beam approach for CT systems (see Fig. 8). For each emitter array position, the receiving array is moved sequentially to cover a chosen angle (Fan-Beam angle) opposite to the emitter. For each position of the receiver, all (or a subset) of the emitter array elements are sequentially used as source, and the signals received by all (or a subset) of the receiving array elements are registered. Then, the emitter array is moved and the fan-beam acquisition is repeated.

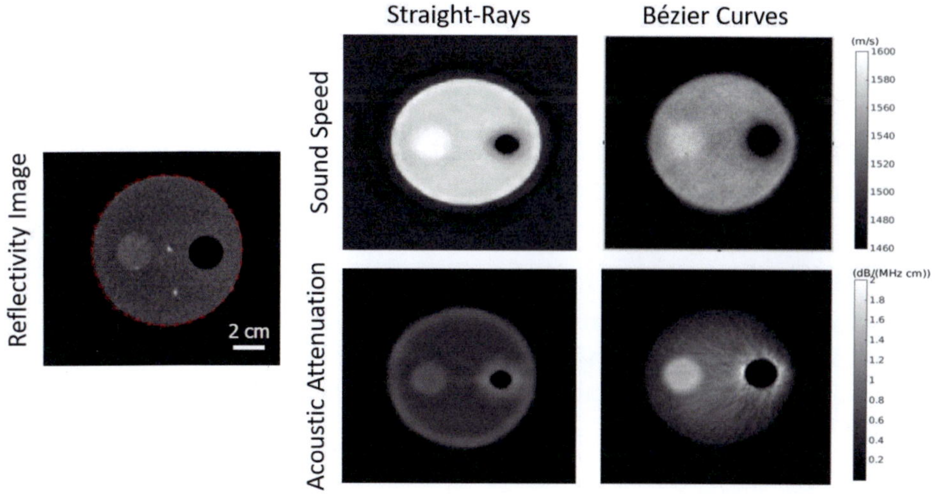

Figure 9: Reconstructed images of the tissue-mimicking phantom acquired with the MUBI scanner. (Left) Reflectivity image. (Center) SS and AA maps obtained with straight rays (i.e. without refraction correction). (Right) SS and AA maps obtained with refraction correction using the proposed method based on Bézier curves.

Reconstruction methods in ultrasound transmission tomography (USTT) are usually very time-consuming, as they usually require to model the full-wave propagation to obtain accurate results [22]. Therefore, approximate methods based on ray-tracing are useful to obtain images with good enough accuracy in a few seconds. In the case of the MUBI scanner, we use a new ray tracing method based on a family of Bézier curves [23] which exploits the large computing capabilities of current GPUs. Bézier curves are able to accurate model the bent paths of refracted rays in the tissues.

Reconstructed SS and AA images of a tissue-mimicking gelatin phantom acquired with the MUBI scanner in transmission mode are shown in Fig. 9. The images obtained with the Bézier curves show less artifacts than the ones obtained using straight-rays.

6 Conclusion

Several ultrasound imaging techniques have been implemented in the MUBI system, some of them quite innovative for breast imaging, as phase coherence processing, full angle spatial compound of ARFI images and UST reconstruction based on Bezier curves.

Phase coherence imaging has the potential of enhancing microcalcifications visibility by increasing their contrast with regard to the surrounding tissue gray level. Some preliminary evidences are presented in this work, and deeper analysis is ongoing by manufacturing phantoms with controlled size and concentration of calcium carbonate grains.

Full angle spatial compound of ARFI images has proven to improve image quality with regard to single-angle images, being a promising technique for breast cancer screening with automated systems. Current work is centered on implementing quantitative elastographic techniques based on measuring the velocity of shear waves, which would also reduce the acquisition time and the risk of thermal increase with regard to ARFI.

The proposed UST reconstruction method based on Bezier curves exploits the large computing capabilities of current GPUs, and images have fewer artifacts than when using straight-rays. The speed-of-sound images, reconstructed in a few seconds with this method, could be used to account for beam refraction inside the breast during the reflectivity image compounding process, without excessively penalizing the execution time.

Some of the acquired datasets are available online at the USCT data exchange and collaboration website (http://ipeusctdb1.ipe.kit.edu/~usct/challenge/) [21].

Acknowledgements

This work was supported by Comunidad de Madrid (S2013/MIT-3024 TOPUS-CM), and Spanish ministry of Economy and Competitiveness, projects FPA2015-65035-P, RTC-2015-3772-1 and DPI2013-42236-R. This is a contribution for the Moncloa Campus of International Excellence. Grupo de Física Nuclear-UCM, Ref.: 910059. This work acknowledges support by EU's H2020 under MediNet a Networking Activity of ENSAR-2 (grant agreement 654002). J. L. Herraiz is also funded by the EU Cofound Fellowship Marie Curie Actions, 7th Frame Program.

References

[1] Y. Zhou, "Ultrasound Diagnosis of Breast Cancer", Journal of Medical Imaging and Health Informatics Vol. 3, 1–14, 2013.

[2] D.A. Berry, K.A. Cronin, S.K. Plevritis, D.G. Fryback, L. Clarke, M. Zelen, J.S. Mandelblatt, A.Y. Yakovlev, J.D. Habbema, E.J. Feuer, "Effect of screening and adjuvant therapy on mortality from breast cancer", The New England Journal of Medicine, 353, 17, 1784-1792., 2005.

[3] M. Nothacker, V. Duda, N. Hahn, M. Warm, F. Degenhardt, H. Madjar, S. Weinbrenner, U. Albert, "Early detection of breast cancer: benefits and risks of supplemental breast ultrasound in asymptomatic women with mammographically dense breast tissue. A systematic review", BMC Cancer, 9,335, 1-9, 2009.

[4] W. Teh., A.R. Wilson, "The role of ultrasound in breast cancer screening. A Consensus Statement by the European Group for Breast Cancer Screening", European Journal of Cancer, 34, 4, 449-450., 1998.

[5] O. Roy, S. Schmidt, L. Cuipin, V. Allada, E. West, D. Kunz, N. Duric, "Breast imaging using ultrasound tomography: From clinical requirements to system design", Ultrasonics Symposium (IUS), IEEE International, 1174 – 1177, 2013.

[6] R. Stozka, J. Würfel, T. Müller, H. Gemmeke, "Medical Imaging by Ultrasound Computer Tomography", Medical Imaging, Proc. SPIE, 4687, 110-119, 2002.

[7] R. Waag, R. Fedewa, "A Ring Transducer System for Medical Ultrasound Research", IEEE Trans. on UFFC, 53, 10, 1707-1718, 2006.

[8] J. Wiskin, D. Borup, S. Johnson, M. Berggren, D. Robinson, J. Smith, J. Chen, Y. Parisky, John Klock, "Inverse scattering and refraction corrected reflection for breast cancer imaging.", Proc. SPIE 7629, Medical Imaging 2010: Ultrasonic Imaging, Tomography, and Therapy, 76290K, 2010.

[9] Ruiter, N.V., Zapf, M., et al.: "First Results of a Clinical Study with 3D Ultrasound Computer Tomography," Proc. IEEE Internat. Ultrasonics Symp., (2013).

[10] Hiller, D., Ermert, H., (1984), System Analysis of Ultrasound Reflection Mode Computerized Tomography, IEEE Trans. Son. Ultrason., 31, 4, 240-250.

[11] Jespersen, S., Wilhjelm J., Sillesen, H., (1998), Multi-Angle Compound Imaging, Ultrasonic Imaging, 20, 81-102.

[12] Medina, L., Camacho, J. & Fritsch, C. (2015). A Characterization of Ultrasonic Full Angle Spatial Compounding as a Possible Alternative for Breast Cancer Screening. Archives of Acoustics, 40(3), pp. 301-310.

[13] L. Medina, N. González-Salido, J. Camacho, M. Pérez-Liva, J. L. Herraiz and J. M. Udías, "Refraction correction in Full Angle Spatial image Compounding," 2016 Global Medical Engineering Physics Exchanges/Pan American Health Care Exchanges (GMEPE/PAHCE), Madrid, 2016, pp. 1-4.

[14] Treeby B.E., Varslot T.K., Zhang E.Z., Laufer J.G., Beard P.C. Automatic sound speed selection in photoacoustic image reconstruction using an autofocus approach. J Biomed Opt. 2011;16(9) 090501–090501-3.

[15] J. Camacho, M. Parrilla and C. Fritsch, "Phase Coherence Imaging," in IEEE Transactions on Ultrasonics, Ferroelectrics, and Frequency Control, vol. 56, no. 5, pp. 958-974, May 2009.

[16] J. Camacho and C. Fritsch, "Phase coherence imaging of grained materials," in IEEE Transactions on Ultrasonics, Ferroelectrics, and Frequency Control, vol. 58, no. 5, pp. 1006-1015, May 2011.

[17] Parker K.J. et al, “A unified view of Imaging the elastic properties of tissue,” J.Acoust. Soc. Am., vol117, no 5, pp. 2705-2712, 2005.

[18] K. Nightingale, M. Soo, R. Nightingale, G. Trahey. Acoustic radiation force impulse imaging: In vivo demonstration of clinical feasibility, Ultrasound Med. Biol, vol. 28, no 2, pp. 227–235, 2002.

[19] González-Salido, Nuria; Camacho, Jorge. Normalization of Multifocal Acoustic Radiation Force Impulse Images. Archives of Acoustics, [S.l.], v. 42, n. 2, p. 321–331, apr. 2017.

[20] Nuria Gonzalez Salido, Luis Medina y Jorge Camacho. .Full Angle Spatial Compound of ARFI Images for Breast Cancer Detection, Ultrasonics, vol 71 pp 161-171. 2016.

[21] Nicole V. Ruiter, Michael Zapf, Torsten Hopp, Koen van Dongen: USCT data challenge, in Proc. SPIE 10139, Medical Imaging 2017: Ultrasonic Imaging and Tomography, 101391N

[22] M. Pérez-Liva, J. L. Herraiz, and J. M. UdíasE. MillerB. T. Cox and B. E. Treeby, Time domain reconstruction of sound speed and attenuation in ultrasound computed tomography using full wave inversion. The Journal of the Acoustical Society of America 141, 1595 (2017);

[23] M. Pérez-Liva, Ph.D. Thesis. University Complutense of Madrid, 2017

First steps towards the Delft Breast Ultrasound Scanning System (DBUS)

L. Heijnsdijk, E. Jansen, U. Taskin, H. den Bok, E. Bergsma, E. Noothout, N. de Jong, and K.W.A. van Dongen

Laboratory of Acoustical Wavefield Imaging, Department of Imaging Physics, Delft University of Technology, Delft, the Netherlands
E-mail: k.w.a.vandongen@tudelft.nl

Abstract

Ultrasound in combination with full-waveform inversion (FWI) is gaining interest as a method to screen breasts for the presence of tumors. FWI has the advantage that is capable in retrieving acoustic medium properties useful for advanced tissue characterization. Many of the existing systems use center frequencies above 2 MHz resulting in sub-millimeter wavelengths. Using FWI in combination with these short wave lengths is challenging due to the computational costs involved. To investigate the applicability of a system with a low-frequency transducer for breast cancer detection, we have built our own two-dimensional circular scanning system. The system contains two 0.5 MHz transducers that are used to make a circular scan of an object. To test the system, several scans of agar phantoms have been made and processed using SAFT. The next step will be to use the acquired data to test the applicability of FWI as a mean to improve breast cancer detection using ultrasound.

Keywords: ultrasound tomography, breast cancer, 2-D scanner, full-waveform inversion

1 Introduction

Ultrasound is gaining interest as an efficient modality to screen for breast cancer[1, 2, 3, 4, 5]. Mainly because it works better than conventional X-ray mammography for dense breasts typical for young women. In addition, it avoids the use of ionizing radiation typical for X-ray mammography, while being relatively cheap compared to MRI. Up to date, ultrasound imaging is most frequently done using synthetic focusing techniques (SAFT). With SAFT, only the echogenicity of the medium is displayed whereas tissue specific information such as speed of sound is not obtained. To obtain these medium properties, ray-based methods have been investigated [6]. However, their success is limited, in particular when using low frequencies. Meanwhile, promising results are obtained with full-wave form inversion (FWI) on both synthetic [7, 8, 9] and measured data [10].

FWI is based on the acoustic wave equation. This way, effects such as multiple scattering, refraction, diffraction and/or dispersion can be accounted for. As all these effects are present in the data to a certain extent, the method has the potential to be more accurate than ray- or eikonal-based methods [6]. A downside of FWI is the computational complexity. As the wave field needs to be modeled at multiple points per wavelength, depending on the applied FWI methods, the computational demand may be come excessive, especially for 3-D inversion. An efficient way to limit this demand is to lower the frequency as this will result in longer wavelengths. For this reason, we are interested in frequencies near 0.5 MHz, which corresponds to wave lengths in the order of 3 mm and hence voxel sizes of 0.5 mm. To test the applicability of FWI at frequencies of 0.5 MHz, we have built a simple 2-D circular scanning system referred to as the Delft Breast Ultrasound Scanner: DBUS.

2 DBUS system

The Delft Breast Ultrasound Scanner (DBUS) is a 2-D circular scanning system. A sketch of the system is shown in figure 1. It contains two circular 0.5 MHz transducers submerged in water (Panametrics V318). The source is mounted on a fixed ruler to allow for varying radii and is standing still during the complete scanning procedure. It is connected via an amplifier (E&I 210L) and an attenuator (JFW 50BR-036) to an arbitrary waveform generator (Agilent 33521A). Meanwhile, the receiver is connected to an analog-to-digital converter (Spectrum M3i.4142-exp). Contrary to the source, the receiver is mounted via a ruler onto the outer-axis of a dual rotary table (LG Motion LGR1090-PD) and can rotate around the phantom. To illuminate the phantom from all sides by the static source, the phantom is attached to the center axis of the rotary table. For each scanning configuration, typically two scans are made; the first scan is made in the presence of the object and is performed for all source/receiver combinations, the next scan is made in the absence of the object and is acquired for a single source position only. The latter scan may be used for transducer characterization.

3 Results

Various objects have been scanned, varying from plastic bottles to agar-based phantoms. A typical example of the latter object is shown in figure 2. For each configuration, two scans are made; one in absence and one in presence of the object. The resulting A-scans together with their spectral profiles are displayed in figure 3. The figure clearly shows that the center frequency of the applied transducers is near 0.5 MHz. Note that the phase shift caused by the object is limited. The resulting B-scans, again in absence and in presence of an object is shown in figure 4. These scans clearly show that the wavefield becomes distorted by the object.

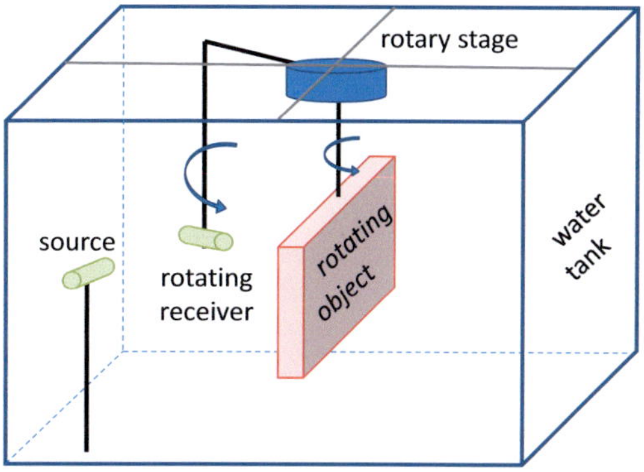

Figure 1: Sketch of the DBUS system. The 0.5 MHz source is located at a fixed location in the corner of the tank, while both the 0.5 MHz receiver and the phantom rotate as they are each separately attached to a dual-stage rotary system.

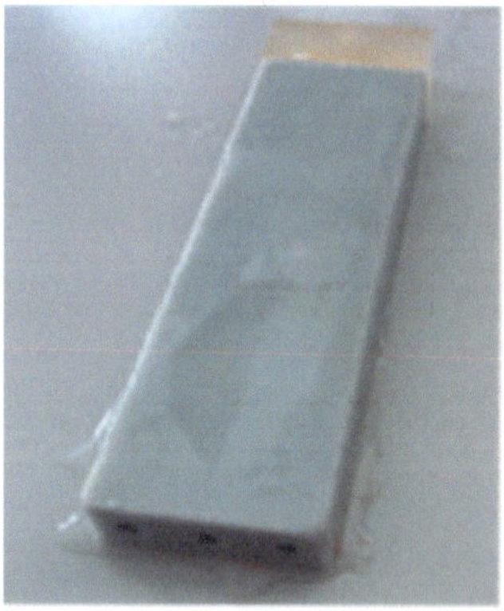

Figure 2: The agar phantom used for testing the system.

By applying SAFT on the measured data, a reconstruction of the phantom is obtained. For this measurement, an agar phantom containing two metal wires with a diameter of 0.75 mm and a nylon straw with a diameter of 6 mm is used. The nylon straw is filled with water. The resulting SAFT image, see figure 5, clearly reveals the boundary of the agar phantom as well as all the inclusions and suggests that the measured data is suitable to start testing FWI on measured data.

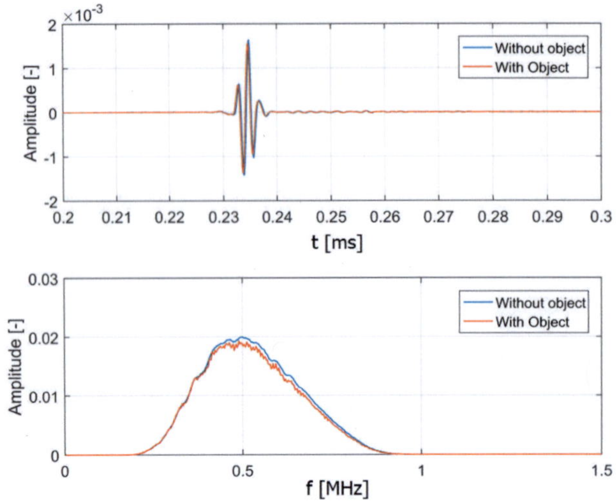

Figure 3: Two A-scans measured by the source and receiver positioned opposite each other; one without object (blue curve) and one with the agar phantom shown in figure 2. (red curve) in both time (top) and frequency domain (bottom).

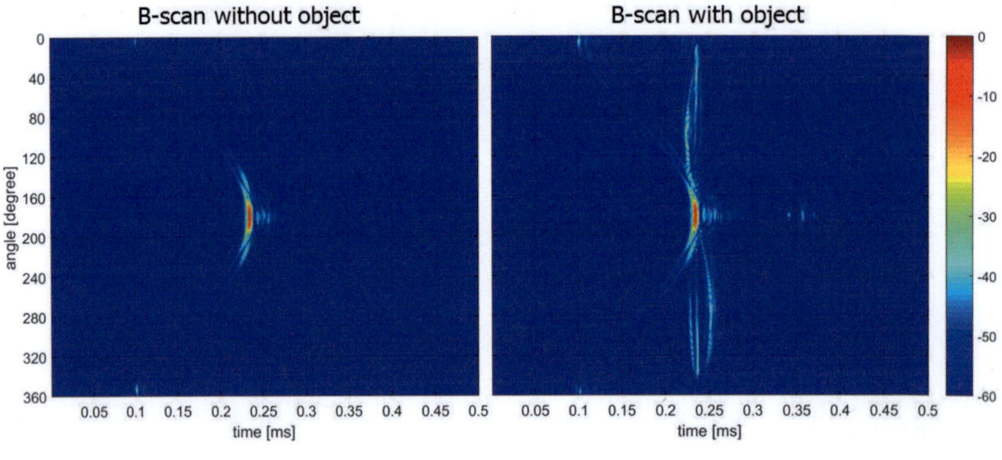

Figure 4: Two normalized B-scans on a dB-scale measured by the system; one without object (left) and one with object (right).

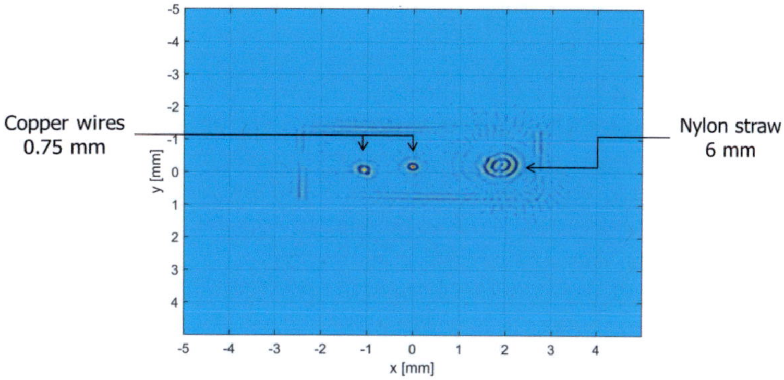

Figure 5: Reconstruction of the object using SAFT.

4 Discussion and conclusion

To meet the demand for a low-frequency scanning system to test FWI, we have a built a 2-D circular scanning system. The main components of the system are a water tank, a dual rotary table for two independent rotations, two single element circular transducers, and electronics to transmit a pulse and to read out the receiver. The center frequency of the transducers are 0.5 MHz. Processing the data acquired with the system using SAFT shows that the system works well. The next step will be to use the acquired data to test FWI on measured data.

References

[1] J. Rouyer, S. Mensah, E. Franceschini, P. Lasaygues, and J.-P. Lefebvre.: Conformal ultrasound imaging system for anatomical breast inspection. IEEE Trans. Ultrason., Ferroelectr., Freq. Control 59(7) (2012) 1457-1469

[2] J. Camacho, L. Medina, J. F. Cruza, J. M. Moreno, and C. Fritsch.: Multimodal Ultrasonic Imaging for Breast Cancer Detection. Archives of Acoustics 37(3) (2012) 253-260

[3] N. V. Ruiter, M. Zapf, R. Dapp, T. Hopp, W. A. Kaiser, and H. Gemmeke.: First results of a clinical study with 3D ultrasound computer tomography. 2013 IEEE International Ultrasonics Symposium (IUS) (2013) 651-654

[4] N. Duric, P. Littrup, S. Schmidt, C. Li, O. Roy, L. Bey-Knight, R. Janer, D. Kunz, X. Chen, Jeffrey Goll, A. Wallen, F. Zafar, V. Allada, E. West, I. Jovanovic, K. Li, and W. Greenway.: Breast imaging with the SoftVue imaging system: first results. SPIE 8675, Medical Imaging 2013. Proc. of SPIE (2013) 86750K86750K8

[5] J. W. Wiskin, D. T. Borup, E. Iuanow, J. Klock, and M. W. Lenox.: 3-D Nonlinear Acoustic Inverse Scattering: Algorithm and Quantitative Results. IEEE Trans. Ultrason., Ferroelectr., Freq. Control 64(8) (2017) 1161-1174

[6] N. Ozmen, R. Dapp, M. Zapf, H. Gemmeke, N.V. Ruiter, and K.W.A. van Dongen.: Comparing different ultrasound imaging methods for breast cancer detection. IEEE Trans. Ultrason., Ferroelectr., Freq. Control 62(4) (2015) 637-646

[7] K.W.A. van Dongen and W.M.D. Wright.: A forward model and conjugate gradient inversion technique for low-frequency ultrasonic imaging. J. Acoust. Soc. Am. 120(4) (2006) 2086-2095

[8] K.W.A. van Dongen, and W.M.D. Wright.: A full vectorial contrast source inversion scheme for three-dimensional acoustic imaging of both compressibility and density profiles. J. Acoust. Soc. Am. 121(3) (2007) 1538-1549

[9] A.B. Ramirez, and K.W.A. van Dongen.: Sparsity constrained contrast source inversion. J. Acoust. Soc. Am. 140(3) (2016) 1749-1757

[10] T.P. Matthews, K. Wang, C. Li, N. Duric, and M.A. Anastasio.: Regularized Dual Averaging Image Reconstruction for Full-Wave Ultrasound Computed Tomography. IEEE Trans. Ultrason., Ferroelectr., Freq. Control 64(5) (2017) 811-825

Upper Bound of Accuracy for Self-Calibration of an 3D Ultrasound Tomography System without Ground Truth

Wei Yap Tan[1], Till Steiner[2], and Nicole V. Ruiter[1]

[1] *Karlsruhe Institute of Technology, Germany*
Email: wei.tan@kit.edu
[2] *Pepperl+Fuchs GmbH, Germany*

Abstract

A self-calibration method was presented for a 3D Ultrasound Tomography System (USCT) in IEEE Ultrasonics Symposium (IUS) 2015 [1]. The method sequentially calibrates a complex USCT system with 2041 transducers based on time-of-flight (TOF) measurements. A direct evaluation of the calibration result was not possible due to unknown ground truth. In this work we present a method to estimate the upper boundary for the calibration accuracy. Evaluation with experiment data shows an estimated upper boundary of the mean error of 0.11 mm, which is smaller than the required accuracy of $\lambda/4 = 0.15$ mm for high quality image reconstruction [2].

Keywords: self-calibration, calibration accuracy, upper boundary

1 Introduction

The current 3D USCT system at KIT has a semi-ellipsoidal arrangement of 2041 ultrasound transducers, which are grouped into 157 transducer arrays (TAS) with four emitters and nine receivers each as shown in Figure 1. These transducers have a center frequency of 2.5 MHz with 50 % bandwidth and an opening angle of approximately 30° at −6 dB.

The semi-ellipsoidal aperture has a diameter of 26 cm and a depth of 18 cm. Additional virtual positions of the ultrasound transducers can be achieved by applying translational and rotational movements to the aperture.

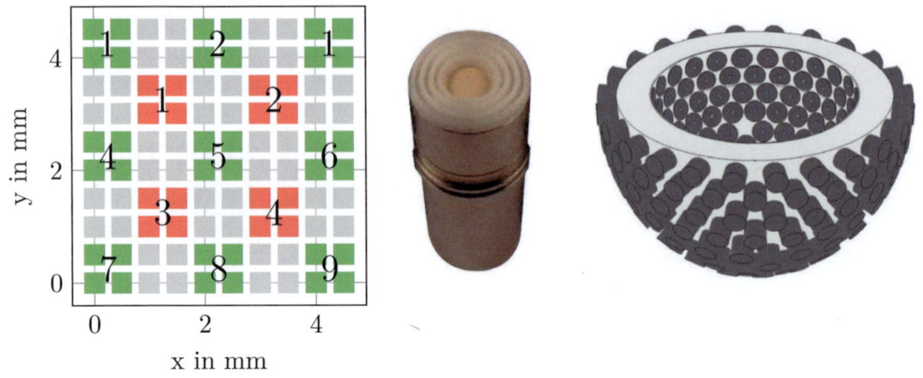

(a) Schematic diagram of a single transducer array

(b) TAS-Array and USCT geometry

Figure 1: The figures shows the current setup of the USCT.

It is a challenging task to manually calibrate the USCT due to the large amount of transducers and data acquisition channels. Possible error sources in USCT are position errors, temperature errors, delay errors and malfunctioning transducers. For high quality reconstruction of objects in the ROI of USCT, a TOF error less than one fourth of the wavelength ($\lambda/4$) is required [2] for the reconstruction of reflectivity image with the synthetic aperture focusing technique (SAFT) [3].

A self-calibration method based on time-of-flights (TOF) between the emitters and receivers was introduced in [1]. The self-calibration method is capable of separating each potential error sources and sequentially calibrate them by solving nonlinear equation systems with the Newton's method.

The proposed method was evaluated with simulated and experiment data. In the simulations, the capability of the method in quantifying and compensating multiple error sources was shown. However, a direct evaluation of the calibration accuracy with the experiment data was not possible due to the unknown ground truth. In this work we present a method to estimate the upper boundary for the calibration accuracy.

2 Methods

The goal of this work is to provide an estimation on the calibration accuracy for USCT under the absence of the ground truth. As the self-calibration method calibrates the USCT based on TOF between emitters and receivers with nonlinear equation systems, the calibration accuracy can be given by investigating the error propagation in these equation systems. The errors considered are errors in the detected TOF as input data of the equation systems.

2.1 Error Propagation in Equation Systems

In numerical mathematics, the condition number κ is used to describe the error propagation in equation systems [4]. The condition number shows how a small change in the input data is reflected in the function values for an equation system. In terms of error propagation, the condition number quantifies the sensitivity of the equation system against errors in the input data.

The determination of the condition number for a nonlinear equation system is performed by applying numerical methods. According to [4], the condition number for a nonlinear equation system is calculated by

$$\kappa = \frac{||J(\mathbf{x})||}{||f(\mathbf{x})||\,||\mathbf{x}||}. \tag{1}$$

For each calibration step, the maximum condition number κ_{max} of the equation systems is estimated by repeated evaluations of the Eq. (1) at a point $\mathbf{x}$ with small changes $\delta\mathbf{x}$. The points $\mathbf{x}$ are for instance the transducer positions and the expected delays in USCT.

In general, an equation system with a condition number $\kappa \geq 1$ is characterized as well conditioned. If κ is much greater than 1, the equation system is considered poorly conditioned. Whereas, for $\kappa = \infty$ the equation system has no solution [4].

The relative error of the solution $\frac{||\Delta\mathbf{x}||}{||\mathbf{x}||}$ of an equation system can be calculated with the maximum condition number κ_{max} and the relative input error $\frac{||\Delta\mathbf{b}||}{||\mathbf{b}||}$ as in Eq. (2).

$$\frac{||\Delta\mathbf{x}||}{||\mathbf{x}||} \leq \kappa_{max} \cdot \frac{||\Delta\mathbf{b}||}{||\mathbf{b}||} \tag{2}$$

The input error $||\Delta\mathbf{b}||$ can be determined from the experimental data of USCT under controlled environment. For example, we conducted in this work a series of consecutive empty measurements of USCT without objects in the aperture. It was assumed that the transducer positions were fixed and the temperature distribution in the water was known. The input error $||\Delta\mathbf{b}||$ is then the maximum deviation of the detected TOF for each emitter-receiver-combination in these measurements.

Since the numerical methods used for solving nonlinear equation systems requires the inversion of the Jacobian matrix, it is important to check the Jacobian matrix for singularity in each iteration step. A Jacobian matrix contains the first-order partial derivatives of an equation system. One method for detecting the singularity is to calculate the determinant of the Jacobian matrix. A Jacobian matrix is singular when the determinant is equal to zero.

2.2 Residual of the Calibration

When solving an equation system $\mathbf{F}(\mathbf{x}) = \mathbf{b}$ with numerical methods such as the Newton's method, the result $\hat{\mathbf{x}}$ is an approximation of the actual solution $\mathbf{x}$. The residual $\mathbf{r}$ is given by

$$\mathbf{r} = \mathbf{b} - \mathbf{F}(\hat{\mathbf{x}}). \tag{3}$$

The minimization of the residual is often used to systematically improve the solution in iterative methods. In addition to the maximum iteration, it can be used as a termination criterion when solving the equation systems.

In the absence of ground truth, the residual can be used to measure the accuracy of the approximated solution. The solution $\hat{\mathbf{x}}$ is considered close to the actual solution $\mathbf{x}$ when the residual is small. In the self-calibration method, the residual of the equation systems is calculated in each calibration step using the unit meter.

2.3 Calibration Accuracy

In this work, the calibration error $\hat{\varepsilon}$ is estimated by

$$\hat{\varepsilon} = \underbrace{|\Delta\mathbf{b}| \cdot c \cdot \sum_{i}^{N} \kappa_{max,i}}_{\text{Error in equation system}} + \overbrace{\sum_{i}^{N} r_i}^{Residual} , \tag{4}$$

with N as the number of calibration steps. The variable c is the speed of sound in the medium. In Eq. (4), the calibration error consists of two terms. The first term contains the amplification of the TOF errors $|\Delta\mathbf{b}|$ through the equation systems. The second term is the residual of the equation systems. Fig. 2 shows an example of the calibration error estimation in one calibration step with an equation system consisting of two unknowns.

In Fig. 2, the upper boundary of the calibration errors due to error propagation in the equation system is plotted with the blue circle around the exact solution $\mathbf{x}_0$. This upper boundary is further enlarged with the residual r of the equation system as shown by the gray dashed circle.

According to Eq. (4), the calibration error can be reduced by minimizing the TOF errors $|\Delta\mathbf{b}|$ and the condition number κ_{max} in each calibration step. The minimization of the condition number can be achieved by maximizing the ratio between the number of equations to the number of unknowns in the equation system. This reduces the contribution of each TOF error in the approximated solution. In the self-calibration method, the number of equations can be increased by including more emitter and receiver combinations.

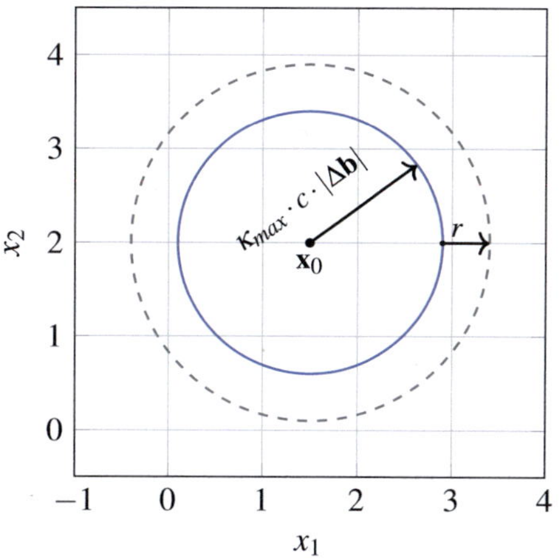

Figure 2: The figure demonstrates the estimation of calibration error for an equation system with two unknowns x_1 and x_2 with one calibration step. The exact solution of the equation system ist $\mathbf{x}_0$.

On the other hand, the TOF errors can be reduced by excluding A-scans with low signal-to-noise ratio (SNR) or malfunctioning transducers and electronics. This strategy contradicts with the idea of minimizing the condition number with more emitter-receiver-combinations. As the ultrasound transducer has a limited opening angle, increasing the emitter-receiver-combinations requires using A-scans from larger transmitting and receiving angles, which have lower SNR.

From this we conclude that the minimization of calibration errors can only be achieved by compromising between minimization of the condition number and TOF errors. Hence, a careful selection of emitter-receiver-combinations for the calibration is crucial for a good calibration result.

3 Evaluation with USCT

In this section, we investigated the relationships between the amount of emitter-receiver-combinations included for the calibration, the condition number in each calibration step and the TOF error. In the self-calibration method in [1], the angle α is used to select receivers with an angle to the normal vector of each emitter smaller than this angle.

A-scans from these selected emitter-receiver-combinations are used for the calibration. Due to the semi-ellipsoidal form of the USCT aperture, TAS in the lower part will not be calibrated. Table 1 shows the calibrated TAS of USCT with different values of the angle α. For a complete calibration of all TAS in USCT, a minimum angle α of 45° is needed.

Angle α	10°	20°	30°	40°	≥50°
Number of calibrated TAS	72	114	138	150	157

Table 1: Number of calibrated TAS in USCT with different values of the angle α

The condition number of each calibration step is computed for the angle $\alpha = 10° \ldots 60°$ and shown in Fig 3. The condition number reduces with more emitter-receiver combinations used for the calibration except for the position calibration. Despite this, the overall condition number improves with larger angle α.

In order to determine the TOF error $|\Delta \mathbf{b}|$, ten consecutive empty measurements were performed with USCT. During the measurements, the positions of the ultrasound transducers were assumed to be constant and the water temperature was monitored. The TOF errors were then computed for angle α from 10° to 60° and plotted in Fig 4.

According to Fig. 4 the maximum TOF error increases rapidly from angle α larger than 20° and reaches the used detection window of 2 µs during the TOF detection with matched filter.

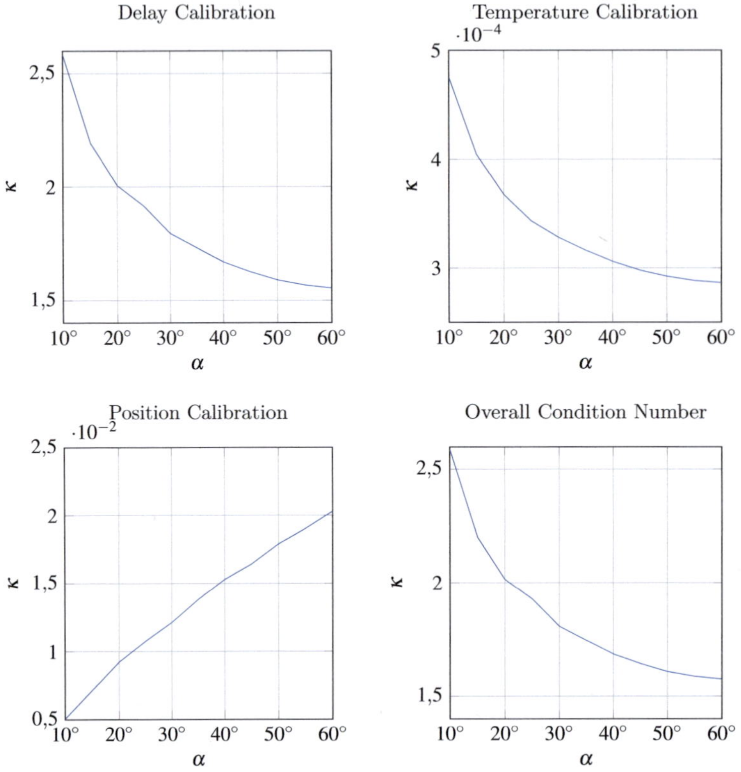

Figure 3: The figure shows the condition number κ_{max} of each calibration step according to the angle α.

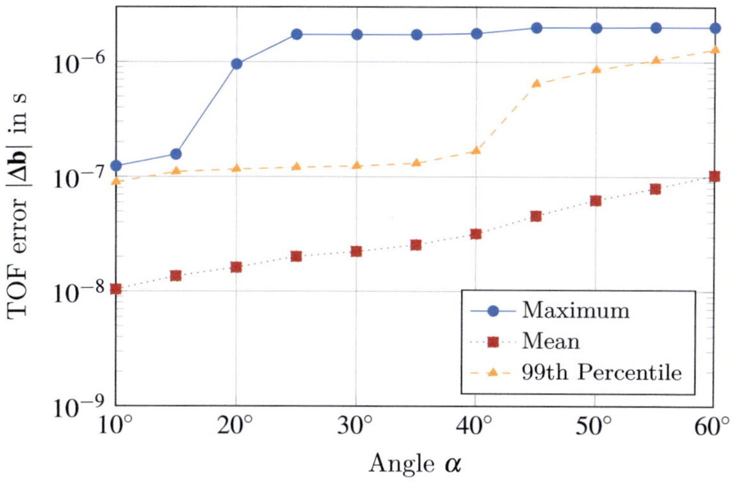

Figure 4: The figure shows the TOF errors for different angles α.

This rapid increase is caused by the fact that some A-scans with bad SNR were not sorted out in the filtering process and appear as outliers in the statistic.

The 99th percentile confirms this assumption as shown in Figure 4. For angles α smaller than 40°, the TOF error was approximately 0.1 µs. Meanwhile, the plotted mean TOF error shows an increase in TOF errors with larger angle α as expected.

The investigation proved that the minimization of both the condition number and the TOF error to be a contradicting process. For the calibration of all TAS in USCT, the angle α was set at 45°. Table 2 lists the estimated calibration errors with a water temperature of 30 °C during the measurements. The total residual was significantly smaller than the TOF error in the order of 1×10^{-7}. A mean calibration error of 0.11 mm was estimated for a total condition number $\kappa_{all} = 1.64$.

	$\lvert\Delta \mathbf{b}\rvert$	$\lvert\Delta \mathbf{b}\rvert \cdot c$	$\lvert\Delta \mathbf{b}\rvert \cdot c \cdot \kappa_{all}$
Mean	45.68 ns	68.95 µm	0.11 mm
0,99-Perzentil	0.64 µs	0.97 mm	1.60 mm
Maximum	1.98 µs	3.00 mm	4.90 mm

Table 2: Calibration error with $\alpha = 45°$

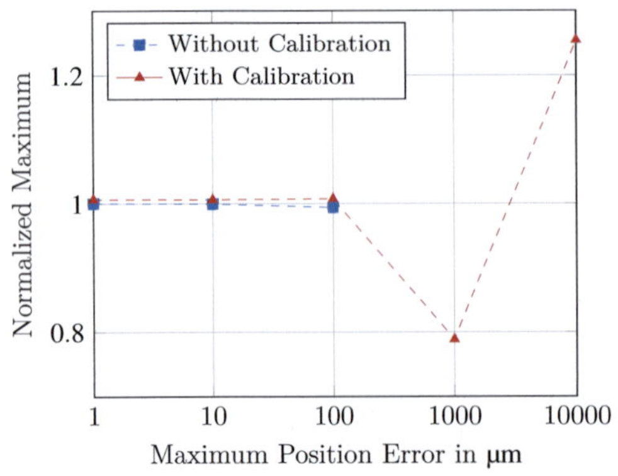

(a) Normalized maximum intensity

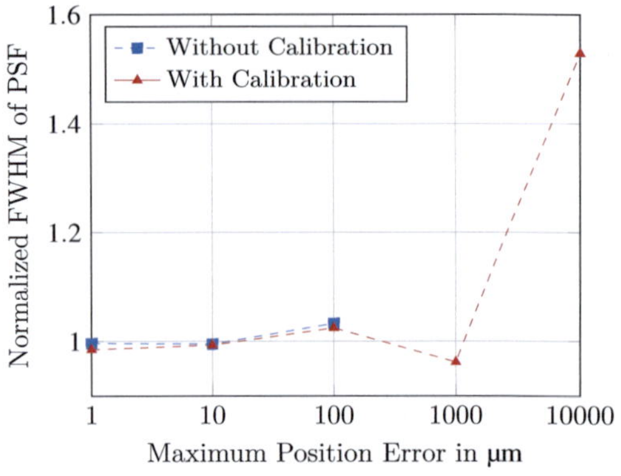

(b) Normalized FWHM

Figure 5: The figure shows the maximum intensity and FWHM of the PSF of the reconstructed point scatter normalized to the ground truth with and without the calibration. The image quality is closest to the ground truth with both normalized value nearest to one. The reconstructions without calibration failed to produce a focused image for errors larger than 1 mm.

4 Improvements in the Image Quality

One critical aspect during the construction of the 3D USCT is the machining accuracy required for the aperture and the transducer arrays. The current version of USCT was built with an accuracy of 10 µm, which implied large technical efforts and costs. The possibility to build the USCT at a coarser accuracy and calibrate the transducer positions will hence be beneficial.

In the following investigation, the USCT was simulated with maximum position errors of individual transducer in a range between 1 µm and 1 cm. For each maximum position error an empty measurement and a measurement with a point scatterer in the middle of the USCT aperture were simulated. The A-scan was sampled at 10 MHz. In order to achieve high accuracy in the simulated TOF of the transmission and reflection signal, fractional delay filter in the Fourier space was used [6]. Other errors sources such as delays and temperature errors were not simulated.

The transmitted coded excitation is a chirp signal with a start frequency at 1.66 MHz and a stop frequency at 3.33 MHz. The TOF detection was performed with a matched filter at 10 MHz sample rate. For the image reconstruction, a SAFT reconstruction with speed of sound and attenuation correction was used [7] and the image resolution was 10 µm.

In Figure 5, the maximum intensity and the full width at half maximum (FWHM) of the point spread function (PSF) [8] of the reconstructed point scatter was normalized to the ground truth. The image quality is closest to the ground truth with both normalized values nearest to one.

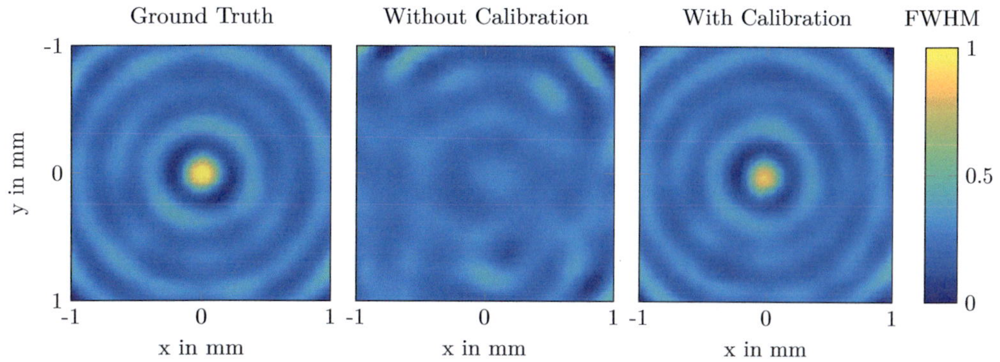

Figure 6: The figure compares the reconstructed point scatterer with and without calibration to the ground truth at maximum position error of 1 mm.

The resulting images were similar to the ground truth for reconstructions with and without calibration for maximum position errors under 100 µm, which is smaller than $\lambda/4 = 152\,\mu$m of the center frequency at 2.5 MHz.

For maximum position errors larger than 1 mm, the reconstruction without calibration failed to produce a focused image of the point scatter as shown in Figure 6. The reconstruction with calibrated USCT at maximum position error of 10 mm has a higher maximum but a larger FWHM than the ground truth.

5 Conclusion

In this work, we proposed a method for estimating the upper boundary of the calibration error of USCT based on the investigation of the error propagation in equation systems. An upper boundary of the mean calibration error of 0.11 mm was estimated with the experiment data of ten consecutive measurements under controlled environment, which is smaller than one fourth of the wavelength used as required for high quality image with USCT [2].

The evaluation also showed that the minimization of the calibration error is a tradeoff between minimizing the condition number κ and the TOF error. The estimation method enables finding the optimal selection of emitter-receiver combinations to obtain the smallest upper boundary of the calibration error.

In Section 4, the simulations of a point scatter with different maximum errors in the transducer positions demonstrates the improvements in the image quality with the self-calibration. It was also showed that for the current USCT system, a machining accuracy of 100 µm would be sufficient for usable image quality when neglecting other error sources such as delays, jitters in the electronics and temperature errors. The investigation also showed that the self-calibration was able to calibrate position errors up to 1 mm and reconstructs focused image comparable to the ground truth as shown in Figure 6.

References

[1] Tan, W. Y., Steiner, T., and Ruiter, N. V. Newton's method based self calibration for a 3D ultrasound tomography system. In *Ultrasonics Symposium (IUS), 2015 IEEE International* (2015).

[2] Schwarzenberg, G. F. *Untersuchung der Abbildungseigenschaften eines 3D-Ultraschall-Computertomographen zur Berechnung der 3D-Abbildungsfunktion und Herleitung einer optimierten Sensorgeometrie*. PhD thesis, Universität Fridericiana zu Karlsruhe (TH), 2008.

[3] Stepinski, T. An implementation of synthetic aperture focusing technique in frequency domain. *IEEE Transactions on Ultrasonics, Ferroelectrics, and Frequency Control 54*, 7 (2007), 1399–1408.

[4] Trefethen, L., and Bau, D. *Numerical Linear Algebra*. Society for Industrial and Applied Mathematics (SIAM, 3600 Market Street, Floor 6, Philadelphia, PA 19104), 1997.

[5] Neuß, N. Einführung in die Numerische Mathematik für Studierende der Fachrichtungen Informatik und Ingenieurwesen, 2011.

[6] Laakso, T., Välimäki, V., Karjalainen, M., and Laine, U. Splitting the unit delay - tools for fractional delay filter design. *IEEE SIGNAL PROCESSING MAGAZINE* (1996), 30–60.

[7] Ruiter, N. V., Kretzek, E., Zapf, M., Hopp, T., and Gemmeke, H. Time of flight interpolated synthetic aperture focusing technique, 2017.

[8] Suetens, P. *Fundamentals of Medical Imaging*. Cambridge medicine. Cambridge University Press, 2009.

Manufacturing Technologies for Ultrasonic Transducers in a Broad Frequency Range

S. E. Gebhardt[1], K. Hohlfeld[2], P. A. Günther[1], and H. Neubert[1]

[1] *Fraunhofer IKTS Institute for Ceramic Technologies and Systems, Dresden, Germany*
E-mail: sylvia.gebhardt@ikts.fraunhofer.de
[2] *TU Dresden, Institute of Materials Science (IfWW), Dresden, Germany*

Abstract

According to the application field, working frequency of ultrasonic transducers needs to be tailored to a certain value. Low frequency ultrasonic transducers with working frequencies of 1 kHz to 1 MHz are especially interesting for sonar applications, whereas high frequency ultrasonic transducers with working frequencies higher than 15 MHz are favorable for high-resolution imaging in biomedical and non-destructive evaluation. Conventional non-destructive testing devices and clinical ultrasound imaging systems are typically operated at frequencies between 1 MHz and 10 MHz. Depending on the operational scenario, thickness, layout, and inner structure of the ultrasonic transducer has to be customized. We here report on different manufacturing technologies for ultrasonic transducers in a broad frequency range. 1-3 piezocomposites based on piezoceramic fibers can be fabricated in almost every thickness allowing for transducer frequencies between 40 kHz and 8 MHz. The soft mold process enables the fabrication of high frequency ultrasonic transducers with potential frequencies of 5 MHz up to 40 MHz. Highly integrated ultrasonic transducers can be prepared by screen-printing a sequence of electrode, piezoceramic, and isolation layers on microelectronic substrates. With that, patterned ultrasonic transducers with working frequencies between 5 MHz and 30 MHz are possible.

Keywords: 1-3 piezocomposite, ultrasonic transducer, piezoelectric fiber, piezofiber composite, piezoelectric thick film, soft mold process

1 Introduction

Ultrasonic transducers are widely used for imaging in sonar, non-destructive testing, and medical diagnostics. They are particularly favorable compared to X-ray imaging, because of their non-ionizing character, low cost and to the fact that from images and measurements physical and structural information of the examined media can be obtained [1]. Whereas for sonar applications ultrasonic transducers with frequencies spanning from 1 kHz to 1 MHz are needed (covering 1-100 kHz for weapons sonar and 100 kHz to 1 MHz for imaging sonar), higher frequencies are necessary for non-destructive testing and medical diagnostics [2]. Conventional non-destructive testing devices and clinical ultrasound imaging systems are typically operated at frequencies between 1 MHz and 10 MHz. To improve the spatial resolution of ultrasonic images, ultrasonic transducers are necessary, which can be operated at higher frequencies. Due to decreasing penetration depth with increasing frequency, high frequency ultrasonic transducers allow for near-surface or intracorporal imaging, for instance in the context of dermatological, ophthalmological, dental or intravascular examinations. They are also interesting for small animal imaging and non-destructive testing of fiber-reinforced plastics, small-sized substance-to-substance bonds, and electronic components.

Designing ultrasonic transducers is always subject of a compromise between high sensitivity for large penetration depth and large bandwith for high axial resolution. These properties are primarily determined by the parameters of the piezoelectric material used, moreover by the backing and the electrical and acoustic impedance matching [3]. 1-3 piezocomposites of piezoelectric rods embedded in a non-piezoelectric and elastic polymer matrix enable transducers of higher sensitivity and bandwith compared to single phase piezoceramic materials because of their approximately 40% to 50% higher electromechanical coupling as well as the tunable and up to the factor of 5 lower acoustic impedance and lower dielectric constant. The weak acoustic coupling between discrete rods in the polymer matrix allows for phased array transducers with acoustically separated elements simply by applying patterned instead of full electrodes. Moreover, soft polymer matrices bring the ability to form curved transducers for focusing.

Due to the periodicity of piezoceramic rods within 1-3 piezocomposites, spurious modes are activated by rod-to-rod interactions [4]. These spurious modes can drastically affect the efficiency of the ultrasonic transducer if they occur near the operational thickness mode [5]. It is thus necessary to shift these modes to frequencies almost twice as high as the thickness mode resonance, which corresponds to a ratio $t/p > 3$ between the thickness of the piezoelectric composite t and its periodicity p [6]. Therefore, 1-3 piezocomposite technologies for transducers in different frequency ranges have to enable not only appropriate composite thickness but in addition a sufficiently fine inner structure. This is challenging especially for frequencies higher than about 15 MHz, which are gaining an increasing interest during the last 20 years driven by the desire for high-resolution imaging.

The dice-and-fill process is a long-established and recognized industrial technology to produce such 1-3 piezocomposites [7]. For this, a series of parallel cuts is made into a bulk piezoelectric plate in two directions perpendicular to each other. The resulting kerfs are than backfilled with a polymer and the base ceramic support as well as the excessive polymer on top removed by grinding and polishing. This method has been approved for the manufacture of ultrasonic transducers with frequencies ranging between 1 MHz and 15 MHz. For frequencies up to 20 MHz, backfilled rod structures are further subdivided to achieve smaller lateral periodicity called pitch. The depth and width of the dicing blade and the brittleness of the piezoelectric material limit the dice-and-fill process. Fine-grained piezoceramics are necessary as a prerequisite for high frequency ultrasonic transducers with small pitches.

For ultrasonic transducers with frequencies lower than 1 MHz, 1-3 piezocomposites with thickness larger than 2 mm are necessary, reaching approximately 15 mm thickness for frequencies of 100 kHz. These requirements are fulfilled by 1-3 piezocomposites based on piezoelectric fibers. They can be fabricated in almost any length. Only the voltage necessary for poling limits the thickness of the piezofiber composit. For piezoelectric materials based on soft PZT (lead zirconate titanate) materials, electric fields of 2 kV/mm are required for poling. A piezofiber composite with 50 mm thickness would thus need a poling voltage of approximately 100 kV.

2 Piezofiber composites based on the arrange & fill method

2.1 Random fiber composites

In 1999 we introduced the arrange & fill process for fabrication of piezocomposites based on piezoceramic fibers [8]. For this, bundles or fixed arrangements of piezoceramic fibers are aligned into a mold and subsequently infiltrated with a polymer matrix. The cured piezocomposite strand can be sliced into plates with a thickness according to the desired resonance frequency. Furthermore, the soft character of the composite material enables CNC (Computerized Numerical Control) machining to virtually any shape or size. Thus, a quick and cost-effective manufacture of large quantities of piezocomposites is possible [9]. Figure 1 shows a selection of possible piezofiber composites and a cross section of a 1-3 piezocomposite with random distribution of fibers with a diameter of 300 μm.

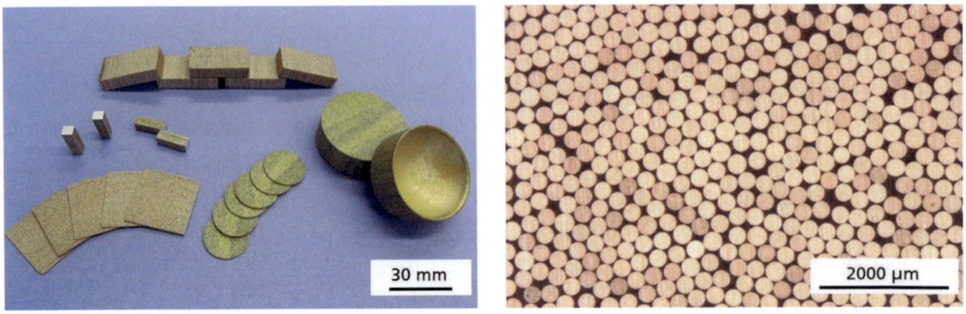

Figure 1: Piezofiber composites (left) and cross section of a 1-3 piezocomposite with random distribution of PZT fibers with a diameter of 300 µm (right).

For fabrication of piezoceramic fibers, different manufacturing technologies have been reported in literature. Piezoceramic fibers with diameters between 100 µm and 1000 µm are typically derived from fiber spinning or extrusion methods. For fiber spinning, piezoceramic powders are dispersed into a binder solution to form a uniform slurry with high solids concentration. The slurry is then spun through a nozzle into a coagulation bath. There, the binder solution precipitates leading to a rigid green fiber, which will subsequently be dried and sintered. Technologies reported in literature are the Viscous Suspension Spinning Process (VSSP), where viscose is used as polymer binder [10] and the ALCERU Process (Alternative Cellulose aus Rudolstadt) based on cellulose binders [11]. We recently introduced the polysulfone spinning process for fabrication of piezoceramic fibers [12]. There, a binder solution of polysulfone binder and N-Methylpyrrolidone (NMP) as solvent is used. For all spinning methods, fiber diameter can be adjusted by the diameter of the spinneret, the slurry discharge velocity and the spinning speed.

Fiber extrusion is a relatively simple method to produce ceramic fibers with different cross sections. First, a feedstock of binder and piezoceramic powder is formed, which is than extruded through a nozzle using a screw extruder [13], [14]. Again, resulting green fibers are debindered and sintered.

Due to the random distribution of the piezoceramic fibers, resulting piezofiber composites are free from spurious modes based on the periodicity of the arrangement. The maximum operation frequency is determined by the diameter and thus the planar mode of the piezoceramic fiber. Moreover, thick piezocomposite blocks with flat or convex/concave formed surfaces can easily be prepared by dicing and CNC machining. This makes piezofiber composites well suited for broadband ultrasonic transducers with frequencies ranging between 40 kHz and 8 MHz.

2.2 Regular fiber composites

For regular piezofiber composites, piezoceramic fibers are positioned into a mask according to the required pattern. The fixed arrangement is than placed into a mold and subsequently infiltrated with a polymer. After curing, the composite strand will be machined into custom shape and sliced into single transducers. A schematic presentation of the process and samples of piezocomposites with regular arrangement of piezofibers are shown in Figure 2.

Piezofiber composites with regular arrangement of fibers are especially interesting for ultrasonic transducers with defined volume fraction of piezoceramic fibers. Beside that, subsections of the transducer with fixed fiber positions can be formed, which allow for acoustically separated array elements.

For a 3-D Ultrasound Computer Tomography (USCT) system, we recently developed piezofiber composites with single fibers located at specific positions of a circular piezocomposite plate [15]. Heart of the USCT system is a 3-D semi-ellipsoidal shaped water filled container with 2041 unfocused ultrasound transducers integrated into the periphery (wall) of the container. Each transducer should exhibit a center frequency of approximately 2.5 MHz, 1 MHz bandwidth and 60° opening angle at -3 dB. Initially, dice-and-fill technique has been used to produce square ultrasonic arrays. 157 ultrasonic transducers with 4 emitting and 9 receiving elements each have been prepared and tested. It turned out, that due to the square shape and the size of 0.81 mm^2 of each element, opening angle as well as sound pressure homogeneity are limited. 3-D simulation of potential transducer designs identified round shaped transducers with active area of 0.16 mm^2 to be ideal in respect of sound pressure and opening angle. Piezoceramic fibers offer the possibility to fabricate round piezoceramic transducers with different diameters. For the considered design, piezoceramic fibers with a diameter of about 460 μm have been arranged in a certain pattern as shown in Figure 2 to improve the signal-to-noise ratio in resulting images by preventing periodic artifacts. Structured electrodes were applied to each single fiber by sputtering gold and connected to the outer control electronics. So each fiber could be addressed individually for emitting and receiving ultrasonic waves.

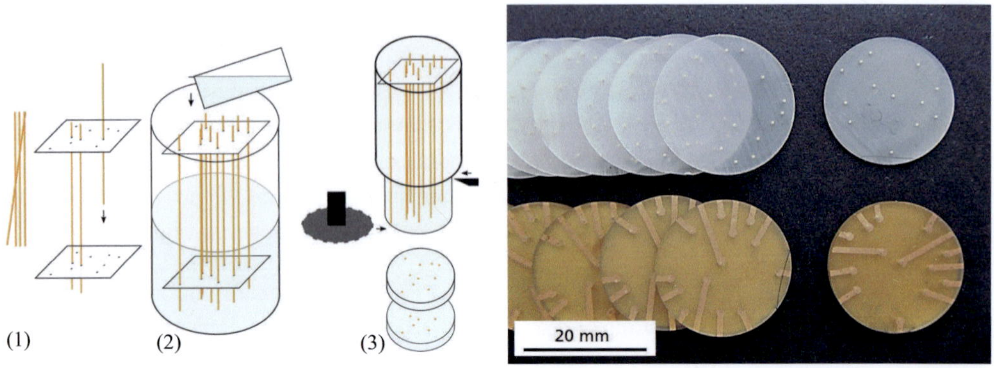

Figure 2: Left: Schematic of piezocomposite fabrication with regular arrangement of fibers: (1) positioning of fibers, (2) polymer infiltration, (3) mechanical machining and dicing. Right: Piezofiber composites with regular arrangement of fibers for integration into a USCT system.

Piezofiber composites with different thickness have been cut from one 150 mm long composite block. Thus, a series of discs with identical position and properties of single fiber transducers was received. Resonance frequency as well as thickness mode coupling coefficient have been measured in dependence of composite thickness. Both are displayed in Figure 3. The coupling coefficient of the piezofiber transducers reached mean values $k_t > 60\%$ for transducers with thickness greater than 0.8 mm. For transducers with smaller thickness the planar mode of the piezofibers interfered with the thickness mode resonance resulting in a reduced coupling coefficient and larger variation of values. In future, fiber diameter has to be reduced in order to obtain highest performance at 2.5 MHz.

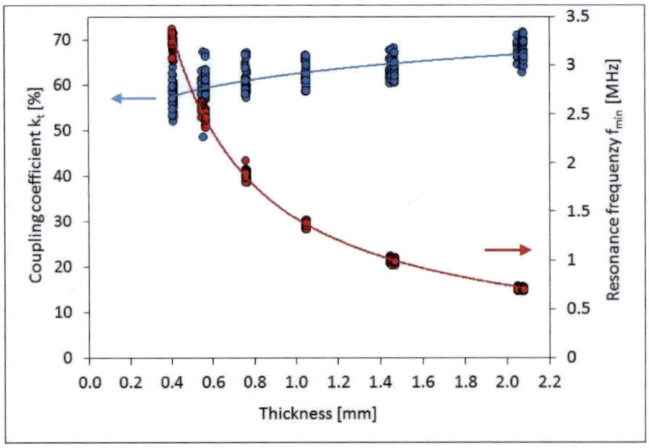

Figure 3: Thickness mode resonance frequency and coupling coefficient in dependence of piezocomposite thickness for a 1-3 piezocomposite with 460 μm fibers.

3 Piezocomposites based on the soft mold process

The soft mold process offers the opportunity for fabrication of fine-scale piezocomposites with free design of ceramic rod geometry and spatial distribution [16]. This makes the process especially interesting for the development of high frequency ultrasonic transducers. Special characteristic of the process is the direct molding of piezoceramic rod arrangements from flexible negatives using slip casting technology. Therefore, soft plastic templates are taken from a positive master mold, which has been structured by microsystems technologies like silicon deep reactive ion etching (DRIE) or LIGA (Lithographie, Galvanik und Abformung) technique. They are filled with a ceramic slurry under vacuum. After drying, ceramic green bodies are demolded and sintered. Thereby the ceramic green body shrinks by approximately 20-25%. The spacings are subsequently filled with a polymer and the base and the top removed by grinding. The process is schematically pictured in Figure 4. In opposite to the dice-and-fill process, rod shape, size, spacing and arrangement can be chosen in a high variety. Master molds as well as soft molds are reusable which makes the process cost-effective. Besides, time and effort for manufacturing becomes independent from rod size and layout.

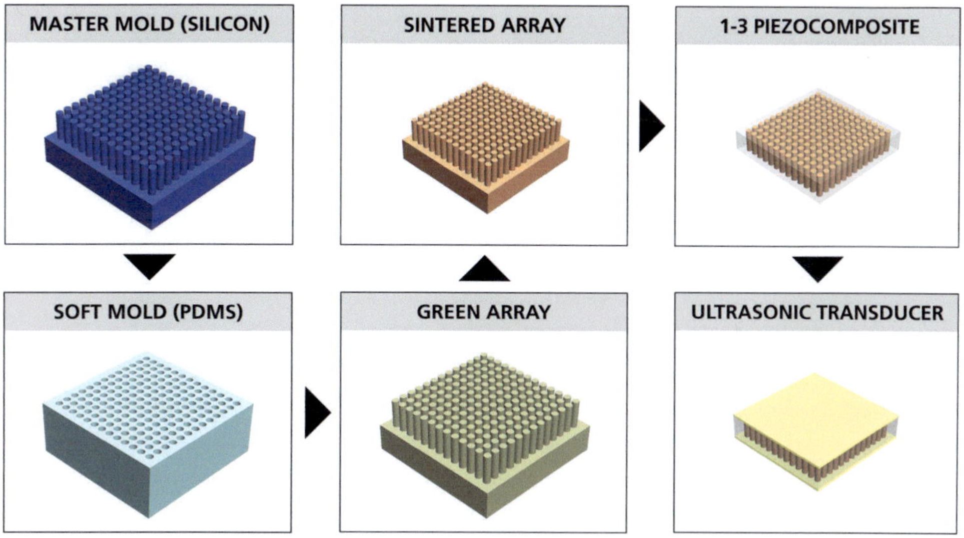

Figure 4: Schematic representation of the soft mold process.

For fabrication of a 20 MHz ultrasonic transducer, we investigated arrangement and spacing of different rod geometries on generation and frequency of spurious modes [17]. Ceramic rods based on triangle and half hexagon cross sections tended to topple during sintering. Best results have been obtained for round rods. Based on those findings, silicon master molds of round rods with 200 μm height, 45 μm diameter, and 55 μm or 60 μm pitch have been prepared. Rod arrangement has been varied between square and hexagonal. Figure 6 shows the layout of the investigated rod structures. After demolding and sintering ceramic rods with 160 μm height, 34 μm diameter and 42 μm or 45 μm pitch could be received. Compared to the conventional dice-and-fill process, unattainable rod spacings of 8 μm or 11 μm are possible using soft mold process. The sintered PZT structures showed a dense, fine grained and homogenous microstructure as can be seen in Figure 5.

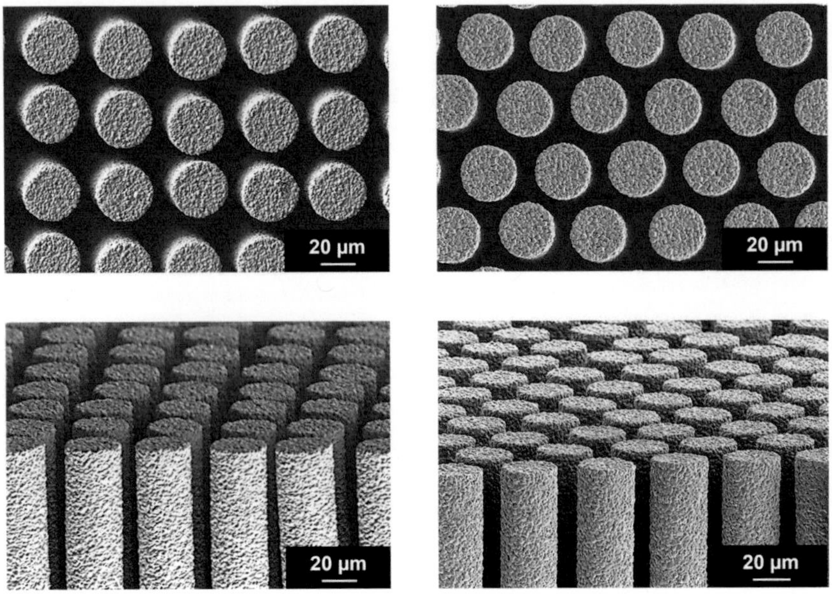

Figure 5: Sintered PZT structures of round rods in square and hexagonal arrangement (Scanning Electron Microscopy images of top and side view)

1-3 piezocomposites derived from the structures A-D were ground to approximately 90 μm thickness in order to reach 20 MHz thickness mode resonance frequency. Depending on rod arrangement and rod pitch, spurious modes occurred at higher frequencies (see Figure 6). For the square arrangement of round rods, first resonance caused by rod-to-rod periodicity was measured at ca. 27 MHz for 42 μm pitch and at ca. 24 MHz for 45 μm pitch. The hexagonal arrangement even improved resonance behavior by shifting spurious modes to higher frequencies of ca. 37 MHz for 42 μm pitch and at ca. 28 MHz for 45 MHz pitch.

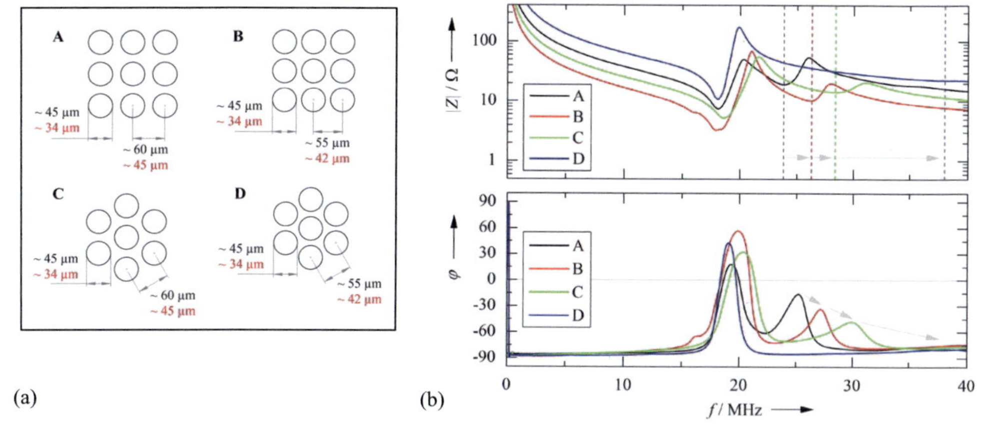

Figure 6: Left: Layout of master molds with circular rods in square and hexagonal arrangement: dimension of master mold (black) and sintered ceramic (red). Right: Electrical impedance $|Z|$ and phase angle φ curves for 1-3 piezocomposites of structure A-D.

The technology has the potential to further reduce rod size and pitch. At present, we are aiming to scale down rod layout for fabrication of ultrasonic transducers with working frequencies up to 40 MHz.

4 Screen-printed ultrasonic transducers

Piezoceramic thick films with typical thickness of 30 µm up to 150 µm offer the opportunity of integrated solutions based on microsystems technologies. Using the screen-printing process, net-shaped structures can easily be applied on flat or tubular substrates without further structuring. We developed a piezoceramic thick film paste based on low sintering PZT powder. It can be printed and sintered on standard electronic substrate materials like alumina (Al_2O_3), low temperature cofired ceramics (LTCC), zirconia (ZrO_2) and selected steel grades. In combination with the stepwise printing and sintering of electrode and isolation layers, compact microsystems are possible.

For a 2-D matrix array transducer a sequence of patterned thick film layers were printed on a 0.25 µm thick Al_2O_3 substrate (99.6%, Rubalit 710, CeramTec, Germany) comprising Au bottom electrode, PZT thick film, Au top electrode, dielectric isolation, and Au electrode fan-out tracks [18]. The thickness of the PZT film was adjusted to 140 µm thickness by repeated printing of PZT thick film layers. 6 x 6 PZT elements of 2 mm x 2 mm size with 1.7 mm x 1.7 mm top electrode were printed with 2.3 mm element pitch. Figure 7 shows the top view of the final device.

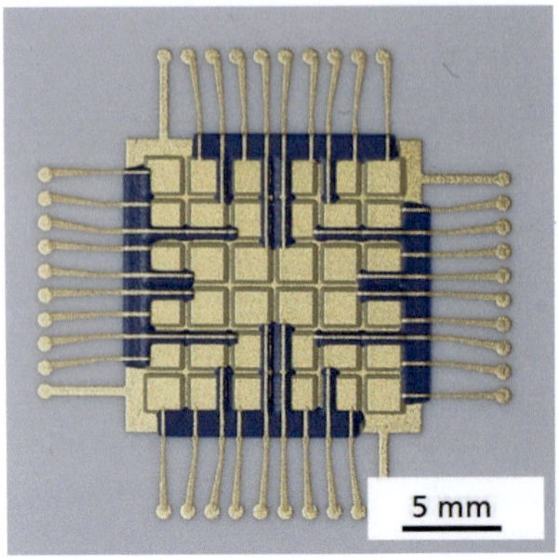

Figure 7: 2-D matrix array on Al_2O_3 substrate comprising screen-printed bottom electrode, PZT thick film, top electrode, dielectric isolation, and electrode fan-out tracks.

The resonance frequencies of printed ultrasonic transducers strongly depend on the substrate thickness and the thickness of the PZT layer. Since the PZT layer is sintered on top of the substrate, a strong bond between the active piezoelectric layer and the substrate material is generated. When thickness of the substrate is small enough, a combined vibration of the PZT thick film and the substrate will occur. In the case of the 2-D matrix array transducer, resonance frequency was measured at 7.4 MHz. This frequency could be used to build a multilayer planar resonant device for particle manipulation. Therefore, a fluid cavity chamber with a glass reflector was attached to the Al_2O_3 substrate. 10 µm fluorescent polystyrene microspheres were used as model structures for particle manipulation. By driving the PZT elements with 7.5 $V_{p\text{-}p}$ sinusoidal signal at the resonant frequency, microparticles within the fluid were levitated and trapped to pressure nodes in the fluid chamber. The experiments proved that screen-printed ultrasonic transducers can generate sufficient acoustic power for ultrasonic manipulation devices.

Depending on the acoustic properties of the substrate material as well as the layout and thickness of the PZT thick film and the substrate, also higher resonance frequencies can be activated. A profound understanding of wave propagation and accurate dimensioning are necessary to construct ultrasonic transducers with resonance frequencies between 5 MHz and 30 MHz.

5 Conclusion

Diverse manufacturing technologies are necessary to produce ultrasonic transducers with different working frequencies. Piezofiber composites are suited for low frequency ultrasonic transducers. Depending on application needs, fiber arrangement can be chosen to be regular or random. A new approach for cost-effective fabrication of 2041 transducers in a USCT system has been developed based on 1-3 piezocomposites with defined position of single piezoceramic fibers. Using structured electrodes, each fiber could be individually addressed and worked as a single transducer. The coupling coefficient of the piezofiber transducers reached mean values $k_t > 60\%$ depending on transducer thickness. The soft mold process allows for the manufacture of 1-3 piezocomposites with a high variety of rod shape, size, spacing and arrangement. For the development of a 20 MHz transducer, square and hexagonal arrangement of round rods with different spacings were investigated. Best results have been achieved from 1-3 piezocomposites made of round rods with 34 µm diameter and 42 µm pitch in hexagonal arrangement. There, spurious modes could be shifted to frequencies up to 37 MHz. Patterned ultrasonic transducers with working frequencies between 5 MHz and 30 MHz are possible by screen-printing a sequence of electrode, piezoceramic, and isolation layers on substrates like Al_2O_3, LTCC, ZrO_2, and selected steel grades. A 2-D matrix array transducer has been developed for a particle manipulation device. Resonance frequency of screen-printed PZT thick film devices strongly depend on acoustic properties of the substrate material as well as the layout and thickness of the PZT thick film and the substrate. The technology can be used to build highly integrated microsystems.

6 Acknowledgement

This work was partly supported by the Deutsche Forschungsgemeinschaft (DFG) in context of the Collaborative Research Centre/Transregio 39 PT-PIESA (subproject A01 and K04) and in context of the Grant GE-2078/5-1.

References

[1] M. Lethiecq, F. Levassort, D. Certon L. P. Tran-Huu-Hue.: Piezoelectric Transducer Design for Medical Diagnosis and NDE. Piezoelectric and Acoustic Materials for Transducer Applications, 1st ed., A. Safari and E. K. Akdogan, Ed. New York, NY, USA: Springer Science+Business Media (2008) 191–215

[2] J. F. Tressler.: Piezoelectric Transducer Designs for Sonar Applications. Piezoelectric and Acoustic Materials for Transducer Applications, 1st ed., A. Safari and E. K. Akdogan, Ed. New York, NY, USA: Springer Science+Business Media (2008) 217-239

[3] J. W. Hunt, M. Arditi, S. Foster.: Ultrasound Transducers for Pulse-Echo Medical Imaging. IEEE Trans. on Biomedical Engng, (8) (1983) 453-481

[4] T. R. Gururaja, W. A. Schulze, L. E. Cross, R. E. Newnham, B. A. Auld, Y. J. Wang.: Piezoelectric composite materials for ultrasonic transducer applications. Part I: Resonant modes of vibration of PZT rod-polymer composites. IEEE Trans. Sonics Ultrason, 19985 (32) (1985) 481-498

[5] R. Rouffaud, F. Levassort, M. P. Thi, C. Bantignies, M. Lethiecq, A.-C. Hladky-Hennion.: Super-Cell Piezoelectric Composite With 1–3 Connectivity. IEEE Trans. Ultrason., Ferroelect., Freq. Control, 12(63) (2016) 2215-2223

[6] J. A. Hossack, G. Hayward.: Finite-element Analysis of 1–3 Composite Transducers. IEEE Trans. Ultrason., Ferroelect., Freq. Control 6(38) (1991) 618–629

[7] H. P. Savakus, K. A. Klicker, R. E. Newnham.: PZT-Epoxy Piezoelectric Transducers: A Simplified Fabrication Procedure. Mater. Res. Bull., 6(16) (1981) 677–680

[8] L. Seffner, A. Schönecker, S. Gebhardt.: Verfahren zur Herstellung eines piezoelektrischen Wandlers (Method for Producing a Piezoelectric Transducer). Patent DE 199 54 020. February 28 (2002)

[9] A. Schönecker.: Piezoelectric Fiber Composite Fabrication. Piezoelectric and Acoustic Materials for Transducer Applications, 1st ed., A. Safari and E. K. Akdogan, Ed. New York, NY, USA: Springer Science+Business Media (2008) 261-287

[10] R. B. Cass.: Fabrication of Continuous Ceramic Fiber by the Viscous Suspension Spinning Process. Ceram. Bulletin 3(70) (1991) 424-429

[11] D. Vorbach, T. Schulze, E. Taeger.: Verfahren zur Herstellung von Cellulose-Filamenten mit sehr hohem Anteil an Zusatzstoffen. Patent DE 4426966. July 29 (1994)

[12] K. Hohlfeld, S. Gebhardt, A. Schönecker, A. Michaelis.: PZT Components Derived from Polysulphone Spinning Process. Advances in Applied Ceramics, 4(114) (2015) 231-236

[13] A. C. Dent, L. J. Nelson, C. R. Bowen, R. Stevens, M. Cain, M. Stewart.: Characterization and Properties of Fine Scale PZT Fibers. Journ. Europ. Ceram. Soc. (25) (2005) 2387-2391

[14] J. Heiber, A. Belloli, P. Ermanni, F. Clemens.: Ferroelectric Characterization of Single PZT Fibers. Journ. Intelligent Material Systems and Structures (20) (2009) 379-385

[15] M. Zapf, K. Hohlfeld, G. Shah, S. Gebhardt, K.W.A. Van Dongen, H. Gemmeke, A. Michaelis, N. V. Ruiter.: Evaluation of Piezo Composite Based Omnidirectional Single Fibre Transducers for 3D USCT. Proc. IEEE International Ultrasonics Symposium, Taipei, Taiwan, October 21-24 (2015) doi 10.1109/ULTSYM.2015.0552

[16] S. Starke, A. Schönecker, W. Gebhardt.: Fine Scale Piezoelectric 1-3 Composites: A New Approach of Cost Effective Fabrication. Proc. 11th IEEE Intern. Symp. Appl. Ferroelectr., Montreux, Switzerland, Aug. 24-27 (1998), 393-396

[17] S. Gebhardt, P. Günther, S. Fröhlich, H. Neubert.: Towards Fabrication of High Frequency Ultrasonic Transducers Using Soft Mold Process. Proc. IEEE International Ultrasonics Symposium, Tours, France, September 18-21 (2016) doi 10.1109/ULTSYM.2016.7728555

[18] Y. Qiu, H. Wang, S. Gebhardt, A. Bolhovitins, C.E.M. Démoré, A. Schönecker, S. Cochran.: Screen-printed Ultrasonic 2-D Matrix Array Transducers for Microparticle Manipulation. Ultrasonics (2015), doi: 10.1016/j.ultras.2015.05.010

Dice-and-fill single element octagon transducers for next generation 3D USCT

Michael Zapf[1], Patrick Pfistner[1], Claudio Imbracio Liberman[1], Koen van Dongen[2], Nico de Jong[2], Benjamin Leyrer[1], Hartmut Gemmeke[1], Nicole V. Ruiter[1]

[1]*Karlsruhe Institute of Technology, Eggenstein-Leopoldshafen, Germany*
E-Mail: michael.zapf@kit.edu
[2]*Delft University of Technology, Delft, Netherlands*

Abstract

At the Karlsruhe Institue of Technology (KIT), a 3D-Ultrasound Computer Tomography (3D-USCT) medical imaging system for early breast cancer detection is currently developed. With the next generation of 3D-USCT 2.5, the current region of interest (ROI) of 10 x 10 x 10 cm³ shall be increased to 20 x 20 x 20 cm³ to allow reliable imaging results also for bigger female breasts. Therefore, the opening angle (OA) of the future transducers should be increased to approx. 60 ° at 3 dB while other characteristics such as bandwidth (BW) and resonance frequency should be preserved or even improved. Based on the current dice-and-fill approach in transducer production, optimization is performed on piezoelectric sensor geometry and size, type and structure of matching and backing layer and interconnection technology of the several parts of the transducer.

Keywords: US transducer, composite materials, SAFT imaging, dice-and-fill

1 Introduction

Breast cancer is the most common cancer in females in the world [1, 2].The spreading probability of the tumor and thus the chances of survival are correlated to its size [3]. Therefore, early detection plays a vital role in reducing the mortality of breast cancer.

KIT developed a 3D USCT imaging system for early breast cancer detection [4] [5] [6]. Imaging is achieved by Synthetic Aperture Focusing Technique (SAFT) using a multistatic setup of 2041 ultrasound transducers, grouped in 157 Transducer Array Systems (TAS) embedded in a semi-elliposoidal aperture (Figure 1). A center frequency of 2.5 MHz is applied. The bandwidth (BW) and opening angle (OA) at 3 dB amount to 1 MHz and 36 °, respectively. The fundamental connection between an ultrasound transducer's emission and reception sensitivity in the azimuth and elevation angle space is the tranducer's aperture size.

Finite element (FE) simulations have shown that a reduction in size of the current generation transducer elements by roughly a factor 2 from 900 µm to 500 µm is required to realize an OA of 60 ° at 3 dB. Wave simulations also revealed that a circular instead of the current rectangular aperture will result in additional homogeneity of the sound field.

As circular sensors are difficult to produce in the dice-and-fill approach, octagon shaped transducers are built for USCT 2.5. The octagon shape can be achieved with the established dice-and-fill technique by adding 2 sawing cuts. Furthermore, inspired by compressive sensing, an irregular distribution of the sensor elements on the TAS is applied which covers almost the full surface area of US transducer. Further improvements are introduced regarding connectivity and bandwidth.

2 Motivation

2.1 3D USCT 2.0 current status

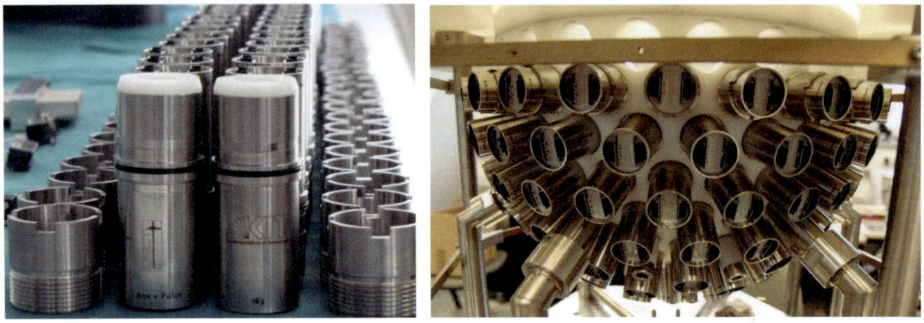

Figure 1: Left: USCT 2.0 TAS systems transducers before assembly in the final system. Right: Semi-ellipsoidal aperture of USCT 2.0

The current USCT 2.0 system covers a ROI of 10 x 10 x 10 cm^3. Results from the clinical trial with the University hospital Jena indicated that a bigger ROI is beneficial to cover a broader range of breasts and adapt also to the buoyance broadening effect of floating breasts [5]. Each of the 157 TAS consists of 13 rectangular transducer elements 0.9 x 0.9 mm in size [7]. One TAS consists of four emitters, nine receivers which are regularly distributed in a square grid, covering just the inner part of the TAS (Figure 2).

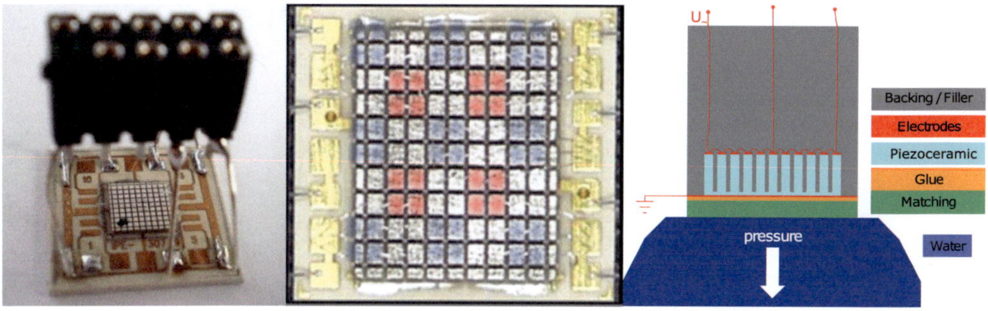

Figure 2: Left: Inner part of one TAS of USCT 2.0. Middle: Closer view on the piezoelectric elements. Four squares are connected to form one receiver (blue) or emitter (red). Right: Schematic side-view on one TAS of USCT 2.0.

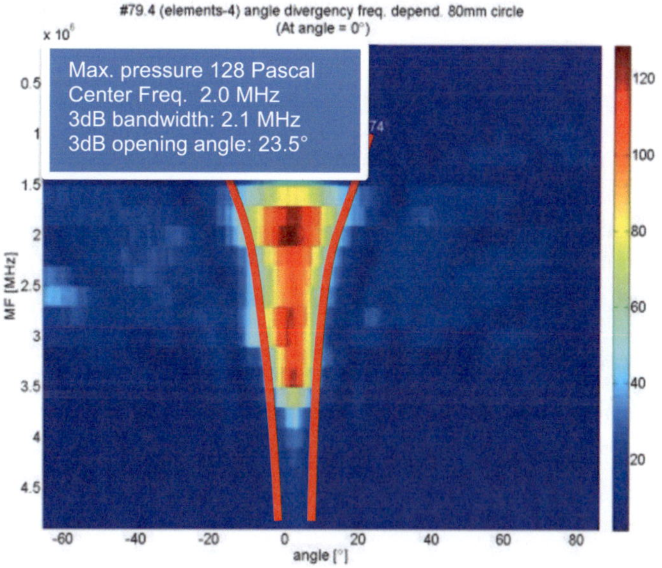

Figure 3: Frequency over angle for one element of one TAS of USCT 2.0. Given with red-lines approx. the frequency dependend 3dB opening angle.

2.2 Design considerations for next generation 3D USCT

For next generation 3D USCT (called 3D USCT 2.5) several should be improved contribute to a homogenous illumination and imaging contrast.

2.2.1 Opening angle (OA)

The benefit of an increased OA is schematically shown in Figure 4.

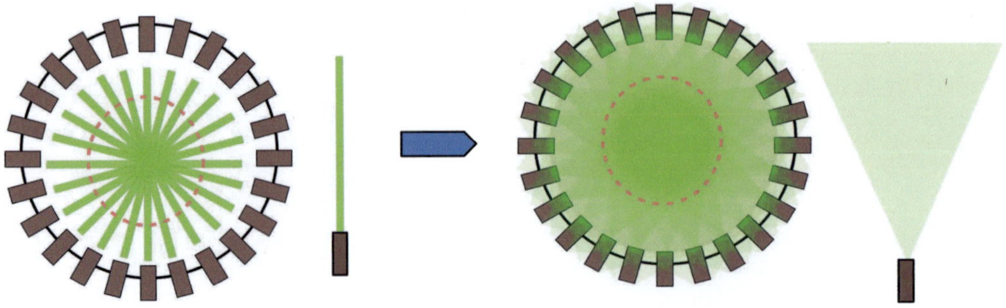

Figure 4: Illumination of an exemplary 3D-USCT system (top down view) for transducers with a small OA (left) compared to transducers with a larger OA (right).

2.2.2 Bandwidth

The BW of the transducers should be increased, as a larger BW better contrast in SAFT images, see Fig. 6. An increased coverage of the K-space, the spatial Fourier domain, can be achieved by broadening the bandwidth of the transducers. [8] Also, full wave inversion schemes and transmission tomography benefits from lower frequency components included in a broader bandwidth which covers also lower frequency down to 0.5 MHz.

2.2.3 Irregular distribution of sensor

An irregular distribution of the elements leads to greater coverage of the ROI and more homogeneous illumination. This is inspired by the "compressive sampling" concept now utilized in many apertures of various imaging systems as also ultra sound imaging systems.

2.2.4 Reduction in sparsity of sampling

An upgrade from 13 to 17 elements is performed. There are still nine receivers but the number of emitters has been doubled from four to eight emitters. Electronic constraints inhibit an upgrade to 9 emitters for symmetric emitter/receiver distribution. More emitters reduce the sparsity in imaging, leading to a more homogeneous coverage of the ROI. The final transducer distribution is shown in Figure 14.

2.3 Simulations

2.3.1 MATLAB

Ultrasound wavefield emission simulations for different surface geometries ("transducer apertures") have been performed as "piston model". As it is well known from antenna and transducer design, there is an reciprocal relationship between the element / aperture size, and the directivity / opening angle of the sound beam. A reduction in transducer sidelength /diameter from 900 µm to 550 µm should lead to an increase in OA to 50 °-60 ° at 3 dB.

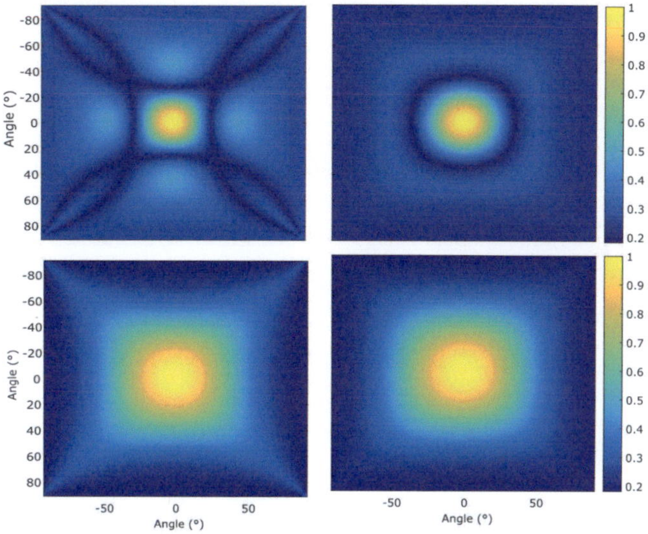

Figure 5: MATLAB aperture piston model simulations: US sound field for rectangular 0.9 mm (upper left), rectangular 0.4 mm (lower left), circular 0.94 mm (upper right) and circular 0.45 mm (lower right).

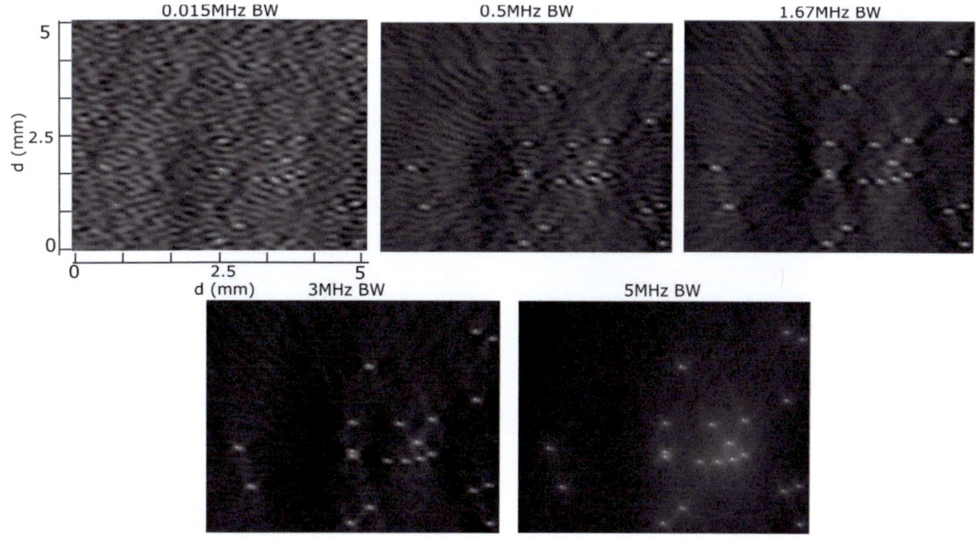

Figure 6: SAFT simulations for many point scatterers for varying BW. Contrast increases for broader bandwidth, while the resolution is more or less retained.

Circular elements express a more homogeneous sound over field compared to rectangular elements. (Figure 5).

SAFT simulations have been performed on point scatterers with varying BW (Figure 6). The results show that for SAFT image reconstruction, more BW leads to higher contrast in the images.

2.3.2 KLM

KLM simulations have been performed to find the ideal matching layer thickness for a broad BW. Simulations on TMM4 as a matching layer are shown in Figure 7. In the given configuration the resonance was the broadest for a 200 μm TMM4 layer due to two resonance peaks.

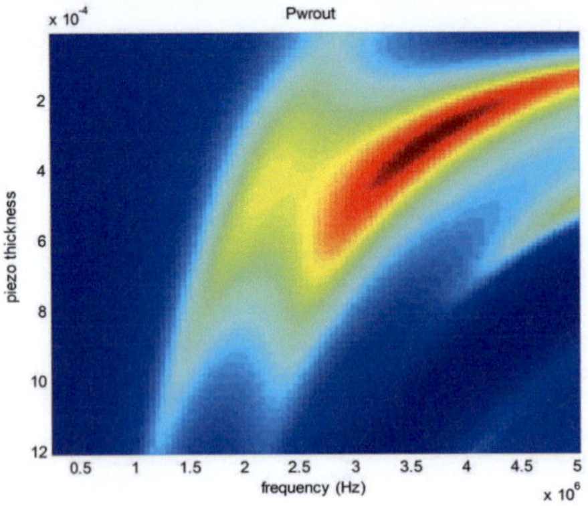

Figure 7: KLM model showing piezo thickness over frequency for a 200μm TMM4 matching layer with varying PZT thickness on the Y axis. X axis give the frequency range.

2.3.3 Finite element simulation

As 1D KLM simulations are insufficient to analyze lateral and shear wave effects of a design, a higher spatial dimensional simulation was utilized. Finite element (FE) simulations in 3D and 2D were performed. Also the impact of various materials on the Transducer performance were analyzed. PZflex was used as standard tool for piezoactive materials and non-piezoactive materials. The spatial properties of the transducer design was meshed with at least 3 times spatial sampling. Temporla sampling was derived automatically by the simulation tool, exported was the sound pressure field in each element in the water in the farfield in 2 to 6 cm distance.

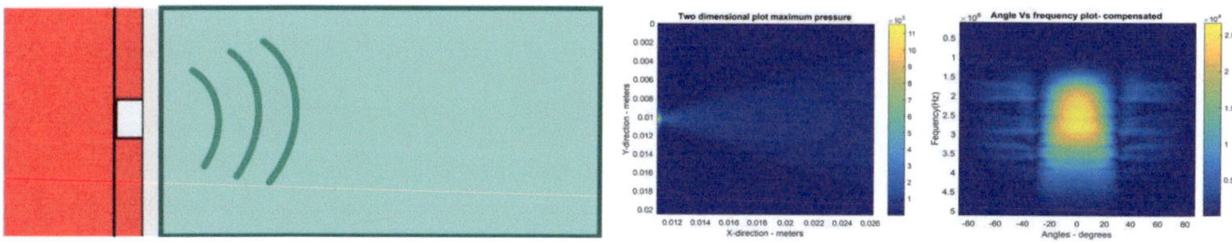

Figure 8: Left: Exemplary 2D PZFlex simulation model spanning 6cm in x and 2 cm in Y: Red: Backing + filling PU + Tungsten (12 MRayl): Red + bright blue: Piezofibrecompositedisc. (CeramTec Sonox 505 14.2 MRayl). Grey: Matching (TMM4 ca. 6.3 MRayl). Blue: Water (1.5 MRayl). Middle: Left: two-dimensional pressure plot X over Y, simulated by PZFlex for the setup described. Right: frequency over angle plot for the same setup.

3 Approach and method

First, the final transducer design approach will be presented. Afterwards, the individual process steps in the complex transducer production and their accompanying challenges and ideas are explained in more detail.

3.1 Transducer design and built up process

The Transducer Array System is built up starting from the backing where a 5 mm thick PVC substrate (Figure 13) with 2mm conical holes at the locations of the sensor elements acts as a base substrate on which top-side a flex-print is glued (Figure 10 right), providing the connectivity for the individual transducer elements. Pin holes guarantee alignment of the flex print and backing PVC.

A PU-tungsten composite material is molded into the holes (Figure 21 left), degassed and cured at room temperature over night.

Small PZT slabs of 700µm x 700µm are glued on copper pads of the flexprint with low temperature curing silver glue. Next, the square elements are shaped into octagons with a width of 550µm with a wafer dicing saw (Figure 16).

On the waterside, a matching layer is glued onto the piezoelectric sensor also with conductive silver-glue providing the common ground connection. Defined distance and parallelism is provided by a precise laser-cut spacer ring (Figure 18).

Two pins fix the rear part of the flex-print. A multi-channel plug ensures easy electrical connection to the back-end electronics (Figure 21 middle). The complete structure is waterproofed and mechanically stabilized with a hard-rubber like PU (Figure 19 left). A schematic side-view of the whole setup is shown in figure 9.

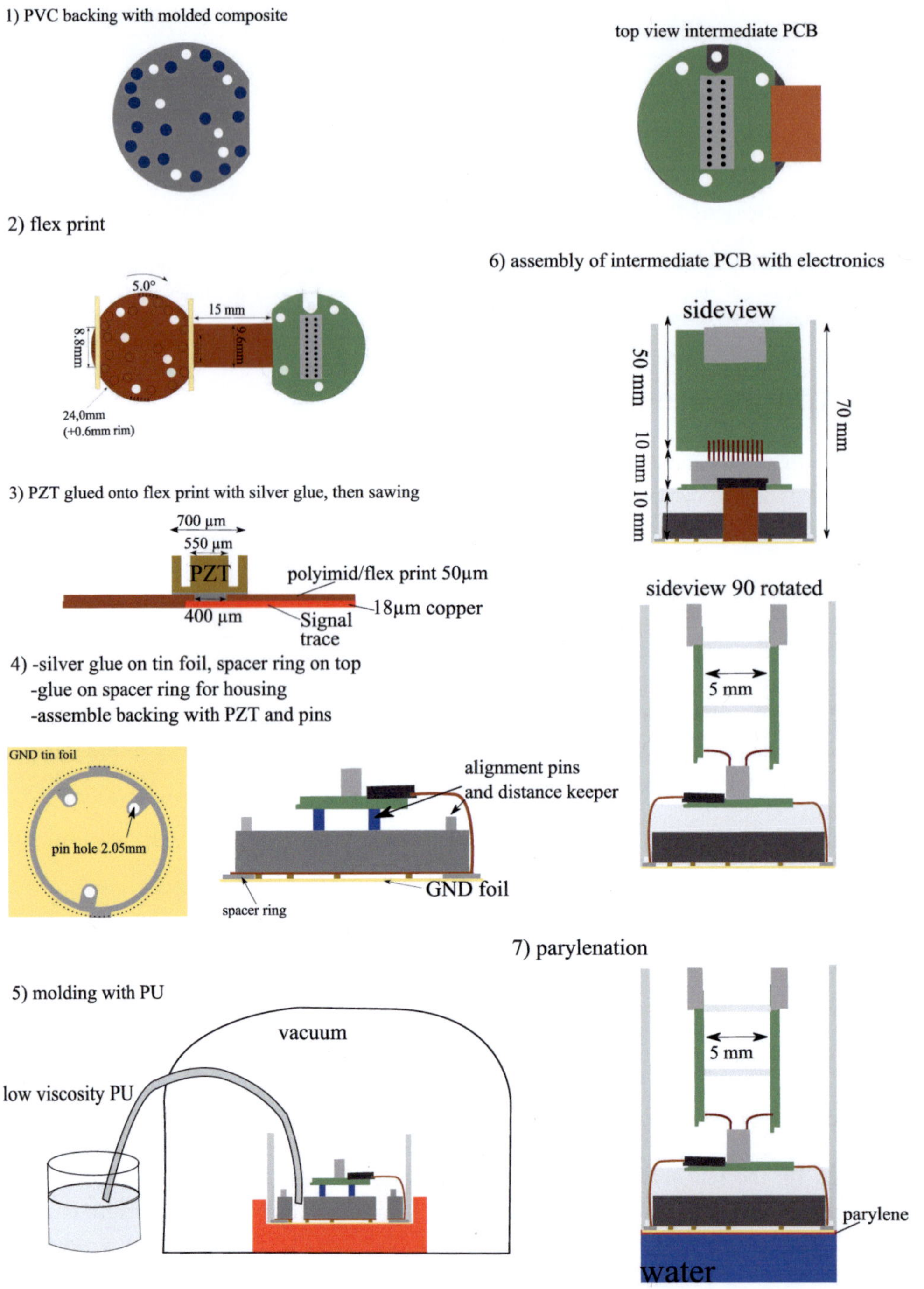

Figure 9: schematic of the whole build-up process for one TAS of next generation.

Electrical characterization was performed with a phase-impedance analyzer for all piezoelectric elements. Ultrasound characteristics were evaluated quantitatively with a hydrophone in a 3-axis water tank for selected sample transducers [8, 9].

3.2 PCB design

A Flexprint design was choosen as PCB base for electrical connectivity for the transducers.

Molding tests with the backing composite material led to bulging of the flex print. In response, four pin holes to span the foil have been added to facilitate molding. The layout and final product are shown in Figure 10.

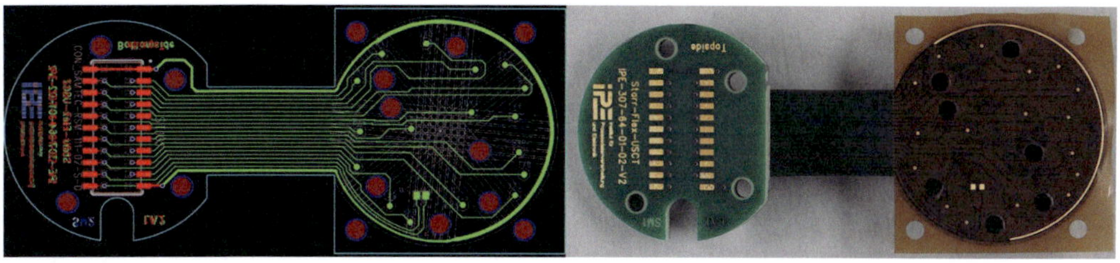

Figure 10: Flexprint PCB layout (left) and flex-print prototype v2 glued on a PVC substrate (right).

3.3 Composite materials

Research was conducted in the field of composite material to find possible matching and backing layers. The focus has been set on backing materials. A strongly attenuating composite of PU and tungsten powder was developed [10]. Acoustic impedance values of up to 11 MRayl are realizable. The improved acoustic matching to the rear improves the BW of the transducer by coupling US energy into the backing and attenuating the sound wave before reentering the piezo element. Degassing of the compound is difficult but possible with addition of a defoamer. Figure 11: 10 cm long rod of developed PU-tungsten composite material (left) and its lower part under the microscope (right). Degassing is possible, no major air inclusions are visible.

3.4 Backing

3.4.1 V1: Completely molded backing

First, tests were performed to investigate the molding ability of the backing composite with integrated pins of 2 mm in diameter. Tests have been successful (Figure 12). Next, a metal form with the actual TAS dimension has been built with alignment pin holes. The molded backing turned out to be not planar enough for the requirement of 20µm tolerancy.

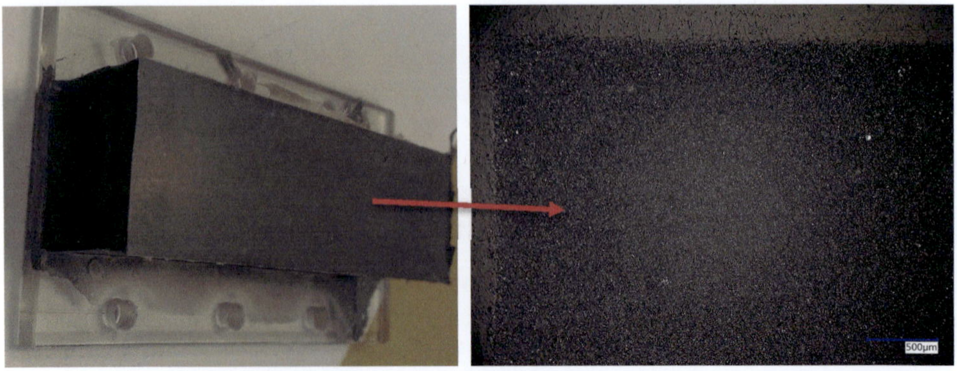

Figure 11: 10 cm long rod of developed PU-tungsten composite material (left) and its lower part under the microscope (right). Degassing is effective; no major air inclusions are visible.

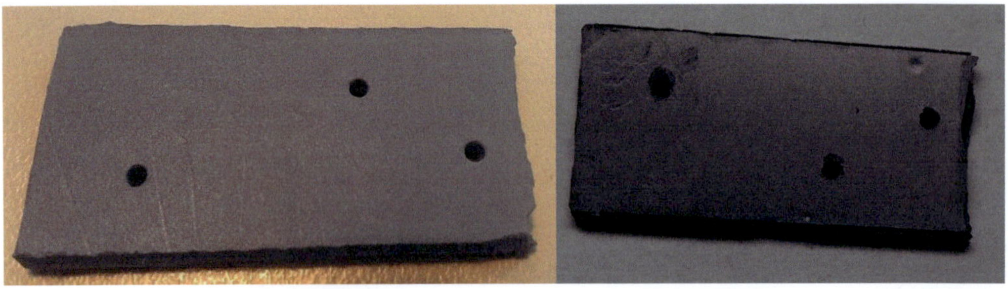

Figure 12: PU-tungsten composite integration test. The material shows surface roughness of the Teflon mold.

3.4.2 PVC substrate with molding of holes

As a completely molded backing proved to be difficult to realize, a combination of a planar backing substrate and molding was proposed. A PVC substrate with 2 mm holes behind the piezo locations was manufactured. The inner walls of the bore holes were parallel. Degassing of the backing composite through the holes was not possible properly.

An improved version with conical holes to the rear side to facilitate degassing (Figure 13) was later done. The end of the bore hole are rounded on the flex print side to facilitate plan parallel gluing of the flex print onto the PVC substrate.

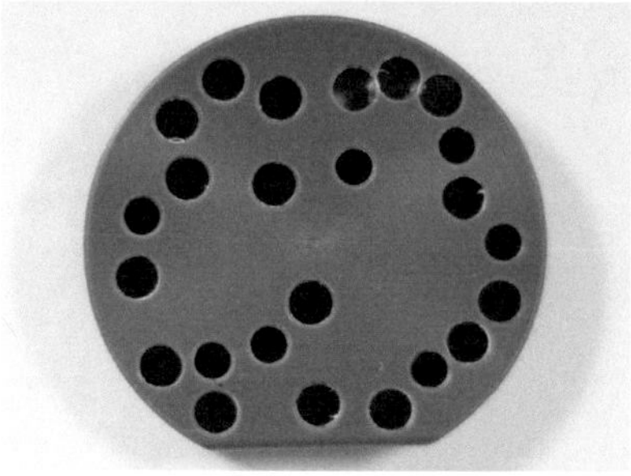

Figure 13: PVC substrate for the rear side for TAS 2.5 with high planarity and conical bore holes.

3.5 Positioning of piezos

3.5.1 V1

To increase the accuracy tolerance in x and y, larger PZT slabs of 1.5 mm side length are positioned onto the target locations with the pick and placer machine. Hereby, the x,y alignment accuracy is increased to ± 500 µm. In this configuration, the piezo has to be cut through completely. As the flex foil is 50 µm in thickness, the tolerance in z is reduced to ± 10 µm to not cut the leads.

3.5.2 V2

In order to increase the z tolerance at the expense of x, y tolerance, the piezos are decreased in side length to 700 µm. This reduces the x, y tolerance to ± 100 µm. Now, the residual piezo parts after sawing are so small that they mostly break during sawing.

In case the residual parts don't break, they are small enough that no complete cut-through is needed. Simulations have shown that sub-structuring to half or three quarter depth does not have a significant influence on acoustic performance of the transducer [11].

3.6 Sawing

The wafer dicing saw needs fiducial marks on opposite sides of the flex print every 45 ° for correct alignment of the sample. They are achieved by generating a regular octagon grid over the whole size of the TAS (Figure 14) and deleting the lines, but leaving the last few millimeters on the edge of the circular aperture. First tests with a fully automatized sawing procedure led to significant deviations from the desired octagon grid.

Therefore, the program has been split into two subprograms for 0 °/90 ° and 45 °/135 °. Before running each of these programs, a manual optical alignment on the fiducial marks or on the sawing traces is performed. These steps comprise possible errors.

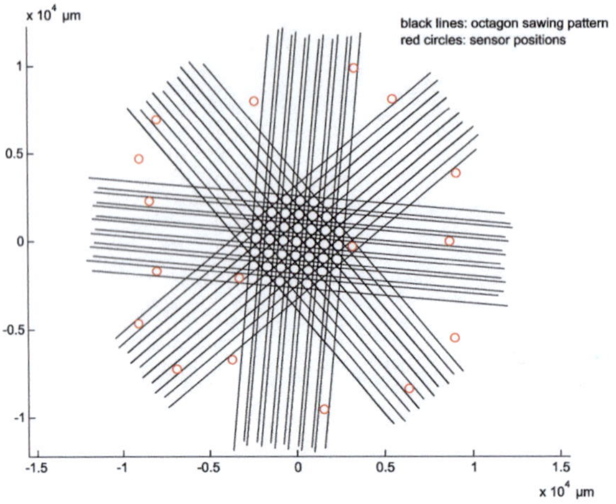

Figure 14: Transducer distribution for USCT TAS 2.5 (red circles). Black lines show the octagon sawing pattern that constrains the available sensor positions to its regular grid.

For a series production of the transducers, a fully automatized sawing process without manual interruption is aimed for. First measurements on the octagon shaped transducers expressed a significantly smaller opening angle than expected by the PZFlex simulations. Lateral waves are suggested to virtually increase the aperture, thereby decreasing the OA.

To reduce the influence of lateral waves, sub-structuring of the octagons into four parts (see Figure 16: Left: Test of additionally sub-structuring octagon. Right: TAS 2.5 prototype assembled with single element octagon dice-and-fill transducers.) is a possible solution. The decreased lateral dimensions of the sensor shift lateral modes to higher frequencies where they do not interfere with the USCT center frequency.

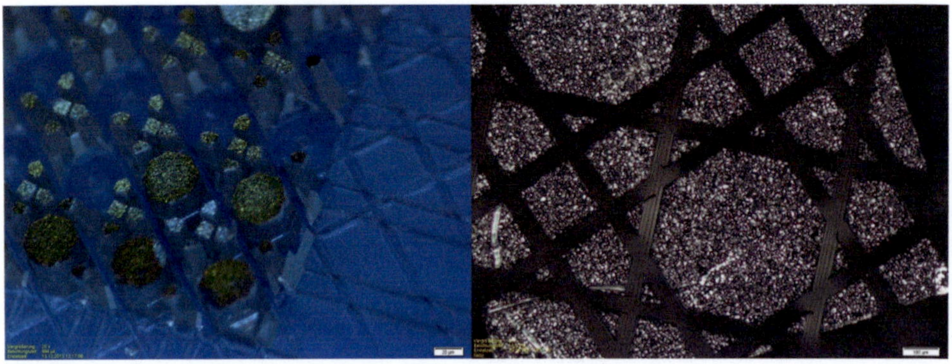

Figure 15: Octagon-shaped sensors after sawing, photos from a microscope.

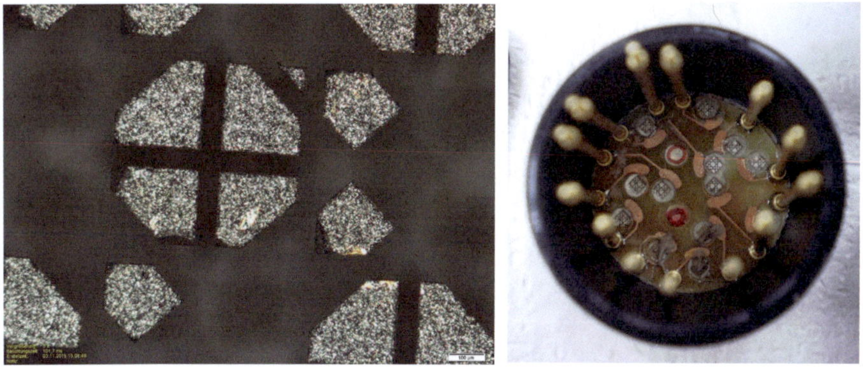

Figure 16: Left: Test of additionally sub-structuring octagon. Right: TAS 2.5 prototype assembled with single element octagon dice-and-fill transducers.

3.7 Gluing

In the first build ups a significant portio, 20-30 % of the sensors fell of during the sawing process. Further tests indicated improper heat curing of the silver glue. An optimized hardware setup improved the temperature profile while curing for one hour. Another improvement of the conductive silver glue utilization was an automated centrifugal mixer which ensured better homogeneity and viscosity. Additionally, quantitative analysis of the mechanical strength of the piezo/flex-print connection is needed to understand the reason for the failures of the piezo elements, to optimize the amount of glue printed, the curing profile and possibly also the type of glue.

In a first test series, PC3000 silver glue was stencil-printed on Cu foil on a 4 mm PVC substrate. Stencil openings varied between 400 µm, 500 µm and 600 µm. The highest shear values have been collected for the 600µm opening. Bigger openings are not used to avoid excessive squeeze-out of the glue while placing the sensors.

To evaluate the mechanical strength of the glued connection between the sensors and the Cu/Polyimide substrate, systematic quantitative analysis has been conducted with an in-house shear tester. A double-sided sheet with copper on one side and PI on the other side was glued onto 4 mm thick PVC substrates. Three samples were prepared for each side facing upwards, combining to six total samples.

A stencil was prepared to print a defined amount of silver glue on the specified piezo positions. Next, square piezoelectric elements (700 x 700 µm, height: 550 µm) were placed into the wet glue with a pick and placer machine. After curing at 120 °C for 20 min in the oven and cool down, the shear tests were conducted. Figure 20 shows images of the several process steps. Curing could to a bulging of the PVC substrate.

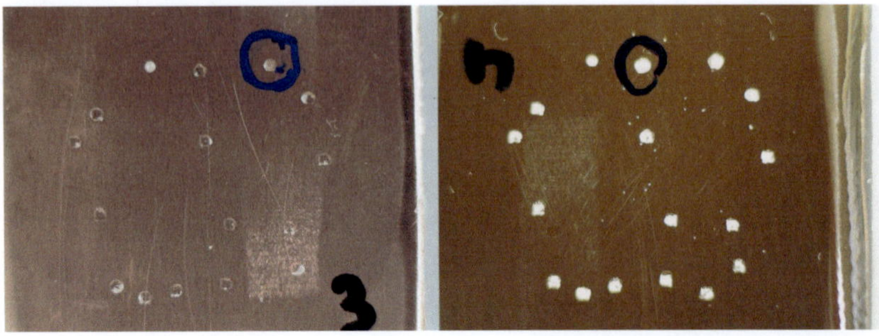

Figure 17: After shearing the piezos on Cu foil (lower left), shearing on the PI side (lower right), more glue is left on the PI surface.

Table 1 shows the mean shear force and the standard deviation for the Cu and the PI substrate. Out of 96 placed elements, four showed significantly lower shear values (<300 g) than the rest. Local impurities of the substrates are assumed to be the reason for this. They are excluded from the mean and standard deviation calculation. The measured shear values have to be scaled down to the final sensor surface area.

The values should guarantee firm mechanical connection that also withstands the forces exerted by the sawing blade.

Sample	Mean (g)	Std (g)	Mean (g)	Std (g)
1 – Cu	1288.6	388.9		
2 – Cu	1261.9	393.9	1330.2	365.5
3 – Cu	1442.7	271.9		
4 – PI	1482.2	213.0		
5 – PI	1933.4	446.5	1743.4	400.6
6 – PI	1802.0	351.9		

Table 1: Mean shear force and corresponding standard deviation of the shear tests performed on PC 3000 silver glue.

3.8 Matching options

3.8.1 TMM4

The acoustic impedance of Rogers TMM4 an aluminum oxide composite with of 6.4 MRayl acoustic impedance is near optimal for a single-layer matching between PZT and water. TMM4 is a very stiff, mechanical mil-and drillable material and exhibits low water absorption. Besides being a strong electrical insulator, thermal conductivity of TMM4 is quite high.

This is helpful for correct water temperature measurements, as the USCT temperature sensors are situated behind the TMM4 plate.

3.8.2 Silver glue and foil as matching

In collaboration with the TU Delft, an alternative design approach was followed with the idea to suppress lateral waves by replacing the stiff matching layer by a composite material of conductive silver glue with a thin sheet of metallic foil as common ground connection and matching layer.

Conductive silver glue, for instance Heraeus PC3000, is available with acoustic impedances suitable as a matching layer for PZT and water.

One approach is the application on the PZT base material, forming here the composite, which can be afterwards structured by sawing. Another approach is to glue a whole disc of the matching layer/PZT composite material onto the flex print. Alternatively, LASER cutting can structure transducers at arbitrary positions and in arbitrary shape. The constraint of the sensor positions to the octagon grid is obsolete. Additionally, LASER cutting results in conical cuts which should lead to varying aspect ratio which should lead to a frequency spreading and damping of unwanted spurious lateral oscillation modes.

Finally, a thin layer of foil is required for common ground connection. Usually, aluminum foil is used while tin was considered as potential option too having a fitting acoustic impedance and a lower better fitting sound speed.

Difficulties in this approach are a planar application of silver glue and a planar application of the ground foil (Figure 18). To provide additional support for the foil, an aluminum spacer ring (Figure 18) with the same thickness as the sensors was designed to be placed on the outside edge of the TAS. Waterproofing is achieved with a thin layer of parylene.

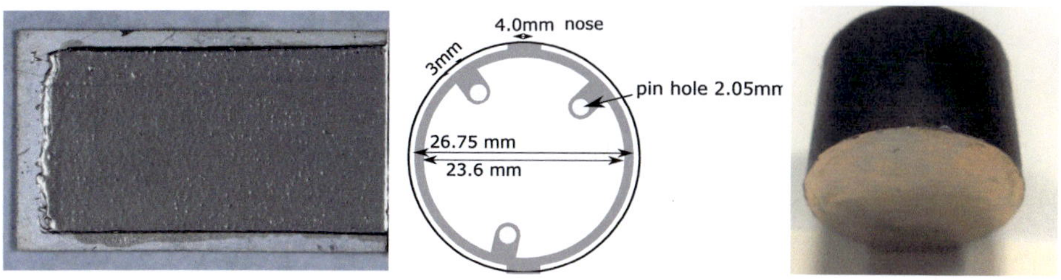

Figure 18: Left: Aluminium foil + PC 3000 silver conductive, middle: stainless steel spacer, right: transducer prototype with aluminum foil as common ground on the front side.

4 Evaluations and results

4.1 TMM4 matching layer

Figure 19 shows the assembled prototype with a TMM4 matching layer from front and rear. Due to process difficulties, 7 out of 17 sensors were working after final assembly. Figure 20 shows a frequency over angle plot from one of the elements and the corresponding pressure over frequency for the main direction perpendicular to the sensor surface. The electrical characterization of the same element can be observed in Figure 20 right.

Mean and standard deviation of important acoustic parameters are given in Table 2.

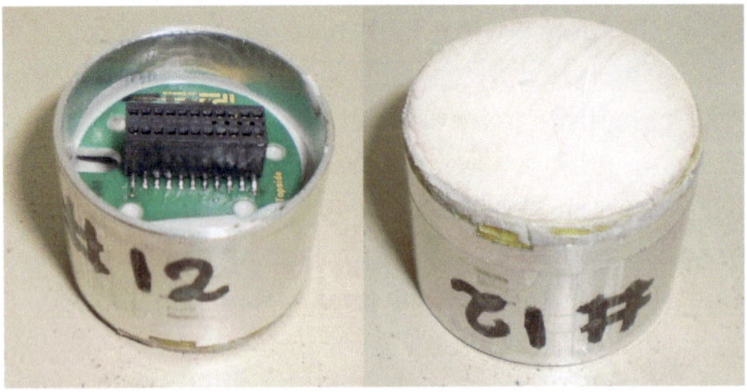

Figure 19: Assembled TAS 2.5 prototype. The rear side is filled with PU for mechanical stabilization (left). A TMM4 plate acts as a matching layer to water (right).

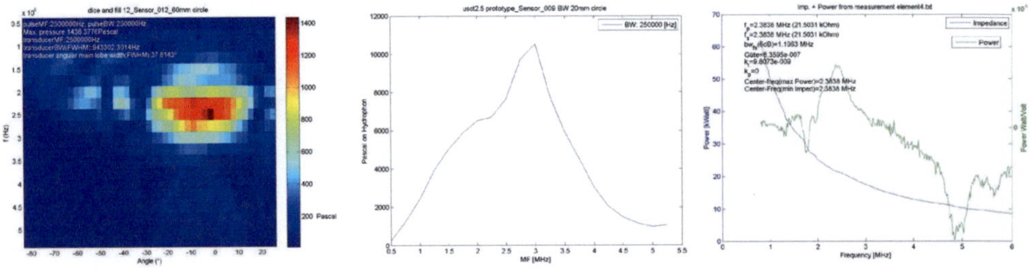

Figure 20: Frequency over angle for one element of transducer 1 (left). Pressure over frequency for main direction (middle). Corresponding electrical characterization from a –Impedance-Phase-analysator with only weakly pronounced serial and parallel resonances from the piezoelectrical material (right).

	BW (MHz)	Opening angle (°)	Pressure (Pa)
Mean	0.82	28.52	532.39
Std Dev	0.18	10.46	617.77

Table 2: Acoustic properties of prototype with TMM4 matching.

4.2 Tin foil matching layer

Figure 21 shows the final assembly steps for the prototype with a tin foil matching layer. Acoustic measurements are performed in the near future. The manufacturing process seems more challenging compared to a stiff matching layer and has to be optimized.

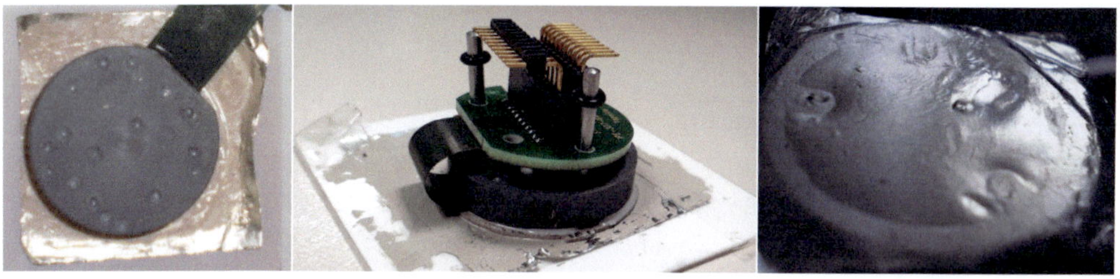

Figure 21: Left: Holes of the PVC substrate filled with PU-tungsten composite backing material. The backing is only applied behind the sensor elements. The backing and flex print are glued onto the tin foil matching. Middle: Pins align the back end of the PCB to fit in the casing later. Right: Tin foil matching layer after application.

4.3 Aluminium + PU matching layer

Figure 22 shows a frequency over angle plot from one of the elements expressing high BW and the corresponding pressure over frequency for the main direction perpendicular to the sensor surface. Figure 23 shows a frequency over angle plot from one of the elements expressing high OA and the corresponding pressure over angle at 2.4 MHz. Mean and standard deviation of important acoustic parameters are given in Table 3.

	BW (MHz)	Opening angle (°)	Pressure (Pa)
Mean	1.55	40.25	2969.86
Std Dev	0.57	21.78	3317.26

Table 3: Acoustic properties of prototype with PU + aluminum matching.

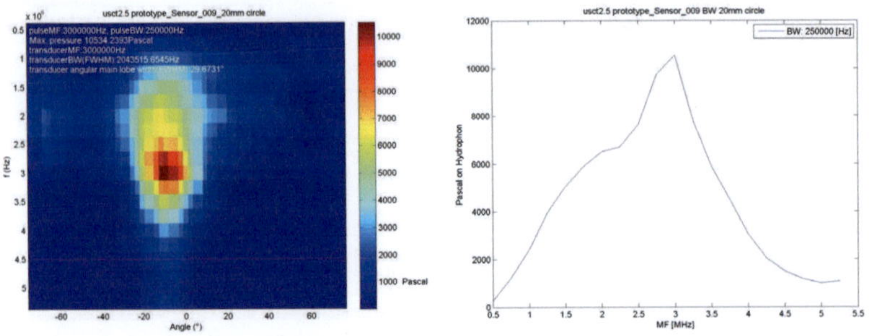

Figure 22: Frequency over angle shown for an element expressing high BW (left). pressure over frequency for emission in normal direction (right).

5 Discussion and conclusion

First prototypes were assembled with a flex print PCB in the described process and first results ares encouraging. The developed PU-tungsten composite backing material led to a significant increase in BW through improved acoustic matching to the rear of the transducer. While a in principle sufficient performance in soundpressure, bandwidth and open angle for the TMM4 + PZT piezo prototyped could be shown, the proution process is currently not finalized and as reliable a aimed for. The curently only semi-automatized process leads still to variations and in result to the failure of a signifcant portion of the transducer elements; especially in the glueing and filling step. This is currently under intensive investigation with further test prototypes. Further shear tests on the piezo have to be conducted to ensure all piezo elements reliable connected to the flex substrate to gain yield >95 % even after the sawing step. To prove the applicability and also potential mass producibility of the new design approach, complete TAS have to be built.

References

[1] [Online]. Available: http : / / www . wcrf . org / int / cancer - facts - figures / data - specific -cancers/breast-cancer-statistics..

[2] [Online]. Available: http://www.who.int/cancer/detection/breastcancer/en/index1.html..

[3] James S Michaelson et al., „"Predicting the survival of patients with breast carcinoma causing tumor size," Cancer, 2002.

[4] Ruiter et al., „Realization of an optimized 3D USCT," SPIE 7968, Medical Imaging 2011: Ultrasonic Imaging, Tomography, and Therapy„ 2011.

[5] T. H. M. Z. C. K. N. R. H. Gemmeke, „3D ultrasound computer tomography. hardware setup, reconstruction methods and first clinical results.".Nuclear Instruments and Methods in Physics Research Section A: Accelerators, Spectrometers, Detectors and Associated Equipment.

[6] Gemmeke et al., „An improved 3D Ultrasound Computer Tomography system". IEEE International Ultrasonics Symposium., 2014.

[7] G. Göbel, „Entwicklung von Ultraschallsensorarrays mit miniaturisierten Komponenten," Diploma, KIT, 2002.

[8] M. Zapf, „Simulation eines Ultraschalltomographen im k-space," in Master thesis for Hochschule Karlsruhe (University of Applied Science), Karlsruhe, 2010.

[9] L. Petzold, „Aufbau eines Messplatzes zur Ermittlung der Schallfeldcharakteristik," Master thesis, KIT, 2006.

[10] G. Shah, „Auto-Calibration of Ultrasound Transducer Characterization Setup," Master thesis, KIT, 2015.

[11] P. Pfistner, „Composite-based ultrasound transducers for a 3D-Ultrasound computer tomograph," Master thesis, KIT, 2017.

[12] B. Kohout, „ Finite Elemente Simulation von Ultraschallwandlersystemen für die Ultraschall Computertomographie," KIT, Diploma , 2010.

[13] G. S. M.Zapf, „Aperture optimization for 3D ultrasound computer," IEEE UFFC Symp., 2007.

[14] N. R. H. Gemmeke, „3D ultrasound computer tomography for medical," Nuclear Instruments and Methods in Physics Research Section A: Accelerators, Spectrometers, Detectors and Associated Equipment, 2007.

Challenges in Breast Ultrasound

H. Madjar

DKD Helios Klinik, Department of Gynecology and Breast Center, Wiesbaden, Germany
E-mail: helmut.madjar@web.de

Abstract

Early detection and curative diagnosis has highly improved with the introduction of ultrasound. Curation concerns symptomatic patients, differentiation of lesions, guided interventions, preoperative staging and follow up after breast cancer treatment. Early detection means population wide screening, but also individualized screening and risk adapted diagnosis. Many screening programmes include only regular mammographic examinations for women above the age of 50 years, where efficacy is proven. However 25-30% of breast cancer occurs in premenopausal woman and 30% of menopausal women have dense breasts where mammography fails in up to 50%. Furthermore, women with dense breasts have higher risk to develop breast cancer. Diagnostic studies using high quality ultrasound technology have proven a 30-40% increased detection rate of small cancers in young women and women with dense breasts. The problem is that ultrasound is operator dependent and requires a systematic examination to cover the whole breast. Reproducibility is problematic with hand-held systems. ABUS technology (Automated Breast Ultrasound Systems) was developed to overcome these problems but requires a number of scan procedures to cover the entire breast, it depends also on operator skills and the static scans do not allow to measure vascularity or elasticity or to perform guided interventions.

Keywords: Breast cancer, Breast ultrasound, Screening, Early detection, Differential diagnosis

1 Introduction

First applications of ultrasound for the examination of the female breast began more than 60 years ago and it took almost 30 years until technical development allowed sufficient use in clinical routine. Although technology is continuously advancing, the indications to use ultrasound for breast cancer diagnosis are under controversial discussion since many years. Its role depends on equipment quality, clinical objectives and skills of medical professionals with different specialisations.

In the early studies, ultrasound was mainly used for circumscribed lumps or mammographic densities to differentiate simple cysts from solid lesions [1]. The development of modern equipment in the past twenty years allowed for accurate detection and differential diagnosis of small lesions [2, 3]. Guidelines for technical standards and quality control in breast Ultrasound were published by the International Breast Ultrasound School [4]. In the USA the critical discussions about breast ultrasound lead to increased acceptance when Stavros, Kolb and other authors published their study results which proved the high accuracy in lesion differentiation and detection [5, 6]. As a result of the newly enhanced attention the American College of Radiology published the first Ultrasound BI-RADS edition [7]. During the following years the attention of clinicians for the extended use of ultrasound to solve breast problems increased all over the world.

2 Breast cancer detection

Mortality reduction by mammographic screening of menopausal women was demonstrated by a number of randomised screening studies in many countries. However, screening was always criticised due to the problems of over diagnosis and a lack of sensitivity in young women and women with dense breasts. During the past 10 to 15 years, ultrasound has been employed as an adjunct to mammography whenever suspicious lesions were detected in order to better characterise lesions and if indicated, to perform an ultrasound-guided interventional procedure to confirm the diagnosis [8].

Ultrasound is widely used in routine diagnostics in order to improve lesion detection and characterization [5, 6, 9, 10, 11, 12]. Several studies have shown that diagnosis of breast lesions with mammography alone is limited in young women and in menopausal women with dense breast tissue [11, 12]. Furthermore, risk of breast cancer development is highly increased in women with dense breasts [13, 14]. A study of more than 200,000 women, showed that breast cancer risk is five times increased in dense breasts compared to women with involutional changes [13]. Our own observations show that dense breast tissue (ACR 3-4) is found in about 30% of menopausal patients. In a clinical setting with curative diagnosis, these patients would routinely receive an additional ultrasound examination. However, in most screening programmes breast density is not even recognized as a predictor for poor mammographic detection and high breast cancer risk. However, the second edition of the German S3 guidelines for early detection of breast cancer strictly recommends the addition of ultrasound in these patients [15].

2.1 Curative diagnosis

Curative diagnosis in non- screening patients refers to individuals with various clinical problems, such as:

- symptomatic patients with palpable lumps, skin changes or pain.
- tumour differentiation if lesions are detected either by palpation or mammography.
- guided intervention by fine needle aspiration, cyst aspiration or core biopsy and preoperative tumour localization to guide surgery in non- palpable lesions.
- preoperative staging, lymph node diagnosis and planning for surgery.
- follow up after breast cancer treatment

2.1.1 Tumor differentiation

The role of breast ultrasound for improved differential diagnosis was investigated over a period of more than twenty years. Equipment quality was variable and the diagnostic criteria for lesion description were not well standardized. Stavros analysed standardized diagnostic criteria in 750 patients using high resolution ultrasound equipment in 625 benign and 125 malignant lesions [17]. Ultrasound differentiated malignant from benign lesions with a sensitivity of 98.4% and a negative predictive value of 99.5%. These results were verified by several other authors [11, 12, 18, 19, 20, 21]. As a result of these results, the American College of Radiology formed an international expert working group in order to evaluate the role of breast ultrasound and to develop standardised diagnostic criteria. In 2003, the first ultrasound BI-RADS catalogue was published [7]. A modification has been published in 2006 by a DEGUM working group together with the German speaking ultrasound societies ÖGUM and SGUMB [21].

The published data show improved differential diagnosis of breast lesions by ultrasound in addition to mammography (Table 1). The sensitivity for cancer diagnosis increases by 10-20% with ultrasound in comparison to mammography alone. Due to the physics of sound propagation ultrasound is superior in dense breasts where mammography shows a lack of contrast between fibroglandular tissue and lesions. Ultrasound shows even small lesions with low echogenicity in highly echogenic dense breast tissue. However, quality assurance, standardization of examination technique and interpretation is essential [4, 22].

			Breast Ultrasound		Mammography	
	N=	Ca's	Sensitivity	Specificity	Sensitivity	Specificity
Stavros 1995	747	125	98.4%	67.8%	76.8%	-
Moss 1999	559	256	88.9%	77.9%	78.9%	82.7%
Rahbar 1999	161	38	95.0%	42.0%	89.0%	42.0%
Zonderland 1999	4728	338	91.0%	98.0%	83.0%	97.0%
Berg 2004	258	177	83.0%	34.0%	67.8%	75.0%

Table 1: Comparison of ultrasound and mammography for breast lesion characterization

2.1.2 Preoperative diagnosis, local staging

If malignant lesions are detected and characterized, preoperative planning is essential. Measurements of tumour size, localization within the breast and skin and nipple distance are relevant information for the surgeon. Also discrimination between unifocal, multifocal and multicentric lesions is important to plan for tumour adapted breast conserving or more radical surgery or neoadjuvant chemotherapy.

Fornage showed that ultrasound provides an accurate measurement of breast cancer size with a correlation coefficient between histopathology and ultrasound of 0.84 and 0.72 for mammography respectively [23].

In order to define the value of ultrasound for local staging we performed a prospective blind study in 100 patients with breast cancer [24]. Breast cancer was palpable in 83%, mammography visualized 96% and ultrasound 98% respectively. Measurement of tumour size showed the highest correlation between histopathology and ultrasound (0.91), for mammography 0.79 and for palpation 0.77. Multifocal and multicentric lesions were found in 39 of the cancer patients where ultrasound detected 34 compared with 13 by mammography.

Similar results were obtained by other studies using ultrasound alone or in combination with MRI with a detection of additional malignant foci in 27%-34% not seen by mammography [19, 24, 25, 26, 27, 28]. The role of second look ultrasound after positive MRI and negative mammography requires further considerations.

The accurate measurement of tumour extension allows also the use of ultrasound for accurate follow up measurements in patients receiving neoadjuvant chemotherapy [29]. Ultrasound is also recognized for its ability to provide accurate guidance for interventional procedures [15].

2.2 Screening

Literature data show that ultrasound is superior compared with mammography in the detection of small lesions in women with dense breasts (ACR 2-4). Therefore, according to the S3 guidelines for early detection ultrasound is recommended in BI-RADS 0 and 3 cases as well as BI-RADS 4-5 and in dense breasts (ACR 3-4) to improve cancer detection and differentiation [15]. The rationale for using ultrasound as an adjunct to mammographic screening to compensate for the reduced sensitivity in dense breasts was described by Berg et al. [30].

Gordon examined a large population of 12,706 women with normal mammograms and normal clinical findings [31]. She detected 1,575 solid tumours which were not palpable or visible by mammography. In 279 patients, (2.2%) an interventional diagnosis was performed and 44 cancers were confirmed.

In a similar population of 11,220 women, Kolb found three occult cancers per 1000 breast ultrasound examinations [6]. He selected only women with ACR breast density 2-4 (n = 3,626) in order to reduce the number of ultrasound examinations. Comparison of tumour size with mammographically detected carcinomas showed a similar distribution of early tumour stages. In a following study with a similar protocol including 13,547 patients he confirmed these results (9). Dividing the patients in groups with breast density 2, 3 and 4, he found a higher sensitivity for ultrasound and a lower sensitivity of mammography in dense breasts. Besides cancers, Kolb detected other lesions in 6% and an interventional diagnosis was required in 2.6%.

Buchberger found additional cancers in 4.1 per 1000 ultrasound examinations among 8,103 patients which were not detected clinically or by mammography [32]. Additional lesions were found in 5% of all examinations and in 3.3% an interventional diagnosis was required.

A multicentric screening study (American College of Radiology Imaging Network - ACRIN) published by Berg compared ultrasound and mammography in 2,637 high risk patients [33]. Forty participants were diagnosed with cancer. Twelve were suspicious on mammography, 8 suspicious on both mammography and ultrasound and 12 on ultrasound alone. In 8.8% of the 2,637 women additional lesions were detected by ultrasound and interventional diagnosis was performed in 5.7%. The rate of additional cancers detected with ultrasound was 4.2/1000.

All these studies prove that a significant number of cancers is detected if whole breast ultrasound is used in addition to mammography in the order of 3-4/1000 women. However, this increases the number of false positives between 0.3% in a single investigator study up to 5.7% in a multicenter study. But compared with a recall rate of 5-6% or higher in mammographic screening this increase is relatively low and may even be lower in follow up examinations.

It may be problematic under the current conditions to implement ultrasound into a nation-wide screening programme due to a wide variation in investigator skills and technical standards. The minimum requirements of official authorities to perform breast ultrasound are far below standards recommended from scientific societies.

3 Discussion

Compared with mammography, ultrasound has advantages in differentiating breast cancer from benign lesions, in preoperative assessment and even in the detection of early cancers which are mammographically and clinically occult. The advantage of breast ultrasound compared to mammography increases with higher breast density and in young women where sensitivity of mammography is low. This is an important issue, as dense breast tissue is very common. More than half of the women younger than 50 years have heterogeneously dense (50-75%) or very dense (¿ 75%) glandular breast tissue [34]. One third of women older than 50 years have also dense breasts [33] and sensitivity of mammography in women with dense breasts is below 50%

[9, 35]. Interval cancer rate is highly increased in this group [13, 35] and furthermore, dense breast tissue is a marker of highly increased risk for breast cancer development [13, 36, 37].

Ultrasound has not yet been proven in randomized screening but the study results are comparable to mammographic screening-detected invasive cancers [14]. In two counties of Austria, Salzburg and Tirol, mammographic pilot screening studies have demonstrated improved tumour detection with the addition of ultrasound in dense breasts and therefor this combination of both modalities was implemented into the nation- wide screening programme.

It is also remarkable that reporting breast density is a legal issue in the USA, which requires that patients are informed about their breast density after mammography. Additional ultrasound or MRI must be offered to avoid delay in breast cancer diagnosis.

The problem of ultrasound is the dependence of different variables [4, 22]. Some operators use ultrasound only in circumscribed areas of mammographic densities or palpable abnormalities, instead of screening the whole breast. Others are willing to perform survey scanning, but due to lack of experience, they overlook small lesions or have a high rate of false positive findings when they cannot distinguish artefacts with sound attenuation from real lesions. Scientific bodies such as the International Breast Ultrasound School (www.ibus.org), the American College of Radiology (www.acr.org) and the German Ultrasound Society (www.degum.de) have published recommendations to improve breast diagnosis, qualification and equipment standards which could provide qualified health service for breast problems in the near future [40].

Indications for breast ultrasound (if quality requirements are met)

- Differentiation of mammographic lesions BI-RADS 0, 3-5
- Palpable lesions: Differentiation between cystic/solid and benign/malignant
- Preoperative planning for breast conservation or mastectomy: tumour size, localization, multifocality and multicentricity
- Follow up measurements of tumour response under neoadjuvant chemotherapy
- Guidance for interventional diagnosis
- Additional breast survey scanning in mammographic dense breasts (ACR 3-4)
- Young women ¡ 40 years and in pregnancy and during lactation
- Additional screening in high risk patients

4 Future aspects

The small field of view with hand- held ultrasound makes whole breast screening difficult, both with 2D and 3D systems. Automated Breast Ultrasound Systems (ABUS) are currently tested in several clinical trials, but this technology does not overcome the problems of investigator dependence. They require several scan procedures for at least the upper and lower outer and inner quadrants which is operator dependent and time consuming. The different volumes cannot be merged together to display the whole breast like on mammograms or MRI images. If suspicious areas are found, Doppler blood flow detection or elastography for measuring tissue stiffness cannot be added and if interventional procedures are indicated, a separate hand held realtime examination is required.

In my opinion as a clinician a whole breast scanner would be desirable to overcome these limitations. The instrument should store volume data of the whole breast and give information about tissue reflectivity as well as other physical information like blood flow, velocity, stiffness or attenuation. It would also be highly useful to merge ultrasound images and mammograms or MRI images together or to combine mammography with ultrasound. This was suggested by K. Richter many years ago who performed exciting studies with a simple prototype [38, 39]. Surprisingly, this simple but effective technique was unfortunately forgotten, may be it finds a come-back.

References

[1] V.P. Jackson: The current role of ultrasonography in breast imaging. Radiol Clin North Am 33 (1995), 1161-1170

[2] J. Jellins: Back to the basic raises quality in ultrasound. Diagnostic Imaging Europe 12-20 (1999)

[3] C.R.B. Merritt: Future directions in breast ultrasonography. Seminars in Breast Disease 2(1) (1999) 89-96

[4] H. Madjar, M. Rickard, J. Jellins, R. Otto: IBUS guidelines for the ultrasonic examination of the breast. Europ J. Ultrasound 9 (1999), 99-102

[5] A.T. Stavros: Breast Ultrasound. Lippcott Williams and Wilkens, Philadelphia (2004)

[6] T.M. Kolb, J. Lichy, J.H. Newhouse: Occult cancer in women with dense breasts: detection with screening US - diagnostic yield and tumor characteristics. Radiology 207 (1998), 191-199

[7] E.B. Mendelson, J.K. Baum, W.A. Berg, C.R.B. Merritt, E. Rubin: Breast Imaging Reporting and Data System, BI-RADS: Ultrasound. Reston, VA: American College of Radiology (2003)

[8] K.D. Schulz, U.S. Albert: Stufe- 3Leitlinie Brustkrebs-Früherkennung in Deutschland. Zuckschwerdt München (2003)

[9] T.M. Kolb, J. Lichy, J.H. Newhouse: Comparison of the Performance of Screening Mammography, Physical Examination, and Breast US and Evaluation of Factors that Influence Them: An Analysis of 27,825 Patients Evaluations. Radiology 225 (2002), 165-175

[10] J.G. Elmore, K. Armstrong, C.D. Lehmann et al. Screening for Breast Cancer. JAMA 293(10) (2005), 1245-1256

[11] E. Baez, K. Strathmann, M. Vetter, H. Madjar, B.J. Hackelöer: Likelihood of malignancy in breast lesions characterized by ultrasound with a combined diagnostic score. Ultrasound Med Biol 31 (2) (2005), 179-184

[12] H.M. Zonderland, E.G. Coerkamp, J. Hermans, J. Van De Vijver, A.E. van Voorthuisen: Diagnosis of breast cancer: contribution of US as an adjunctive to mammography. Radiology 213 (1999), 412-422

[13] N.F. Boyd, H. Guo, L.J. Martin, L. Sun, J. Stone, E. Fishell, R.A. Jong, G. Hislop, A. Chiarelli, S. Minkin, M.J. Yaffe: Mammographic Density and the Risk and Detection of Breast Cancer. Engl J Med 356(3) (2007) 227-236

[14] M. Nothacker, V. Duda, M. Hahn, M. Warm, F. Degenhardt, H. Madjar, S. Weinbrenner, U.S. Albert: Early detection of breast cancer: benefits and risks of supplemental breast ultrasound in asymptomatic women with mammographically dense breast tissue. A systematic review. BMC Cancer 20(9) (2009), 335-342

[15] U.S. Albert (ed): Stufe-3-Leitlinie Brustkrebs-Früherkennung in Deutschland 1. Aktualisierung 2008, Zuckschwerdt, München (2008)

[16] A.T. Stavros, D. Thickman, C.L. Rapp et al.: Solid breast nodules: use of sonography to distinguish between benign and malignant lesions. Radiology 196 (1995), 123-134

[17] P. Skaane, K. Engedal: Analysis of sonographic features in the differentiation of fibroadenomas and invasiv ductal carcinoma. AJR 170 (1998), 109-114

[18] G. Rhabar, A.C. Sie, G.C. Hansen, J.S. Prince, M.L. Melany, H.W. Reynolds, V.P. Jackson, J.W. Syre, W. Bassett: Benign versus malignant solid breast masses: US differentiation. Radiology 213(3) (1999), 889-894

[19] W.A. Berg, L. Gutierrez, M.S. NessAiver, W.B. Carter, M. Bhargavan, R.S. Lewis, O.B. Ioffe: Diagnostic Accuracy of Mammography, Clinical Examination, US, and MR Imaging in Preoperative Asessment of Breast Cancer. Radiology 233 (2004), 830-849

[20] H.A. Moss, P.D. Britton, C.D. Flower et al: How reliable is modern breast imaging in differentiating benign from malignant breast lesions in the symptomatic population?. Clin Radiol 54 (1999), 676-682

[21] H. Madjar, R. Ohlinger, A. Mundinger, D. Watermann, J.P. Frenz, W. Bader, R. Schulz-Wendtland, F. Degenhardt: BI-RADS-analogue DEGUM criteria for findings in breast ultrasound consensus of the DEGUM Committee on Breast Ultrasound. Ultraschall Med 27(4) (2006), 374-379

[22] H. Madjar: The Practice of Breast Ultrasound. Thieme, Stuttgart, New York (2008)

[23] W.D. Fornage, O. Toubas, M. Morel: Clinical, mammographic and sonographic determination of preoperative breast cancer size. Cancer 60 (1987), 765-771

[24] H. Madjar, H.A. Ladner, W. Sauerbrei, A. Oberstein, H. Prömpeler, A. Pfleiderer: Peroperative staging of breast cancer by palpation, mammography and high-resolution ultrasound. Ultrasound Obstet Gynecol 3 (1993), 185-190

[25] W.A. Berg, P.L. Gilbreath: Multicentric and multifocal cancer: whole breast US in preoperative evaluation. Radiology 214 (2000), 59-66

[26] W.K. Moon, D.Y. Noh, J.G. Im: Multifocal, multicentric and contralateral breast cancers: bilateral whole-breast ultrasound in the preoperative evaluation of patients. Radiology 224 (2002), 569-576

[27] A. Hlawatsch, A. Teifke, M. Schmidt, M. Thelen: Preoperative assessment of breast cancer: sonography versus MR imaging. AJR Am J Roentgenol 179 (2002), 1493-1501

[28] L. Liberman, E.A. Morris, D.D. Dershaw, A.F. Abramson, L.K. Tan: MR imaging of the ipsilateral breast in women with percutaneously proven breast cancer. AJR Am J Roentgenol 180 (2003), 901-910

[29] M.T. Seymour, E.C. Moskovic, G. Walsh, P. Trott, I.E. Smith: Ultrasound assessment of residual abnormalities following primary chemotherapy for breast cancer. Brit J Cancer 76(3) (1997), 371-376

[30] W.A. Berg: Rationale for a trial of screening breast ultrasound: American College of Radiology Imaging Network (ACRIN) 6666. AJR 180(5) (2003), 1225-1228

[31] P.B. Gordon, S.L. Goldenberg: Malignant breast masses detected only by ultrasound: a retrospective review. Cancer 76 (1995), 626-630

[32] W. Buchberger, A. Niehoff, P. Obrist, P. Koekkoek-Doll, M. Dunser: Clinically and mammographically occult breast lesions: detection and classification with high-resolution sonography. Semin Ultrasound CT MR 21(4) (2000), 325-336

[33] W.A. Berg, J.D. Blume, J.B. Cormack, E.B. Mendelson, D. Lehrer et al.: Combined screening with ultrasound and mammography vs mammography alone in women at elevated risk of breast cancer. JAMA 299(18) (2008), 2151-2163

[34] P.C. Stomper, D.J. D'Souza, P.A. DiNotto, M.A. Arrendondo: Analysis of parenchymal density on mammograms in 1353 women 25-79 years old. AJR Am J Roentgenol 167(5) (1996), 1261-1265

[35] M.T. Mandelson, N. Oestreicher, P.L. Porter et al.: Breast density as a predictor of mammographic detection: comparison of interval- and screen-detected cancers. J Natl Cancer Inst 92(13) (2000), 1081-1087

[36] J.A. Harvey, V.E. Bovbjerg: Quantitative assessment of mammographic breast density: ralationship with breast cancer risk. Radiology 230(1) (2004), 29-41

[37] K. Kerlikowske: The mammogram that cried Wolfe. N Engl J Med 356(3) (2007), 297-300

[38] K. Richter: Clinical amplitude/velocity reconstructive imaging (CARI) a new sonographic method for detecting breast lesions. Brit. J. Radiol. 68 (1995), 375384.

[39] K. Richter: Detection of diffuse breast cancer with a new sonographic method. J. clin. Ultrasound 24 (1996), 157168

[40] M.O. Müller-Schimpfle, V.C. Brandenbusch, F. Degenhardt, V. Duda, H. Madjar, A. Mundinger, R. Rathmann, M. Hahn: The problem of mammographic breast density the position of the DEGUM Working Group on Breast Imaging Ultraschall in Med. (2016)

Ultrasound Tomography for Breast Cancer Screening

Neb Duric[1,2], Peter Littrup[2,3], Cuiping Li[1,2], Mark Sak[2], Yash Sandhu[2], Ken Bergman[2], Michael Boone[2], Di Chen[1,2]

[1] *Karmanos Cancer Institute, Wayne State University, Detroit, MI 48201, USA*
E-Mail: duric@karmanos.org
[2] *Delphinus Medical Technologies, Inc, Novi, MI 48374*
[3] *Ascension Crittenton Hospital, Rochester, MI*

Abstract

Both mammography and standard ultrasound (US) rely upon subjective criteria within the breast imaging reporting and data system (BI-RADS) to provide more uniform interpretation of outcomes, as well as differentiation and risk stratification of associated abnormalities. We have been developing a new technique for breast imaging that is based on ultrasound tomography which has the potential to provide extended detection and/or diagnostic criteria. Informed consent was obtained from all patients, prospectively recruited in an IRB-approved protocol following HIPAA guidelines. Images were produced by tomographic algorithms for reflection, sound speed and stiffness, then reviewed by a board-certified radiologist. In the first phase of the study, UST images were compared to multi-modal imaging to determine the appearance of lesions and breast parenchyma. In the second phase of the study, correlative comparisons with MR breast imaging were used to establish basic operational capabilities of the UST system including the identification and characterization of parenchymal patterns. Our study demonstrated a high degree of correlation of breast tissue structures relative to fat subtracted contrast enhanced MRI. With a scan duration of ~1-3 minutes, no significant motion artifacts were observed. Initial clinical results suggest an ability to characterize masses. Experience with the SoftVue system indicates that rendering of parenchymal structures and masses is similar to MRI while providing unique metrics for lesion characterization.

Keywords: Breast, Ultrasound, 3-D Imaging, Tomography, Cancer

1 Introduction

In the USA, breast cancer is the most common cancer among women, accounting for 1/3 of cancers diagnosed. Statistically, ~230,000 new cases of invasive breast cancer and ~63,000 in situ breast carcinomas are diagnosed annually in the US; breast cancer is the third leading cause of cancer death among women, causing ~40,000 deaths in the US every year [1]. According to SEER statistics, approximately 61% of women are found to have localized breast cancers at the time of diagnosis; about 31% are found to be regional disease; another 5% are diagnosed with distant metastases while about 3% are unstaged [2]. The 5-year survival rate for women with localized cancer is 98%; for those with regional disease, it drops to 84%; for those diagnosed with distant stage, the survival rate drops dramatically to 23%; while for unstaged cancers the 5-year survival rate is about 58%. Figure 1 illustrates the dependence of survival on cancer stage.

Improved breast cancer detection would have the greatest effect on the statistic of nearly 1 in 3 women who are diagnosed each year with later stage (regional or greater) breast cancer, totaling approximately 60,000 women per year in the United States. The net effect would be an increase in survival time and a corresponding decrease in mortality rates. This is also suggested in a recent meta-analysis, whereby increased participation and sensitivity lead to additional invasive cancer detection and greater mortality reduction [3].

Limited performance of mammography. For women with dense breast tissue, who are at the highest risk for developing breast cancer [4-7], the performance of mammography is at its worst [8]. Consequently, many cancers are missed at their earliest stages when they are the most treatable. Improved cancer detection for women with denser breasts would decrease the proportion of breast cancers diagnosed at later stages, which would significantly lower the mortality rate.

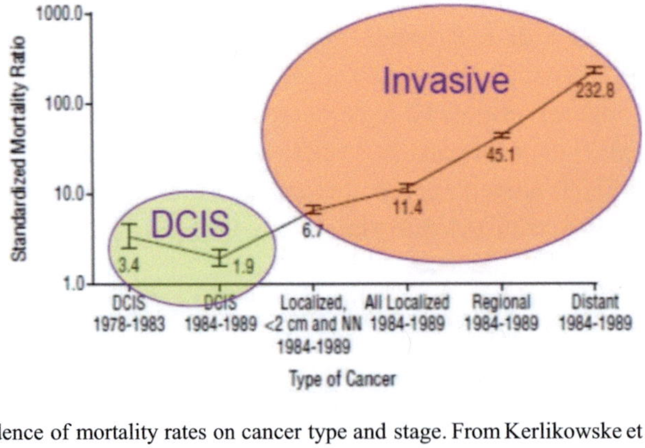

Figure 1: The dependence of mortality rates on cancer type and stage. From Kerlikowske et al, Arch Intern Med/Vol 160, April 10, 2000.

The Breast Screening Challenge. X-ray mammography detects about 5 cancers per 1000 screens [9]. However, its positive predictive value (PPV) is low and its sensitivity is greatly reduced in women with dense breast tissue [9]. Although digital breast tomosynthesis (DBT) may improve upon some of the limitations of standard mammography, it is unlikely to create a paradigm shift in performance [10] while generating potentially higher levels of ionizing radiation [11]. MRI can significantly improve on these limitations by its volumetric, radiation-free imaging. Studies have shown that MRI can have a positive impact in the breast management continuum ranging from risk assessment to diagnosis and treatment monitoring [11-22]. However, MRI can have a high false positive rate, requires contrast injection and the exams can be both long and costly [13]. Furthermore, MR has long been prohibitively expensive for routine use and there is a need for a low-cost equivalent alternative.

Recent studies have demonstrated the effectiveness of hand held ultrasound imaging in detecting breast cancer, particularly for women with dense breasts [23-33]. We have examined the data from these studies to extract the statistics of cancer detection by imaging mode. The results are summarized in Figure 2. It is striking to note that ultrasound (US) almost doubles the detection rate of invasive cancers in dense breasts. However, despite these successful study outcomes, handheld ultrasound is unlikely to be adopted for screening because it is operator-dependent, and its imaging aperture is small, which hinders whole breast imaging. Furthermore, ultrasound's increased sensitivity to invasive cancer is offset by lowered sensitivity to DCIS since mammography detects more microcalcifications [34]. Although such a trade-off may be justified by the fact that mortality from invasive cancers is much higher than that from DCIS, a combined screening (mammography plus US) would provide a comprehensive screen. It has therefore been proposed that US be used for screening, supplemental to mammography.

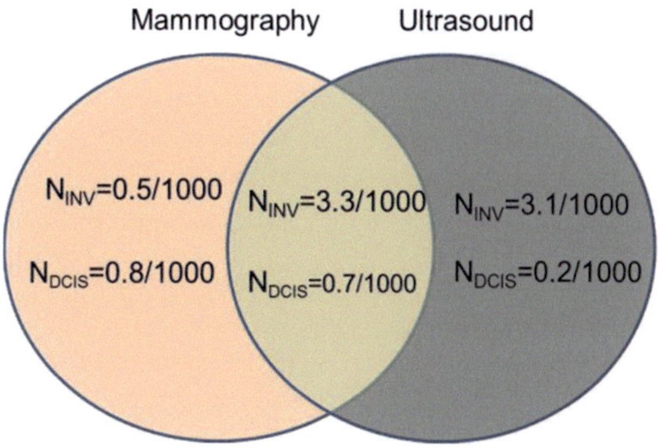

Figure 2: Venn diagram summarizing comparative cancer detection rates for screening mammography and ultrasound.

To that end, automated breast ultrasound (ABUS) has been introduced as a way of overcoming these issues, mainly by reducing operator dependence and increasing the field of view. For example, the GE Invenia ABUS ultrasound system for breast cancer screening, originally developed by U-Systems., recently received screening approval, adjunctive to mammography, from the FDA, because it demonstrated an ability to detect cancers missed by mammography in dense breasts. The SomoInsight screening study [23], indeed showed that ABUS plus mammography outperformed mammography alone, leading to the first FDA approval for ultrasound screening for breast cancer.

The fundamental quandary of breast screening today is the knowledge that (i) mammography misses cancers in dense breasts, (ii) that Automated Breast ultrasound (ABUS) detects cancers that mammography misses and yet (iii) screening continues largely with mammography only. This paradox is amplified even further by the proliferation of state breast density notification laws in the USA which mandate that this information be available to women undergoing breast cancer screening. The primary reason this paradox exists today is that ABUS screening increases call back rates (up to a factor of 2 in case of the SomoInsight study [22]). The improvement in classification performance, measured by the area under the ROC curve, is modest because the increase in sensitivity is partially offset by an increase in false positives thus slowing its adoption. Technically, with its basic B-mode capability, ABUS has the same issue with false positives as hand held ultrasound. It is therefore unlikely that ABUS will be widely adopted for screening in the foreseeable future without more tissue-specific imaging capability. Improved lesion characterization would help lower the barriers to adoption of screening ultrasound.

Ultrasound Tomography (UST) is an emerging technique that has the potential for quantitative, tissue specific imaging and characterization, by virtue of its transmission imaging capability [35-60]. Improved specificity would lower call back rates and lower barriers to adoption. An adjunctive use of UST would have the potential to improve specificity relative to current ABUS and provide a comprehensive screen that would uncover invasive cancers otherwise missed by mammography. Detection of such early stage invasive cancers would provide women with curative treatment, the opportunity for which might be otherwise lost.

2 Methods and Materials

In an initial attempt to assess the potential of UST in breast imaging, studies were carried out at the Karmanos Cancer Institute, Detroit, MI, USA. Informed consent was obtained from all patients, prospectively recruited in an IRB-approved protocol following HIPAA guidelines. Patients were scanned at the Alexander J Walt Comprehensive Breast Center. Standard multi-modality imaging was available for all patients. The Walt Breast Center houses SoftVue, a UST system manufactured by Delphinus Medical Technologies, Inc (Novi, MI). SoftVue was used to scan the recruited patients for this study. Coronal image series were produced by tomographic algorithms for reflection, sound speed and stiffness. All images were reviewed by a board-certified radiologist with more than 20 years of experience in breast imaging and US-technology development. Symptomatic study participants were scanned with a SoftVue UST system. Pathological correlation was based on biopsy results and standard im- aging (e.g., US-definitive cyst). Tomographic algorithms were used to generate images stacks of reflectivity, sound speed and stiffness for each patient. Lesions were identified based on correlation with standard imaging so that the tumor sound speed (SS) and stiffness could be assessed. An example of each type of image is shown in Figure 3.

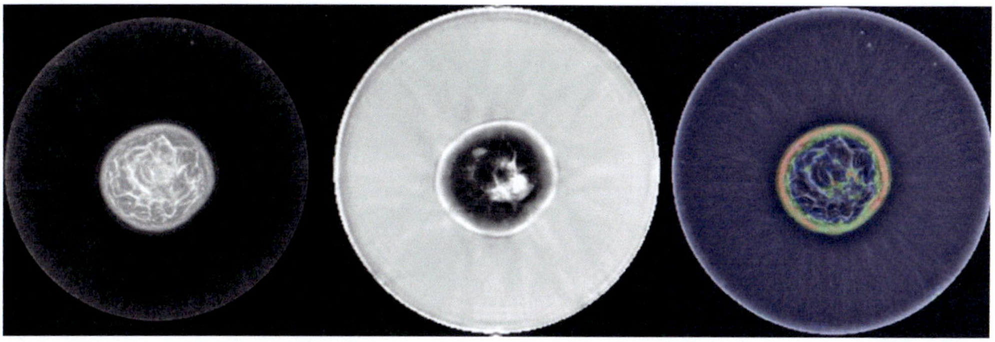

Figure 3: From left to right, reflection, sound speed and stiffness image slices depicting breast parenchyma

In the first phase of the study, correlative comparisons with multi-modal imaging were carried out to assess lesion properties relative to mammography, US and MR. In the second phase, comparison with MR breast imaging was used to establish basic operational capabilities of the UST system including the identification and characterization of parenchymal patterns and determination of the spatial resolution of UST. The third phase of the study focused on lesion characterization using standard BIRADS criteria.

3 Results and Discussion

3.1 Multi-modal comparison

Figure 4 shows a 9mm IDC at 3 o'clock. CC and MLO mammographic views of the affected breast are shown on the left with the lesion identified by arrows. The UST views corresponding to the coronal planes that contain the lesions are across the top with reflection, sound speed and stiffness images laid out from left to right. The corresponding ultrasound and MR images are shown along the bottom. Inspection of the images shows good correspondence in shape and location of the lesion. The greatest similarity is between the UST images and fat-subtracted, enhanced MRI. IDC is generally hypoechoic in reflection and has high sound speed and stiffness. An IDC in a heterogeneously dense breast is shown in Figure 5.

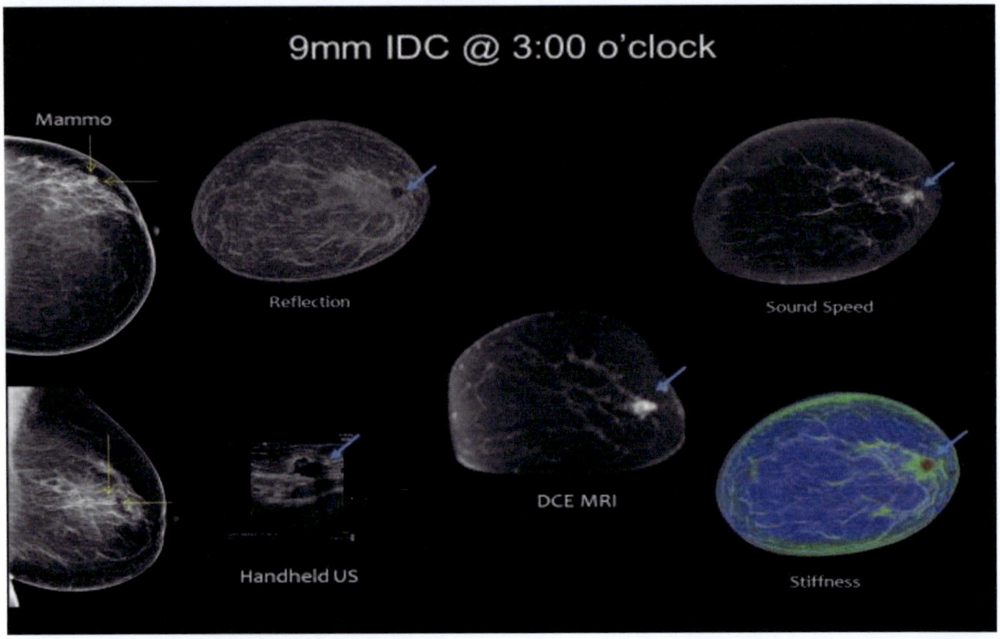

Figure 4: A 9mm IDC at 3 o'clock. CC and MLO mammographic views of the affected breast are shown on the left with the lesion identified by arrows. The coronal UST views are shown in the form of reflection, sound speed and stiffness images. The corresponding ultrasound and MR images are also shown.

3.2 MR Concordance

UST and MR imaging were performed within weeks of each other. UST imaging was carried out with the SoftVue system (Delphinus Medical Technologies) and the MR exams with a Philips Achieva 3T system. As discussed above, UST images correlate best with MR images. Further inspection shows that of the three UST image types, the sound speed image correlates best with MR. Figure 6 shows a coronal view comparison between UST speed of sound and MR contrast enhanced fat subtracted images of representative parenchyma.

The parenchymal patterns are very similar with the only major difference relating to the shape of the breast. This difference can be explained by the fact that the SoftVue system utilizes water so that buoyancy foreshortens the breast while with MR, gravity lengthens the breast in the AP dimension (i.e. prone).

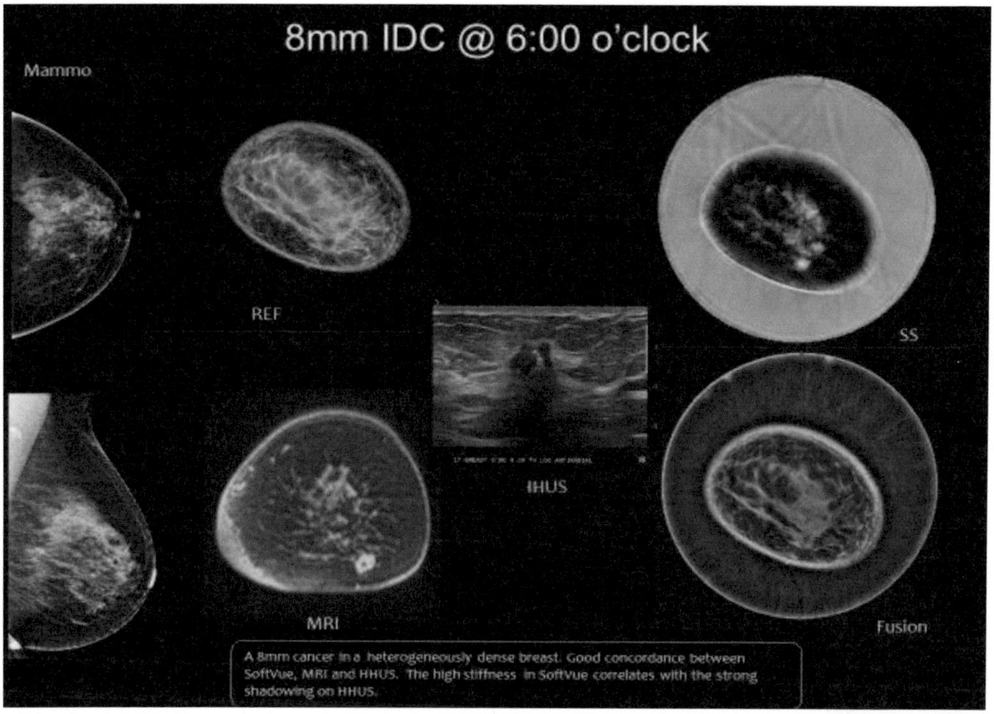

Figure 5: A 8mm IDC at 6 o'clock showing concordance with other modalities.

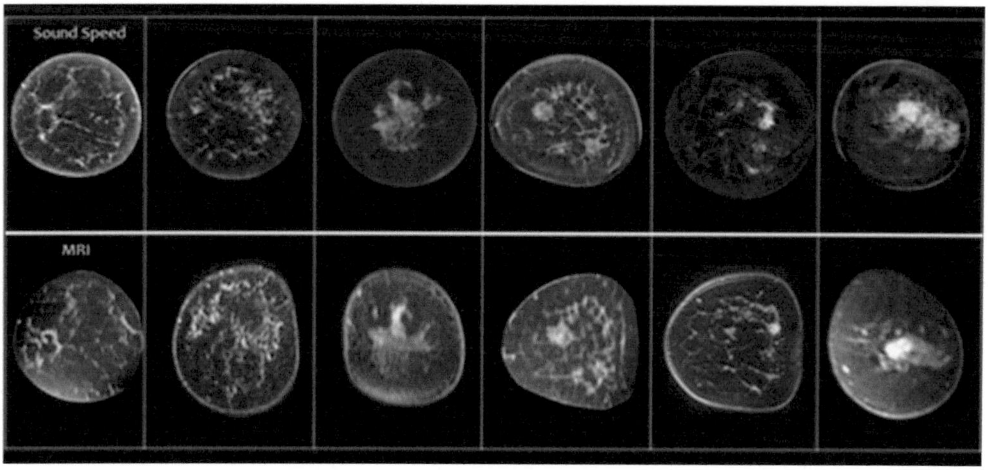

Figure 6: Top: Coronal UST sound speed images for 6 different patients. Bottom: Corresponding fat subtracted contrast enhanced MR images.

3.3 Mass characterization using BIRADS

Characterization of Cancer. Figures 7, 8 and 9 show three examples of breast cancer. The three cancers range in size from 7 to 15mm. The left side of each image provides a coronal view of tumor location and extent of accompanying dense tissue. The right side shows a zoomed-in view of each tumor showing more detailed morphology. Visual inspection using the standard BIRADS lexicon suggests that the cancers can be characterized as being irregular in shape in all three modalities, hypoechoic in reflection and spiculated in reflection and sound speed. Furthermore, the tumors have high sound speed and stiffness.

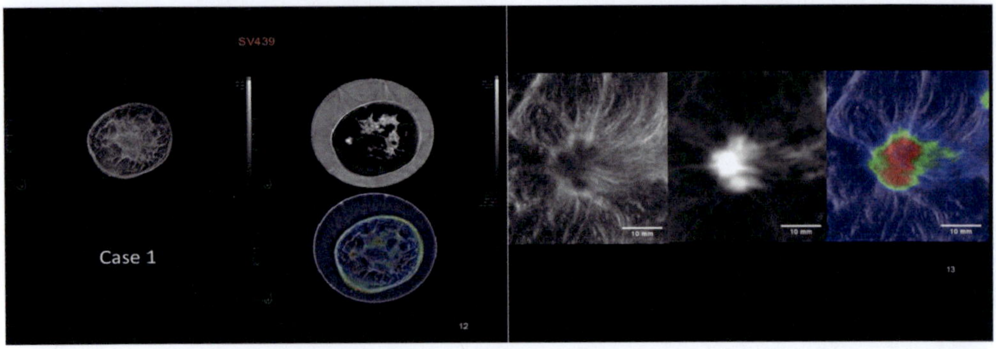

Figure 7: Left: A cancer at 9 o'clock. Right: Zoomed in views

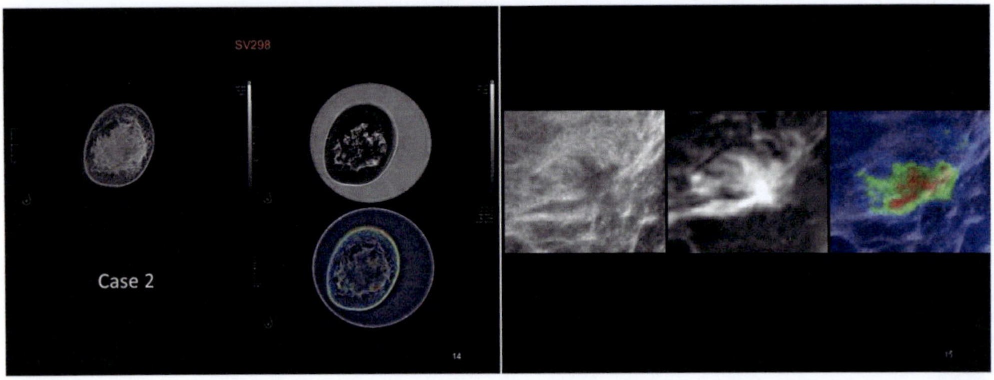

Figure 8: Left: A cancer at 4 o'clock. Right: Zoomed in views.

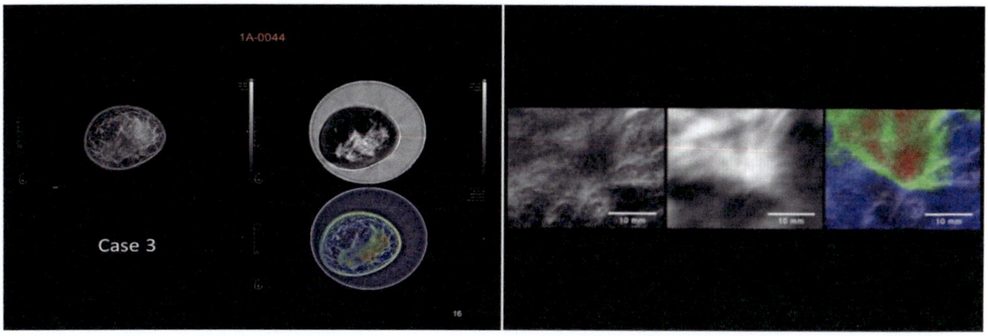

Figure 9: Left: A cancer at 5 o'clock. Right: Zoomed in views.

Characterization of benign lesions. Figures 10, 11, 12 and 13 show examples of benign masses, ranging in size from 4 to 20mm. The left side of each image provides a coronal view of tumor location and extent of accompanying dense tissue. The right side shows a zoomed-in view of each mass for more detailed morphology. Visual inspection using the standard BI-RADS lexicon suggests that cysts can be characterized as being well circumscribed in all three modalities and anechoic in reflection (Figure 10). Furthermore, the cysts have sound speeds similar to water and no stiffness signature. Fibroadenomas (FAs) are characterized as being well circumscribed in all three modalities and hypoechoic in reflection (Figure 10). Furthermore, FAs have sound speeds higher than that of water and have variable stiffness. Some FAs are stiff (Figure 11), some have mixed stiffness (Figure 12) and some are very soft (Figure 13).

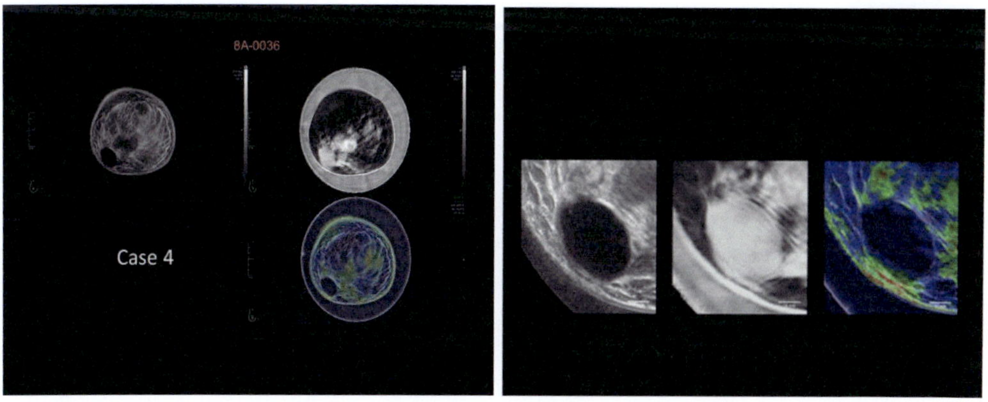

Figure 10: Left: A cyst at 7 o'clock. Right: Zoomed in views.

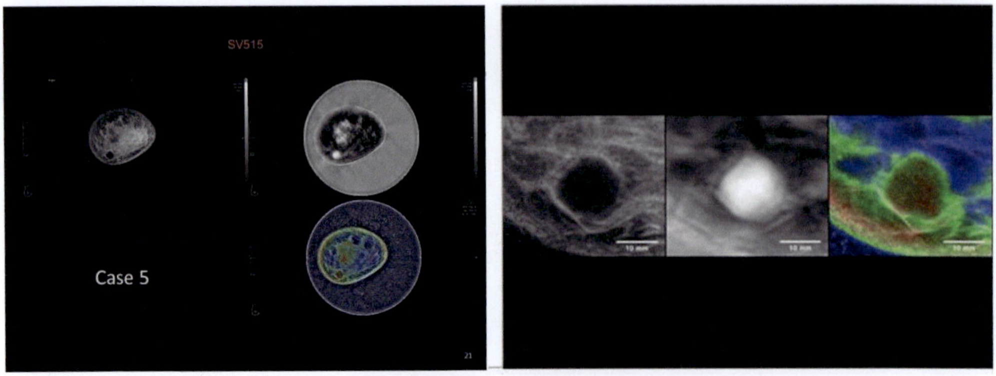

Figure 11: Left: A fibroadenoma at 7 o'clock. Right: Zoomed in views

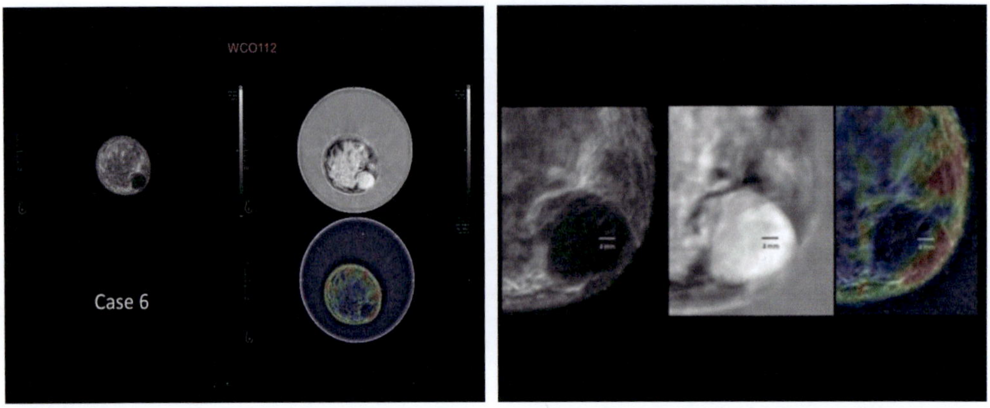

Figure 12: Left: A 5mm cyst inside a fibroadenoma at 5 o'clock. Right: Zoomed in views.

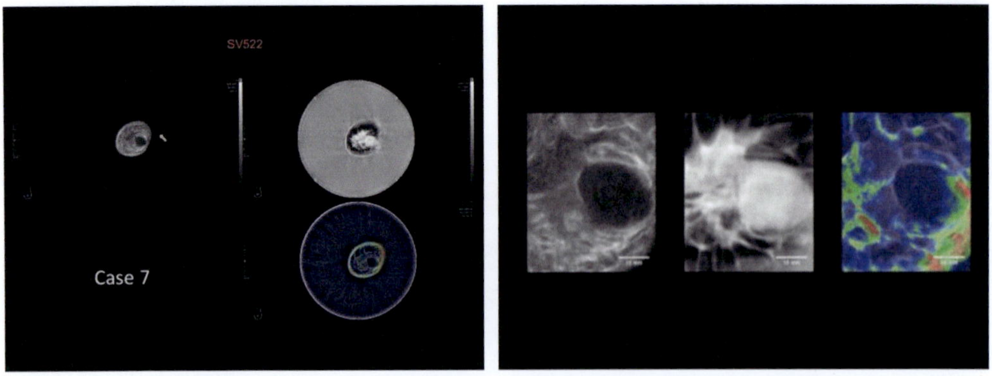

Figure 13: Left: A fibroadenoma at 3 o'clock. Right: Zoomed in views

US-BI-RADS criteria are predominantly devoted to assessment of tumor shape, margins and interaction with adjacent tissue [61, 62]. However, criteria such as shadowing or enhanced through transmission are not applicable to UST's circular geometry. UST, operating at 3 MHz, appears more sensitive to specular reflectors of benign mass capsules, or the spiculations and/or architectural distortions of many cancers. Measurement of physical properties like sound speed are unique to UST [63-68]. Moreover, the whole-breast feature of localized tissue stiffness also opens the possibility of improved cancer detection for screening. These differences in characterization are being investigated as part of a predictive model to determine how much improvement in specificity over conventional ultrasound can be expected.

4 Conclusions

In this study we reviewed the status of breast cancer screening and the potential role that ultrasound tomography (UST) could play in breast imaging. Several results from recent ongoing UST studies were used in this review. The main conclusions from those studies are:

(i) UST sound speed demonstrated a high degree of correlation of breast tissue structures relative to fat-subtracted, contrast enhanced MRI. This correlation of structures was most evident in coronal plane comparisons.

(ii) UST demonstrated a spatial resolution of 0.7mm in the coronal plane, similar to MRI.

(iii) Initial clinical results suggest an ability to characterize lesions using Standard BI-RADS criteria of visual assessment of margins (in all 3 UST modalities), in combination with relative stiffness values. These parameters leverage all three imaging modes of UST (reflection, sound speed and stiffness).

UST is a promising new modality that has the potential to complement existing breast imaging methods to aid in lesion detection and characterization. Future larger scale studies will assess UST's role in diagnostic and screening settings.

Acknowledgments

The work presented in this paper was supported by NIH grant 5R44CA165320-05.

References

[1] SEER website. http://seer.cancer.gov/

[2] American Cancer Society. Cancer Prevention & Early Detection Facts & Figures 2009. Atlanta, GA: American Cancer Society, 2009; 34-37.

[3] Chen TH, Yen AM, Fann JC, Gordon P, Chen SL, Chiu SY, Hsu CY, Chang KJ, Lee WC, Yeoh KG, Saito H, Promthet S, Hamashima C, Maidin A, Robinson F, Zhao LZ. Clarifying the debate on population-based screening for breast cancer with mammography: A systematic review of randomized controlled trials on mammography with Bayesian meta-analysis and causal model. Medicine (Baltimore) 2017; 96:e5684.

[4] Boyd NF, Guo H, Martin LJ, Sun L, Stone J, Fishell E, Jong RA, Hislop G, Chiarelli A, Minkin S. et al.: Mammographic density and the risk and detection of breast cancer. N Engl J Med 2007, 356:227-236.

[5] Chen J, Pee D, Ayyagari R, Graubard B, Schairer C, Byrne C, Benichou J, Gail MH: Projecting absolute invasive breast cancer risk in white women with a model that includes mammographic density. J Natl Cancer Inst 2006, 98:1215-1226.

[6] Ursin G, Hovanessian-Larsen L, Parisky YR, Pike MC, Wu AH: Greatly increased occurrence of breast cancers in areas of mammographically dense tissue. Breast Cancer Res 2005, 7:R605-R608.

[7] Martin LJ, Boyd N: Potential mechanisms of breast cancer risk associated with mammographic density: hypotheses based on epidemiological evidence. Breast Cancer Res 2008, 10:1-14.

[8] Armstrong K, Moye E, Williams S, Berlin JA, Reynolds EE. Screening mammography in women 40 to 49 years of age: a systematic review for the American College of Physicians. Ann Intern Med. 2007; 146:516-26

[9] http://www.cancer.gov/cancertopics/pdq/screening/breast/healthprofessional/page7

[10] Friedewald, S. M., Rafferty, E. A., Rose, S. L., Durand, M. A., Plecha, D. M., Greenberg, J. S., ... & Conant, E. F. (2014). Breast cancer screening using tomosynthesis in combination with digital mammography. Jama, 311(24), 2499-2507.

[11] Hendrick, R. E. (2010). Radiation doses and cancer risks from breast imaging Studies 1. Radiology, 257(1), 246-253.

[12] Turnbull, LW. Dynamic contrast-enhanced MRI in the diagnosis and management of breast cancer. J NMR Biomed 2008.

[13] Jansen, SA,Fan, X, Karczmar, GS, Abe, H, Schmidt, RA, Newstead, GM. Differentiation between benign and malignant breast lesions detected by bilateral dynamic contrast-enhanced MRI: A sensitivity and specificity study. MAGNETIC RESONANCE IN MEDICINE. 59, 4, 747, 2008. John Wiley & Sons, Ltd

[14] Kuhl CK, Schrading S, Bieling HB, Wardelmann E, Leutner CC, Koenig R, Kuhn W, Schild HH. MRI for diagnosis of pure ductal carcinoma in situ: a prospective observational study. Lancet. 2007; 370:485-92.

[15] Saslow D, Boetes C, Burke W, Harms S, Leach MO, Lehman CD, Morris E, Pisano E, Schnall M, Sener S, Smith RA, Warner E, Yaffe M, Andrews KS, Russell CA; American Cancer Society Breast Cancer Advisory Group. American Cancer Society guidelines for breast screening with MRI as an adjunct to mammography. CA Cancer J Clin. 2007; 57:75-89.

[16] Chen, J.H., et al., MRI evaluation of pathologically complete response and residual tumors in breast cancer after neoadjuvant chemotherapy. Cancer, 2008. 112(1): 17-26.

[17] Sharma, U., et al., Longitudinal study of the assessment by MRI and diffusion-weighted imaging of tumor response in patients with locally advanced breast cancer undergoing neoadjuvant chemotherapy. NMR Biomed, 2009. 22(1): p. 104-13.

[18] Bando, H., et al., Imaging evaluation of pathological response in breast cancer after neoadjuvant chemotherapy by real-time sonoelastography and MRI. European Journal of Cancer-Supplement, 2008. 6(7): p. 66-66.

[19] Bhattacharyya, M., et al., Using MRI to plan breast-conserving surgery following neoadjuvant chemotherapy for early breast cancer. Br J Cancer, 2008. 98(2): p. 289-93.

[20] Partridge, S., Recurrence Rates After DCE-MRI Image Guided Planning for Breast-conserving Surgery Following Neoadjuvant Chemotherapy for Locally Advanced Breast Cancer Patients. Breast Diseases: A Year Book Quarterly, 2008. 19(1):p. 91- 91.

[21] Tozaki, M., Diagnosis of breast cancer: MDCT versus MRI. Breast Cancer, 2008. 15(3): p. 205-211.

[22] Partridge, S., et al., Accuracy of MR imaging for revealing residual breast cancer in patients who have undergone neoadjuvant chemotherapy. 2002, Am Roentgen Ray Soc. p. 1193-1199.

[23] Brem RF, Tabár L, Duffy SW, Inciardi MF, Guingrich JA, Hashimoto BE, Lander MR, Lapidus RL, Peterson MK, Rapelyea JA, Roux S, Schilling KJ, Shah BA, Torrente J, Wynn RT, Miller DP. Assessing improvement in detection of breast cancer with three-dimensional automated breast US in women with dense breast tissue: the SomoInsight Study. Radiology. 2015 Mar; 274(3):663-73.

[24] Berg WA, Zhang Z, Lehrer D, Jong RA, Pisano ED, Barr RG, Böhm-Vélez M, Mahoney MC, Evans WP 3rd, Larsen LH, Morton MJ, Mendelson EB, Farria DM, Cormack JB, Marques HS, Adams A, Yeh NM, Gabrielli G; ACRIN 6666 Investigators. Detection of breast cancer with addition of annual screening ultrasound or a single screening MRI to mammography in women with elevated breast cancer risk. JAMA. 2012 Apr 4;307(13):1394-404

[25] Hooley RJ, Greenberg KL, Stackhouse RM, Geisel JL, Butler RS, Philpotts LE. Screening US in patients with mammographically dense breasts: initial experience with Connecticut Public Act 09-41. Radiology. 2012 Oct; 265(1):59-69.

[26] Kelly KM, Dean J, Comulada WS, Lee SJ. Breast cancer detection using automated whole breast ultrasound and mammography in radiographically dense breasts. Eur Radiol. 2010 Mar; 20(3):734-42.

[27] Corsetti V, Houssami N, Ferrari A, Ghirardi M, Bellarosa S, Angelini O, Bani C, Sardo P, Remida G, Galligioni E, Ciatto S. Breast screening with ultrasound in women with mammography-negative dense breasts: evidence on incremental cancer detection and false positives, and associated cost. Eur J Cancer. 2008 Mar;44(4):539-44

[28] Crystal P, Strano SD, Shcharynski S, Koretz MJ. Using sonography to screen women with mammographically dense breasts. AJR Am J Roentgenol. 2003, 181(1):177- 82.

[29] Leconte I, Feger C, Galant C, Berlière M, Berg BV, D'Hoore W, Maldague B. Mammography and subsequent whole-breast sonography of non palpable breast cancers: the importance of radiologic breast density.AJR Am J Roentgenol. 2003 Jun; 180(6):1675-9.

[30] Kolb TM, Lichy J, Newhouse JH. Comparison of the performance of screening mammography, physical examination, and breast US and evaluation of factors that influence them: an analysis of 27,825 patient evaluations. Radiology. 2002 Oct;225(1):165-75.

[31] Kaplan SS. Clinical utility of bilateral whole-breast US in the evaluation of women with dense breast tissue. Radiology. 2001 Dec; 221(3):641-9.

[32] Buchberger W, Niehoff A, Obrist P, DeKoekkoek-Doll P, Dünser M. Semin. Clinically and mammographically occult breast lesions: detection and classification with high-resolution sonography. Ultrasound CT MR. 2000 Aug;21(4):325-36.

[33] Gordon PB, Goldenberg SL. Malignant breast masses detected only by ultrasound. A retrospective review. Cancer. 1995 Aug 15;76(4):626-30.

[34] Ernster VL, Ballard-BarbashR, Barlow WE, Zheng Y, Weaver DL, et al. Detection of Ductal Carcinoma In Situ in Women Undergoing Screening Mammography. J Natl Cancer Inst 2002, 94:1546-1554.

[35] Johnson, S., et al., From laboratory to clinical trials: An odyssey of ultrasound inverse scattering imaging for breast cancer diagnosis. The Journal of the Acoustical Society of America, 2006. 120: p. 3023.

[36] Johnson SA and Tracy ML. Inverse scattering solutions by a sinc basis, multiple source, moment method. Part I: Theory, Ultrasonic Imaging, 5:361-375, 1983.

[37] Schreiman JS, Gisvold JJ, Greenleaf JF, Bahn RC. Ultrasound transmission computed tomography of the breast. Radiology 1984; 150:523-30.

[38] Natterer FA. Propagation backpropagation method for ultrasound tomography, Inverse problems 1995; 11:1225-1232.

[39] Carson PL, Meyer CR, Scherzinger AL, Oughton TV. Breast imaging in coronal planes with simultaneous pulse echo and transmission ultrasound. Science 1981 Dec 4; 214(4525):1141-3.

[40] M. P. Andre, H.S. Janee, P. J. Martin, G. P. Otto, B. A. Spivey, D. A. Palmer, "High-speed data acquisition in a diffraction tomography system employing large-scale toroidal arrays," International Journal of Imaging Systems and Technology 8, pp.137-147, 1997.

[41] Johnson S. A., Borup, D. T., Wiskin J. W., Natterer F., Wuebbling F., Zhang Y., Olsen C. Apparatus and Method for Imaging with Wavefields using Inverse Scattering Techniques. United States Patent 6,005,916 (1999).
[42] Marmarelis, V.Z., Kim, T., Shehada, R.E. Proceedings of the SPIE: Medical Imaging 2003; San Diego, California; Feb. 23-28, 2002. Ultrasonic Imaging and Signal Processing – Paper 5035-6.
[43] Liu, D.-L., and Waag, R. C. "Propagation and backpropagation for ultrasonic wavefront design," IEEE Trans. on Ultras. Ferro. and Freq. Contr. 44(1):1-13 (1997).
[44] Liu, D. and R. Waag, Harmonic amplitude distribution in a wideband ultrasonic wavefront after propagation through human abdominal wall and breast specimens. The Journal of the Acoustical Society of America, 1997. 101: p. 1172.
[45] Duric N, Littrup PJ, Poulo L, et al. Detection of breast cancer with ultrasound tomography: First results with the Computed Ultrasound Risk Evaluation (UST) prototype. Med. Phys. 2007; 34: 773-785
[46] Boyd, N. F. et al. (2010). "Breast Tissue Composition and Susceptibility to Breast Cancer". JNCI : Journal of the National Cancer Institute (0027-8874), 102 (16), p. 1224, 2010. (Review Article).
[47] Glide C, Duric N, Littrup P. Novel approach to evaluating breast density utilizing ultrasound tomography. Med Phys 2007; 34(2):744-753.
[48] Glide-Hurst CK, Duric N, Littrup P. Volumetric breast density evaluation from ultrasound tomography images. Med Phys 2008; 35(9):3988-3997.
[49] L. Myc, N. Duric, P. Littrup, C. Li, B. Ranger, J. Lupinacci, S. Schmidt, et al., "Volumetric breast density evaluation by Ultrasound Tomography and Magnetic Resonance Imaging: A preliminary comparative study", Proceedings of SPIE Vol. 7629, 76290N (2010).
[50] C. Li, N. Duric,; L. Huang. Clinical breast imaging using sound-speed reconstructions of ultrasound tomography data. Proc. SPIE 6920, 6920-09 (2008)
[51] C. Li, N. Duric, L. Huang. Comparison of ultrasound stiffness tomography techniques for breast cancer diagnosis. Proc. SPIE 6920, 6920-49 (2008).
[52] C. Li, L. Huang, N. Duric, H. Zhang, C. Rowe. An improved automatic time-of-flight picker for medical ultrasound tomography. Ultrasonics. (Accepted).
[53] Duric N, Littrup P, Li C, Rama O, Bey-Knight L, Schmidt S, Lupinacci J, (2009) Detection and characterization of breast masses with ultrasound tomography: Clinical results. Proc. of SPIE: Medical Imaging 2009. Vol. 7265 72651G-1-8.
[54] F Simonetti, L Huang, N Duric. "A multiscale approach to diffraction tomography of complex three-dimensional objects". Applied physics letters (0003-6951), 95 (6), p. 061904. 2009.
[55] F Simonetti, L Huang, N Duric, P Littrup. "Diffraction and coherence in breast ultrasound tomography: A study with a toroidal array. Medical Physics, 36(7):2955-65, 2009

[56] N. Duric, P. Littrup, P. Chandiwala-Mody, C. Li, S. Schmidt, et al., "In-vivo imaging results with ultrasound tomography: Report on an ongoing study at the Karmanos Cancer Institute", Proceedings of SPIE Vol. 7629, 76290M (2010).

[57] Ranger B, Littrup P, Duric N, Li C, Lupinacci J, Myc L, Rama O, Bey-Knight L, (2009) Breast imaging with acoustic tomography: a comparative study with MRI. Proc. of SPIE: Medical Imaging 2009. Vol. 7265 726510-1-8

[58] B. Ranger, P. Littrup, N. Duric, C. Li, S. Schmidt, et al., "Breast imaging with ultrasound tomography: a comparative study with MRI", Proceedings of SPIE Vol. 7629, 76291C (2010).

[59] Ranger, B., Littrup, P. J., Duric, N., Chandiwala-Mody, P., Li, C., Schmidt, S., & Lupinacci, J. (2012). Breast ultrasound tomography versus magnetic resonance imaging for clinical display of anatomy and tumor rendering: Preliminary results. AJR. American journal of roentgenology, 198(1), 233.

[60] S. Schmidt, Z. Huang, N. Duric, C. Li and O. Roy. "Modification of Kirchhoff migration with variable sound speed and stiffness for acoustic imaging of media and application to tomographic imaging of the breast: Med. Phys. 38, 998 (2011).

[61] Entrekin RR, Porter BA, Sillesen HH, Wong AD, Cooperberg PL, Fix CH. Real-time spatial compound imaging application to breast, vascular, and musculoskeletal ultrasound.Semin Ultrasound CT MR 2001; 22:50-64.

[62] Stavros, A.T., Thickman, D., Rapp, C.L., Dennis, M.A., Parker, S.H., Sisney, G. Solid breast nodules: Use of sonography to distinguish between benign and malignant lesions. Radiology, Volume 196, Issue 1, 1995, Pages 123-134.

[63] Greenleaf JF, Johnson SA, Bahn RC, Rajagopalan B.: Quantitative cross-sectional imaging of ultrasound parameters. 1977 Ultrasonics Symposium Proc., IEEE Cat. # 77CH1264-1SU, pp. 989- 995, 1977.

[64] Goss SA, Johnston RL and Dunn F. Comprehensive compilation of empirical ultrasonic properties of mammalian tissues. J Acoust Soc AM 1978; 64: 423-457.

[65] Duck FA. Physical properties of tissue. Academic Press, London, 1990.

[66] Edmonds PD, Mortensen CL, Hill JR, Holland SK, Jensen JF, Schattner P and Valdes AD. Ultrasound tissue characterization of breast biopsy specimens. Ultrasound Imaging 1991; 13:162-185.

[67] Weiwad W, Heinig A, Goetz L, Hartmann H, Lampe D, Buchman J, et al. Direct measurement of sound velocity in various specimens of breast tissue. Invest Radiol 2000; 35:721-6.

[68] Littrup PJ, Duric N, Brem RF, Yamashita MW. Improving specificity of whole breast ultrasound using tomographic techniques. Paper SSA02-05. Presented at Radiology Society of North America, 11/27/2016.

3D Ultrasound Computer Tomography for Breast Cancer Diagnosis at KIT: an Overview

N.V. Ruiter[1], T. Hopp[1], M. Zapf[1], A. Menshikov[1], C. Kaiser[2], H. Gemmeke[1]

[1] *Karlsruhe Institute of Technology, Karlsruhe, Germany*
E-mail: nicole.ruiter@kit.edu
[2] *University Medical Center, Mannheim, Germany*

Abstract

3D Ultrasound Computer Tomography (USCT) emitting and receiving spherical wave fronts overcomes the limitations of 2D systems by offering a nearly isotropic 3D point spread function, a large depth of field, less loss of out-of-plane reflections, and fast 3D data acquisition. 3D devices for clinical practice require a more complex hard- and software due to the huge data rate, time-consuming image reconstruction, and large number of small transducers. The here reviewed KIT 3D USCT is a prototype for clinical studies, which realizes for the first time the full benefits of a 3D system.

Keywords: Ultrasound Computer Tomography, clinical application

1 Introduction

Ultrasound computer tomography (USCT) was first investigated in the 1970s, see e.g. the work by Schomberg [1]. The main advantages of such USCT systems for breast cancer detection and diagnosis are simultaneously recordings of reflection, attenuation and speed of sound images, high image quality, fast data acquisition, and no use of ionization radiation.

Building such a device for clinical practice was not successful for a long time - mostly due to the huge data rate and the time-consuming image reconstruction. Yet, promising ex-vivo results have been archived by numerous groups, e.g. [2]–[5]. Currently, the first 2D and 2.5D systems have become available for clinical evaluation [6], [7]. Usually USCT systems implement unfocused ultrasound emission and reception to reconstruct optimally focused reflection images by synthetic aperture post-beamforming. However, in most systems post-beamforming is only applied in one imaging plane. This leads to large slice thickness with limited depth of field, loss of out-of-plane reflections, and large number of movement steps to acquire a stack of images of the whole volume [7]. 3D USCT, using spherical wave fronts for imaging, overcomes these limitations [8].

However, a 3D system requires a large number of transducers approx. two orders of magnitude larger than in a 2D system to fulfil the sampling theorem. In order to approximate a spherical wave front, the individual transducer area has to be small, which leads to low sound pressure and low signal-to-noise ratio (SNR). For in-vivo imaging, the data acquisition time has to be short to prevent image degradation by patient movement. Also, the image reconstruction using post-beamforming is very time consuming.

The current prototype for 3D USCT, the KIT 3D USCT II, is the first full 3D system for in-vivo imaging. It demonstrates that imaging with a sparse transducer setup it is possible. First clinical data showed that 3D acquisition and reconstruction of speed of sound and attenuation images give a direct access to tissue types and cancer detection as proposed by Greenleaf [9]. The prototype, the hardware setup, the image reconstruction methods and experimental and clinical results are described in this overview paper.

2 Methodology

2.1 Device and hardware setup

The KIT 3D USCT prototype is shown in Fig.1. The patient is lying in a prone position on the patient bed. The breast is imaged in a fixed setup in a water bath. The aperture with 2041 transducers surrounds the breast. Due to no breast deformation and defined patient positioning, the volume images of the female breast are reproducible.

The device has a semi-ellipsoidal aperture with 628 emitters and 1413 receivers. Approx. spherical wave fronts are generated by each emitter at 2.5 MHz (approx. 50% bandwidth). Rotational and translational movement, so-called aperture positions, of the complete sensor system creates further virtual positions of the ultrasound transducers. The aperture in form of a semi-ellipsoid was optimized in respect to the isotropy of the 3D point spread function (PSF), the image contrast and the illumination [8]. An overview of the specifications of the KIT 3D USCT is given in Table 1 (all errors are given as standard deviations).

Sound pressure is generated and received using lead-zirconate titanate (PZT) composites. One quadratic module of PZT composite contains nine receivers and four emitters. Each transducer array is embedded including its pre-amplifier and control electronics in a Transducer Array System (TAS) casing. Each TAS contains a temperature sensor for tracking the temperature distribution and shift at 157 positions during measurements.

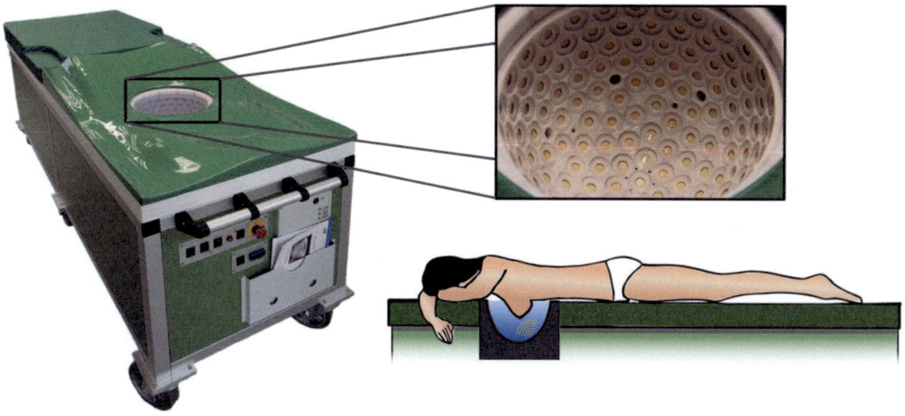

Figure 1: Left: KIT 3D USCT patient bed. Top right: Detail view of transducer aperture with 157 transducer array systems (TAS) containing 4 emitters and 9 receivers each. Bottom right: patient positioning on the patient bed during data acquisition. The breast is suspended freely in a water bath.

Type of specification	Value
No. parallel channels	480
Digitization	20 MHz @ 12 bit
On-board memory	80 $GByte$
Multiplex factor	3
Multiple sampling	1 to 128
No. TAS	157
No. emitters	628
No. receivers	1,413
Diameter TAS	28 mm
Emitters / TAS	4
Receivers / TAS	9
Receiver channels / TAS	3
Area individual transducer	$(0.9\ mm)^2$
No. sub-elements / transducer	2 x 2
Area sub-element	$(0.4\ mm)^2$
Max. excitation voltage	80 V
Opening angle	$38.2° \pm 1.5°$ @ $-6\ dB$
Resonance frequency	$2.7 \pm 0.08\ MHz$
Bandwidth	$1.5 \pm 0.15\ MHz$ @ $-6\ dB$
Sound pressure	$5.9 \pm 0.63\ kPa$ @ 12 cm

Table 1: Specification of KIT 3D USCT

Additionally, two calibrated PT100 temperature sensors are embedded in the TAS holder to enable increased accuracy. The measured temperature distribution can be applied during the image reconstruction to estimate the distribution of the speed of sound in the contact medium water.

The data acquisition is carried out with an FPGA based system, which can store up to 80 $GByte$ of A-scans [10]. The system is housed in a 19" crate with a central processing board containing the control of the transducers, free programmable pulse shape of the transducer, and control of the system by a PCI Mezzanine Card (PMC) handling all input and output tasks of the crate. The PMC is a 1.4 GHz Pentium M board running Linux as operational system and supports a fast Ethernet interface and has a SATA interface to a solid state drive for storage of the measured data. The crate contains beside the central processing board 20 data acquisition boards (FLT). Each FLT contains 24 receiver channels, summing up to 480 channels processed simultaneously in the system and enabling data acquisition at one aperture position in approx. ten seconds. The digitalization is performed by three 8-fold (12 Bit @ 20 MHz) ADCs per board. After digitization, the parallel data streams are processed by FPGAs. The data streams are bandpass filtered (1.67 to 3.33 MHz @ $-60\ dB$) and the data rate is reduced by a factor of 6, performing bandpass undersampling. Using this approach, it is possible to store up to 47 data sets at different aperture positions in one data acquisition process in the internal memory buffer.

The aperture is realized as semi-elliptical TAS holder. The TAS holder is the container for the contact medium water and has several openings for water supply and drainage. The semi-elliptical aperture has a diameter of 26 cm and a height of 18 cm. The whole device is embedded in a patient bed as shown in Fig. 1 with a length of 2 m, a width of 70 cm and a height of 90 cm. It holds the aperture connected to the data acquisition hardware, translation- and rotation mechanics and motors, power supplies, water reservoir and heating, and disinfection system. It is covered by a mattress and serves as examination couch.

A 3D system requires a large number of transducers approx. two orders of magnitude more than a 2D system. The technical feasibility limits the number of transducer positions resulting in a sparse aperture and causing artefacts due to grating lobe effects in the resulting images [11]. A ring aperture requires a transducer distance smaller than $0.5\,\lambda\,R/r$, where R is the radius of the ring and r the radius of the ROI [12]. A semi-spherical aperture leads to an upper limit of $(2\,\pi\,r/\lambda)^2$ transducers [13], if a uniform 1D sampling for the azimuth and elevation angles is applied.

For an exemplary ring system with radius 11.5 cm (see Table III) 103 $GByte$ of raw data per breast have to be processed. To record, store and process this data is certainly challenging but feasible today. For a fully sampled sphere of this size the number of transducers, i.e. 10^5, and the amount of data, i.e. 40 *TByte*, to be processed are no longer feasible.

Therefore, a compromise between the number of transducers and the image quality has to be made, i.e. contrast between image content and grating lobe artefacts. A quantification of the signal-to-artefact ratio for the KIT 3D USCT can be found in [11].

2.2 Image reconstruction

The applied reconstruction algorithm for reflectivity images is the 3D synthetic aperture focusing technique (SAFT). SAFT calculates at each image point the mean of all reflections which might originate from this position. For the simplest reconstruction, the harmonic mean of the speed of sound may be assumed to be constant, e.g. the speed of sound of water at the temperature measured during image acquisition. Alternatively, more accurate estimations of the speed of sound distributions, e.g. a speed of sound map calculated from the recorded transmissions, can be applied [14]. Correcting for the attenuation can be similarly estimated from the attenuation map of the breast [15].

The speed of sound and attenuation are reconstructed using a ray-based approach. The transmission signals are detected and the time-of-flight and relative signal energy, respectively, are applied in an algebraic reconstruction technique (ART) to calculate the resulting images. A compressive sensing algorithm, i.e. a 3D adaption of total variation minimization (TVAL3) is employed for optimization [16].

The computing system for reconstruction consists of a reconstruction PC (4 x AMD Opteron Octacore, 2.3 *GHz*, 256 *GB* RAM) and an external crate for Graphical Processor Units (GPU) (One Stop Systems) is connected via a second-generation PCI-Express bus. The external GPU crate is equipped with four Nvidia Geforce GTX 590 cards, with two GF100 GPUs per card. This results in a total number of eight separate GPUs for image reconstruction [17]. A time of flight interpolation based GPU implementation (TOFI-SAFT) [18] was developed which accelerates our previous GPU implementation of speed of sound corrected SAFT by a factor of 7 with only minor reduction of image quality. The approximation allows reconstructing speed of sound and attenuation corrected SAFT images as fast as non-corrected SAFT. A speed of sound and attenuation corrected SAFT volume of 444^2 x 266 voxels, with 128^3 resolution of the attenuation and SOS maps and 10^7 A-scans can be calculated in 9 min. on eight GPU Titan.

The resulting reflectivity, speed of sound and attenuation images can be viewed separately, directly overlaid or overlaid with an applied threshold. The direct overlay codes the speed of sound or attenuation in a color map and the reflectivity as grey values. The overlay is done by adding the color-coded image to the grey image with an adjustable degree of transparency. The thresholded-fused image follows the method in [6], where a color image only marks image areas where the speed of sound and attenuation are above given thresholds, and then is overlaid on top of the reflectivity volume.

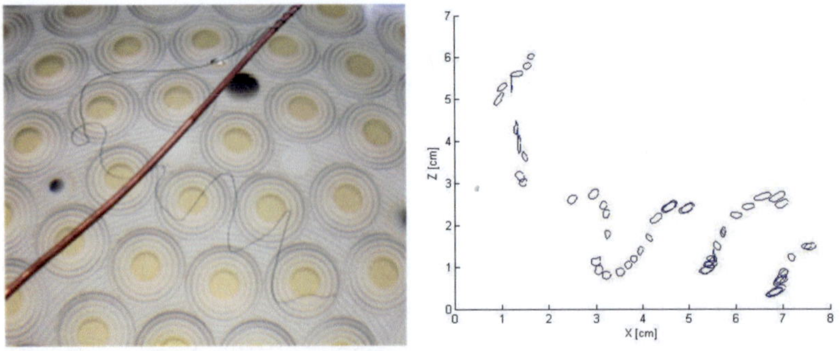

Figure 2: Bonding wire for PSF assessment. Left: photo. Right: 2D profiles at the evaluation points and their direction and position in space. Scaled up to a factor 3 for better visibility.

For comparison with other breast imaging modalities image registration may be applied. This enables direct comparability on a voxel to voxel basis, either for convenient viewing by radiologists or even for automatic analysis. Examples of MRI to USCT registration [19] are given in the results section, results of an evaluation of tissue classification using USCT to X-ray mammography registration is given in [20].

3 Imaging properties and clinical study

The predicted performance of the system, i.e. low spatial variance and isotropy of the 3D PSF, was evaluated in terms of FWHM [21]: A bonding wire with a diameter of 0.07 *mm*, i.e. much thinner than the theoretical resolution of the system, was manually twisted into a helical structure within a bounding box of 5.2 *cm* x 4.3 *cm* x 6.5 *cm*, so that the FWHM could be measured from many directions, see Fig. 2. The overall mean of the measured FWHMs was 0.24 *mm* ± 0.05 *mm*, fitting very well the predicted resolution of 0.22 *mm*. The spatial variability was low, i.e. the standard deviation of the mean FWHM was measured at 36 *μm* (predicted: 35 *μm*). The 3D global point spread function was measured with nearly isotropic diameters of dx,y,z = (0.2, 0.26, 0.24) mm, (predicted: (0.2, 0.2, 0.25) mm).

The influence of a sparse 3D aperture on the contrast of reflectivity images was tested on simulated and real data in [11]. The main results were that the background noise due to grating lobes is mainly influenced by the sparsity of the aperture and the imaged object. For experimental data with the 3D USCT II prototype the amount of data acquired at ten aperture positions were empirically found to be a good compromise between data acquisition time and contrast. Fig. 3, left, shows example reconstructions for a healthy volunteer: whereas the contrast of the images increases from adding more data up to eight aperture positions, the increase of contrast using data from 16 aperture positions is only small. Fig. 3, right, shows a comparison of reconstructions of a breast phantom with the same amount of data, but different transducer combinations. Whereas the left slice was reconstructed using transducers in a regular sampling pattern, the reconstruction of the right slice used from a large amount of different aperture positions the most irregularly spaced transducer combinations. The increase in contrast is significant. This property of a sparse aperture will be applied in the next generation system [21].

The first clinical study with the 3D USCT II device was conducted at the University Hospital in Jena (Germany). Ten patients were images. The primary aims of the study were to test the data acquisition and image reconstruction protocols, the fused display of the multimodal USCT images and the process of data acquisition and its optimization.

The patients included in the study were acquired during the standard MRI examination at the University Hospital Jena. The average age of the ten patients was 55.6 years (±13.5years). The youngest patient was 37 years and the oldest 78 years. They first had their scheduled MRI examination and were then - if they met the inclusion criteria - asked to participate in the study. If they agreed, the USCT image acquisition was carried out directly after the MRI, so that the MRI images could be used as ground truth for comparison to the USCT volumes. The patient was asked to disinfect her breasts. Then she lay on the patient mattress and positioned the first breast into the USCT device. The central positioning of the breast was monitored and corrected using a B-scan like preview. Then the data acquisition for this breast was started. The same process was, if applicable, repeated for the second breast. At the end the patient was asked to fill a questionnaire to rate the imaging procedure. Before the next patient was examined, the data was read out onto a hard disc, the water was exchanged and the device disinfected.

For emission a linear frequency coded chirp with 2.5 *MHz* center frequency, 1 *MHz* bandwidth and 12.8 μs duration was employed. Patients with breast lesions were imaged with ten aperture positions. For two patients, who were diagnosed with large cancer masses, the breasts with lesions were imaged with 13 aperture positions.

During the pilot study we could image approximately one patient per hour, which fitted quite well into the clinical process. For preparation of the device and patient information we needed between 15 and 30 *min*. The patient positioning took approx. 2 to 5 *min.* per breast and the image acquisition in sum 11 *min*.

In the meantime, the data was read out (14 *min*), the device was disinfected and the water was exchanged, sterilized and heated (approx. 15 *min*). The data acquisition time is mainly dominated by the time to move the aperture between different aperture positions. This time is depending on the path to be travelled. The mean time for DAQ with one movement during the pilot study was 50 *s*, i.e. 10 *s* DAQ plus 40 *s* aperture motion. In the meantime patient positioning and aperture movement could be accelerated by a factor two.

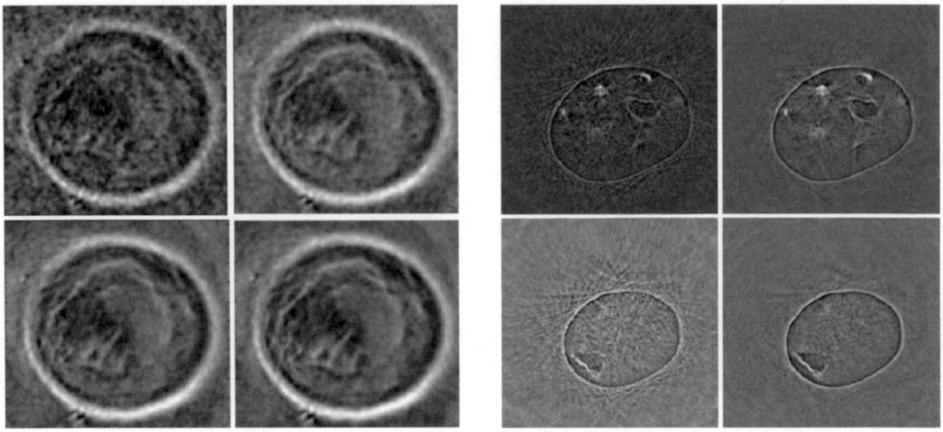

Figure 3: Left: 38-year-old healthy volunteer with an A cup: reconstructions of a frontal slice for one, four, eight and sixteen aperture positions from top left to bottom right. The slices are 11 *cm* by 12 *cm* and 3 *cm* inside the breast measured from the nipple position. Right: Slices of a CIRS multimodality breast phantom with the same amount of data, but with regular (left) and irregular (right) transducer spacing.

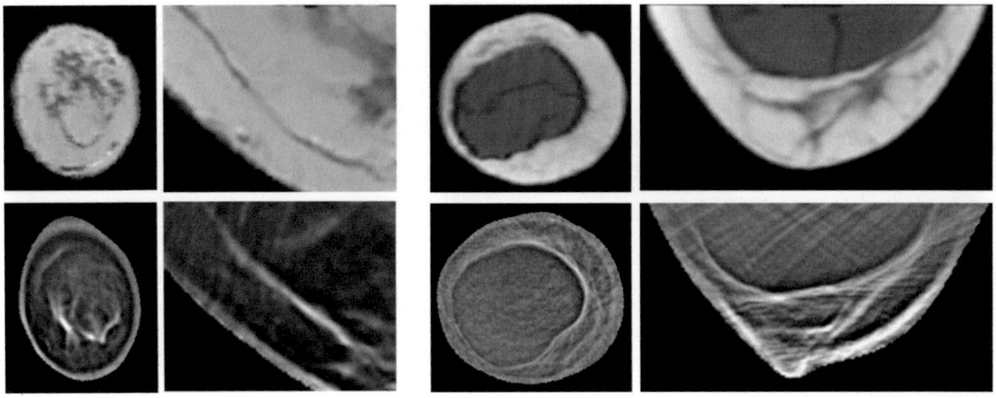

Figure 4: Top row: Registered native MRI in planar and transversal planes. Bottom row: USCT reflectivity slices at same positions. Left: Healthy patient. Right: 58-year-old patient with intact silicone implants (right breast).

Patient motion [23] was tracked in successive reflectivity reconstructions of full breast volumes for each aperture position. The mean distance between initial and final position was 2.2 *mm* (± 0.9 *mm*) and the average sum of all moved distances was 4.9 *mm* (± 1.9 *mm*). The tracked movement was corrected by summing successive images, which were transformed according to the detected motion.

Clinical data is shown in Fig. 4 and 5. All MRI volumes were registered to the USCT results so that direct spatial correspondence of the slices was archived [24].

Fig. 4 (left) shows native MRI slices and USCT reflectivity slices of a healthy patient to indicate the similarities of some tissue structures, Fig. 4 (right) the comparison of MRI and USCT reflectivity of a breast with an intact silicone implant. Fig. 5 shows cancer cases: for both cases registered MRI subtraction volumes are shown, indicating the tumor positions by a high content of contrast agent. The left case shows USCT reflectivity superposed with color-coded speed of sound and the right superposed with speed of sound tresholded at 1500 *m/s*. In both cases areas of high speed of sound in red are present at the approximaly same positions as high amounts of contrast agent in the MRIs.

4 Conclusion and future work

We developed an optimized, unfocused 3D USCT with approximately isotropic 3D PSF and presented first images which demonstrate the performance of the system. We realized a sparse 3D USCT setup, resulting in homogeneous illumination, and nearly isotropic 3D PSF.

Image reconstructions with a wire and a clinical phantom confirm this: Currently, the mean FWHM in three dimensions is 0.24 *mm* with low dimensional and spatial deviation. The contrast of the reconstructed 3D volume of a breast phantom is very satisfactory in spite of our sparse aperture. The resolution is comparable to the high-quality MRI volume.

It seems that speed of sound is at the current state the most indicating modality for cancer. The spatial resolution of speed of sound and attenuation is currently limited by the ray based reconstruction algorithm in the range of 5 to 12 *mm*. Yet, this needs further evaluation. More complex reconstruction methods for transmission tomography leading to higher resolution are under development.

Patient positioning is crucial for imaging with our system. Displacements in the (transversal) $x - y$ plane cause the illumination of the breast to vary strongly. Displacement in z (antero-posterior) direction leads to suboptimal coverage of the breast; the proximal part of the breast is then not imaged. Patient motion seems to be a minor problem; no definite movements between reconstructions of the single aperture positions could be detected. Breathing movement of the patients seems to have no effect on the images of the breast. The duration of the now improved data acquisition to 6 min per breast seemed to be acceptable for the patients. The process of breast examination with USCT was described as relatively comfortable by the patients.

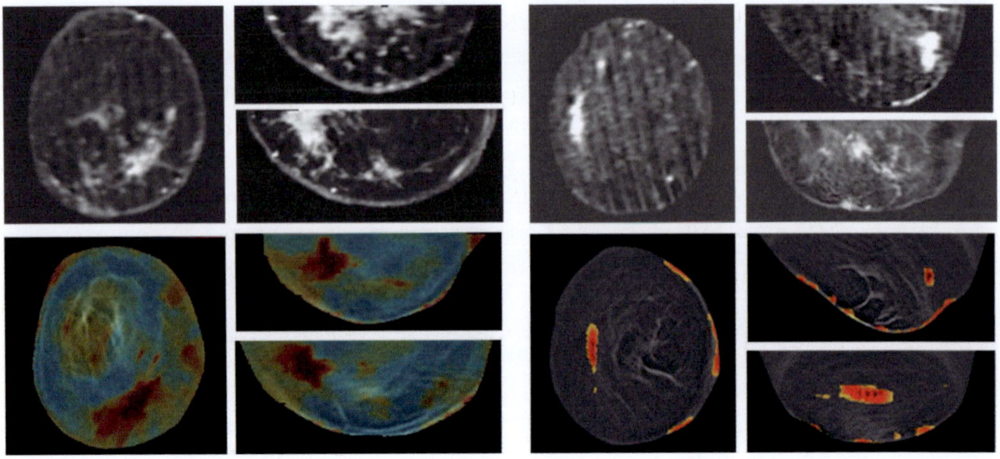

Figure 5: Top row: Registered MRI subtraction slices in planar, sagittal and transversal planes. Bottom row: USCT fusion slices at same positions. Left: 64-year-old patient with a large breast cancer in the left breast. Speed of sound is color coded and superposed on the reflectivity volume. Red colors indicate high speed of sound. Right: 74-year-old patient with breast cancer in the left breast. Speed of sound is thresholded at 1500 *m/s* and overlaid on the reflectivity volume.

The next step in this work is to carry out a large clinical study and built a new 3D USCT system with higher contrast for reflection and position resolution for transmission tomography, shorter data acquisition time and a better access to the chest wall.

References

[1] H. Schomberg, *An improved approach to reconstructive ultrasound tomography*, J. Phys. D: Appl. Phys. 11, 1978.

[2] M. Nguyen, H. Bressmer, et al., *Improvements in ultrasound transmission computed tomography*, Proc. European Conference on Engineering and Medicine, pp. 189190, 1993.

[3] M. Ashfaq, and H. Ermert, *A new approach towards ultrasonic transmission tomography with a standard ultrasound system*, Proc. IEEE UFFC Symp., vol. 3, pp. 184851, 2004.

[4] S. Mensah, P. Lasaygues, E. Debieu, and E. Franceschini, *ANAIS: An ultrasound mammograph*, Journal of the Acoustical Society of America, vol. 123, no. 5, pp. 30023002, 2008.

[5] R. Stotzka, J. Würfel, T.O. Müller, and H. Gemmeke, *Medical imaging by ultrasound computer tomography*, Proc. SPIE Med. Imag., pp. 110-119, 2002.

[6] N. Duric, P. Littrup, P. Chandiwala-Mody, C. Li, S. Schmidt, L. Myc, O. Rama, L. Bey-Knight, J. Lupinacci, B. Ranger, A. Szczepanski, and E. West, *In-vivo imaging results with ultrasound tomography: Report on an ongoing study at the Karmanos Cancer Institute*, Proc. SPIE Med. Imag., vol. 7629, pp. 76290M, 2010.

[7] J. Wiskin, D. Borup, S. Johnson, M. Berggren, D. Robinson, J. Smith, J. Chen, Y. Parisky, J. Klock, *Inverse scattering and refraction corrected reflection for breast cancer imaging*, Proc. SPIE Med. Imag., vol. 7629, pp. 76290K, 2010.

[8] G. Schwarzenberg, M. Zapf, and N.V. Ruiter, *Aperture optimization for 3D ultrasound computer tomography*, Proc. IEEE UFFC Symp., pp. 1820-1823, 2007.

[9] J.F. Greenleaf, R.C. Bahn: *Clinical Imaging with Transmissive Ultrasonic Computerized Tomography*, IEEE Transactions on Biomedical Engineering 28(2), 177–185, 1981.

[10] A. Kopmann, T. Bergmann, H. Gemmeke, M. Howe, M. Kleifges, A. Menshikov, D. Tcherniakhovski, J.F. Wilkerson, and S. Wuestling, *FPGA-based DAQ system for multi-channel detectors*, Proc. IEEE NSS MIC, 2008.

[11] N.V. Ruiter, M. Zapf, T. Hopp, and H. Gemmeke, *Experimental evaluation of noise generated by grating lobes for a sparse 3D ultrasound computer tomography system*, Proc. SPIE Med. Imaging, 2013.

[12] F. Simonetti, L. Huang, and N. Duric, *On the sampling of wave fields with circular ring apertures*, Journal of applied physics, vol. 101, 2007.

[13] F. Simonetti, and L. Huang, *Synthetic aperture diffraction tomography for three-dimensional imaging*, Proc. R. Soc. A, 465, 2009.

[14] E. Kretzek, and N.V. Ruiter, *GPU based 3D SAFT reconstruction including phase aberration*, Proc. SPIE 9040, Medical Imaging 2014: Ultrasonic Imaging and Tomography, pages 90400W (2014).

[15] E. Kretzek, T. Hopp, and N.V. Ruiter, *GPU-based 3D SAFT reconstruction including attenuation correction*, Proc. SPIE 9419, Medical Imaging 2015: Ultrasonic Imaging and Tomography, pages 94190E (2015).

[16] R. Dapp, M. Zapf, and N.V. Ruiter, et al., *Geometry Independent Speed of Sound Reconstruction for 3D USCT Using Apriori Informatio*n, Proc. IEEE UFFC Symp., pp. 1403-1406, 2011.

[17] E. Kretzek, M. Zapf, M. Birk, H. Gemmeke, and N.V. Ruiter, *GPU based acceleration of 3D USCT image reconstruction with efficient integration into MATLAB*, Proc. SPIE Med. Imag. 8675 (2013) 86750O.

[18] N.V. Ruiter, E. Kretzek, M. Zapf, T. Hopp, and H. Gemmeke, *Time of flight interpolated synthetic aperture focusing technique*, Proc. SPIE 10139, Medical Imaging 2017: Ultrasonic Imaging and Tomography, 101390Q (2017).

[19] T. Hopp, R. Dapp, M. Zapf, E. Kretzek, H. Gemmeke, and N.V. Ruiter, *Registration of 3D ultrasound computer tomography and MRI for evaluation of tissue correspondences*, Progress in Biomedical Optics and Imaging - Proceedings of SPIE, 2015.

[20] T. Hopp, N. Duric, and N.V. Ruiter, *Image Fusion of Ultrasound Computer Tomography Volumes with X-Ray Mammograms using a Biomechanical Model Based 2D/3D Registration*, Computerized Medical Imaging and Graphics, 40, 2014.

[21] N.V. Ruiter, M. Zapf, and H. Gemmeke, *Evaluation of 3D point spread function of a semi-ellipsoidal ultrasound computer tomography system*, Proc. IEEE UFFC Symp., 2011.

[22] N.V. Ruiter, M. Zapf, T. Hopp, R. Dapp, and H. Gemmeke, *Optimization of the aperture and the transducer characteristics of a 3D Ultrasound Computer Tomography System,* Proc. SPIE Medical Imaging: Ultrasonic Imaging and Tomography, 2014.

[23] N.V. Ruiter, T. Hopp, M. Zapf, E. Kretzek, H. Gemmeke, *Analysis of patient movement during 3D USCT data acquisition*, Proc. SPIE Med. Imag. 9790, 97900A, 2016.

[24] T. Hopp, L. Sroba, M. Zapf, R. Dapp, E. Kretzek, H. Gemmeke, and N.V. Ruiter, *Breast Imaging with 3D Ultrasound Computer Tomography: Results of a First In-vivo Study in Comparison to MRI Images*, H. Fujita, T. Hara, and C. Muramatsu (Eds.): IWDM 2014, LNCS 8539, pp. 72–79, 2014.

Breast Tissue Characterization with Sound Speed and Tissue Stiffness

Cuiping Li[1,2], Gursharan Singh Sandhu[1], Michael Boone[1], Neb Duric[1,2], Peter Littrup[1-4], Mark Sak[1], Kenneth Bergman[1]

[1]*Delphinus Medical Technologies, Inc., Novi, MI, USA,*
E-Mail: cli@delphinusmt.com
[2]*Department of Oncology, Wayne State University, Detroit, MI., USA,*
[3]*Department of Radiology, Wayne State University, Detroit, MI., USA,*
[4]*Ascension Crittenton Hospital, Rochester, MI, USA*

Abstract

Mammography is not sufficiently effective for women with dense breast tissue. At least in North America and Europe, womenwith dense breasts appear to be at much higher risk for developing breast cancer. Consequently, many breast cancers go undetected at a treatable stage. Improved cancer detection and characterization for women with dense breast tissue is urgently needed. Our clinical study has shown that ultrasound tomography (UST) is an emerging technique that moves beyond B-mode imaging by its transmission capabilities. Transmission ultrasound provides additional tissue parameters such as sound speed, attenuation, and tissue stiffness information. For women with dense breasts, these parameters can be used to assist in detecting malignant masses within glandular or fatty tissue and differentiating malignant and benign masses. This paper focuses on the use of waveform ultrasound sound speed imaging and tissue stiffness information generated using transmission data to characterize different breast tissues and breast masses. In-vivo examples will be given to assess its effectiveness.

Keywords: Sound speed, stiffness, spiculation, BIRADS category

1 Introduction

SomoInsight was a breast screening study that used whole breast ultrasound as a supplement to mammography. It demonstrated that whole breast ultrasound plus mammography outperformed mammography alone [1], leading to the first FDA approval for ultrasound screening for breast cancer. However, one drawback of ultrasound screening is that the call back rate increases significantly (up to a factor of 2 in case of the SomoInsight study) due to lack of efficient lesion characterization [2].

Ultrasound tomography (UST) is an emerging technique that moves beyond B-mode imaging by its transmission capabilities [3-18]. Complementary to B-mode imaging that uses pulse echo signals, transmission ultrasound takes advantage of transmitted signals to provide additional characterization by measuring tissue parameters such as sound speed (SS), attenuation and stiffness which not only can potentially improve detection of subtle suspicious masses but also can help differentiate lesions.

In this study, we are going to illustrate the ability of SoftVue's waveform SS and stiffness image to render a variety of breast tissue and masses. We analyzed in vivo breast sound speed and tissue stiffness images to demonstrate SS and stiffness features for different breast tissues and unique signatures for a variety of breast masses. We present results from our analysis and discuss the implications of these results for clinical breast imaging.

The purpose of this study is to demonstrate the efficacy of SoftVue to characterize breast masses with SS and tissue stiffness color mapping, aiming at additional lesion characterization for possible reduction in call back rates.

2 Method

The SoftVue system utilizes a ring-shaped ultrasound transducer that acquires both backscattered signals and transmitted signals [19]. Backscattered signals are used to produce SoftVue reflection images (B-mode), while transmission signals are used to reconstruct tissue SS, attenuation and stiffness distribution. The resulting tissue stiffness images are color coded and overlaid on the reflection images. All these parameters can be used to assist characterization of breast tissue and breast masses.

Validation of SoftVue tissue stiffness images to assist breast mass characterization has been shown [2], where one anthropomorphic breast phantom was used for initial technique validation, and 11 in vivo breast masses' stiffness images were compared with the standard elastography measurements. In this study, we focused on using SoftVue's SS image and tissue stiffness images to help detection and characterization of breast tissue and masses. Our measuring metric for SS imaging are based on both the quantitative SS values and BI-RADS criteria (Table 1) [19]. Different mass boundary scores are sketched in Figure 1. We use stiffness imaging to addresses potential improved characterization of subtle suspicious masses. The method is illustrated in Table 2. A total of 15 in vivo breasts were imaged, representing a variety of breast lesions in patients whose breast density ranges from fatty to dense.

Mass/Tissue Type			
	Mass/Tissue Shape	**Mass Margin**	**SS Value**
Cyst	Oval/round	Well circumscribed with distinct margin	Cyst: similar to water SS
Fibroadenoma	usually oval	Usually circumscribed	Fibroadenoma: similar or higher than water SS
Cancer	Irregular	Microlobulated, Indistinct, angular, spiculated	Cancer: Varies, usually greater than water SS and dense parenchyma.
Fat	Any shape	n/a	Less that water SS

Table 1: Quantative SS and BI-RADS Criteria for Different Masses

Mass/Tissue Type	Possible measurements
Cyst	Soft (bluer than background on average)
Fibroadenoma	Mixed (can be stiff or soft)
Cancer	Stiff (redder than background on average)
Fatty Tissue	Soft (blueish)
Dense Parenchyma	Stiff (generally not as stiff/red as cancer)

Table 2: SoftVue Stiffness Signatures for Different Masses

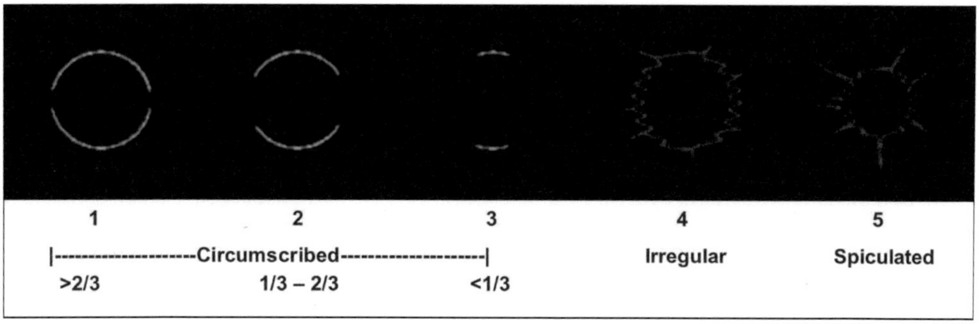

Figure 1: Mass boundary scores: 1-3: well to partially circumscribed; Score 4-5: irregular and spiculated, respectively.

SoftVue's SS and color stiffness images for the selected masses were analyzed and compared to the corresponding mammogram, standard ultrasound, and/or MRI, depending on their availability. A semi-transparent overlay of the SoftVue color stiffness images on the reflection image of the same coronal slice was used to ease the identification of the region of interest.

3 Results

The above metrics were applied to 15 in vivo breast images reconstructed with the SoftVue system. Results are summarized in Table 3. All 5 cancers were characterized as stiff or moderately stiff (red) with mean SS range from 1530-1571 m/s. Four fibroadenomas showed mixed stiffness (range of colors), one was stiff. Average SS for these 5 fibroadenomas spans from 1534 m/s to 1563 m/s, which is greatly overlapping with the above cancers' SS. All 4 cysts had mean SS from 1520 to 1534, which is very close to water bath SS.

A few examples are presented below. A highly spiculated IDC is shown at 6 o'clock in figure 2 with an average SS of 1550 m/s and is stiffer than the surrounding dense breast tissue (Figure 2d). Spiculations of this IDC are better presented in the zoom-in view (figure 2c). In standard B-mode (figure 2a), this mass shows strong shadowing, which indicates high attenuation. Figure 3 shows a dense breast slice with a well circumscribed oval shaped fibroadenoma at 10:00 o'clock. In figure 3c we can clearly see the wall of the fibroadenoma. Figure 3d shows moderate stiffness compared to adjacent dense parenchyma and an average SS of 1552 m/s. Again, standard B-model image is presented in figure 3a for reference. An extremely dense breast slice is presented in figure 4, which has a well circumscribed cyst at 1:00 o'clock with an average SS of 1528 m/s. The stiffness image in figure 4d indicates that it is soft. In all three examples, fatty breast tissue has the lowest SS among normal breast tissue and breast masses, while breast parenchyma generally has higher SS than cyst.

4 Discussion

The stiffness distribution of breast masses shows that cancers are generally stiffer compared to surrounding tissue, while cysts appear soft. Fibroadenomas can be either soft, stiff or mixed of both. This trend is consistent with properties shown in other modalities. SS values for cancers and fibroadenomas are greatly overlapping, while, as expected, cyst SS is consistently similar to water SS. The combination of SS, stiffness and mass margin values demonstrates great potential to characterize benign from malignant breast masses.

However, there are some outlier cases that suggest we need additional pathology correlations. In this study, we analyzed two outlier cases. One case has scar tissue in the breast and the other case has benign non-fibroadenoma and non-cystic findings. The scar tissue demonstrates spiculated boundary with high SS and stiffness. The benign finding in case 9 in Table

3 shows well circumscribed boundary, high SS and stiffness. SS and stiffness images for both cases are presented in figure 5a and 5b, respectively.

Case #	Breast Density	Lesion Pathology	Average Lesion Size (cm)	Clock position	Mass Margin	Average Lesion SS compared to water SS	SoftVue stiffness assessment
1	Hetero-geneous	Cancer (ILC)	0.93	5:00	5	greater	Stiff
2	Scattered	Cancer (IDC)	3.0	11:00	4	greater	Stiff
3	Dense	Cancer (IDC)	2	3:00	4	greater	Moder-ately Stiff
4	Heteroge-neous	Cancer (IDC)	1.23	6:00	5	greater	Stiff
5	fatty	Cancer (DCIS)		11:00	4	Moderately greater	stiff
6	Scattered	Fibroadeno-mas	0.97, 1.38	4:00, 11:00	2, 1	Greater, moderately greater	Mixed, Stiff
7	Dense	Fibroadenoma	1.89	10:00	1	greater	Mixed
8	Heteroge-neous	Scar		4:00	5	greater	Stiff
9	Heteroge-neous	Solid Benign Mass		12:00	2	greater	Stiff
10	Dense	Fibroade-noma	2.19	3:00	2	moderately greater	Mixed
11	Dense	Fibroade-noma		6:00	2	greater	mixed
12	Dense	Cyst		10:00	2	similar	soft
13	Extremely dense	Cyst		1:00	2	similar	Soft
14	Heteroge-neous	Cyst	1.66, 1.53	6:00, 9:00	2, 3	similar, slightly greater	Moderately soft
15	Heteroge-neous	Cyst	3.7	8:00	2	similar	Soft

Table 3: Summary table for all 15 cases

5 Conclusions

Our in vivo analyses show that, in addition to standard reflection ultrasound and margin-boundary considerations, combinations of SS and tissue stiffness information provide unique metrics to assist detection and characterization of different breast tissue and masses.

We have established detection/diagnosis metrics for waveform breast SS and through-transmission rendered tissue stiffness. A few examples demonstrate that a combination of SS and tissue stiffness has great potential to assist detection and characterization of different breast tissues and breast masses.

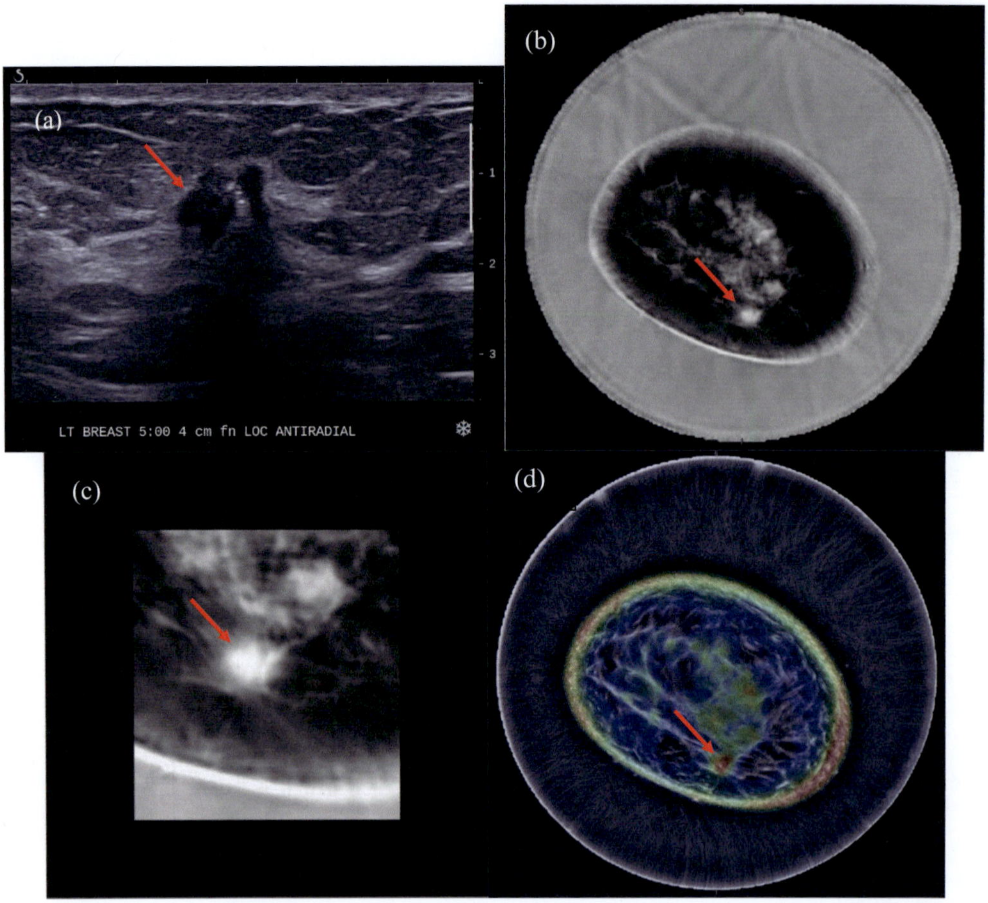

Figure 2: Coronal slice with an IDC at 6:00 o'clock (red arrows). (a) Standard B-mode image for the IDC; (b) SoftVue SS image; (c) Zoomed-in SS view for the IDC; (d) Corresponding color-coded tissue stiffness overlay on reflection image (from blue to red color ~ soft to stiff).

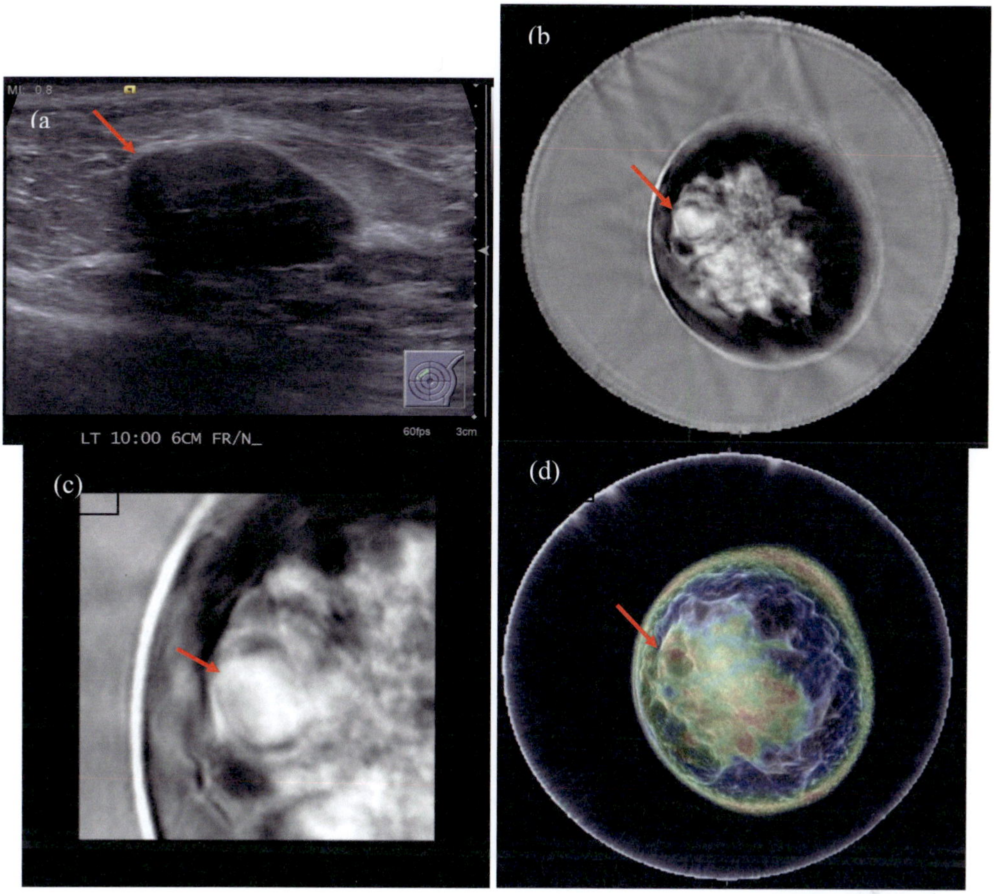

Figure 3: Coronal slice with a fibroadenoma at 10:00 o'clock (red arrows). (a) Standard B-mode image for the Fibroadenoma; (b) SoftVue SS image; (c) Zoomed-in SS view for the fibroadenoma; (d) Corresponding color-coded tissue stiffness overlay on reflection image.

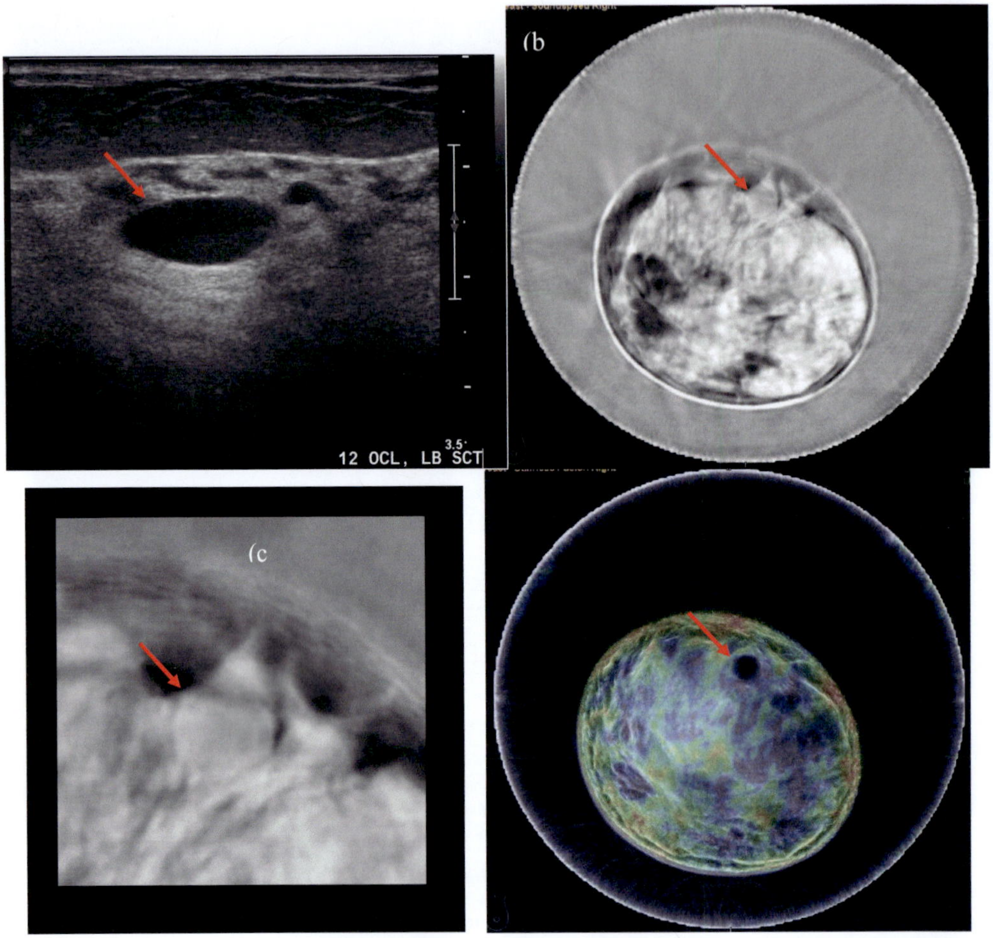

Figure 4: Coronal slice with a cyst at 1:00 o'clock (red arrows). (a) Standard B-mode image for the cyst; (b) SoftVue SS image; (c) Zoomed-in SS view for the cyst; (d) Corresponding color-coded tissue stiffness information overlay on reflection image.

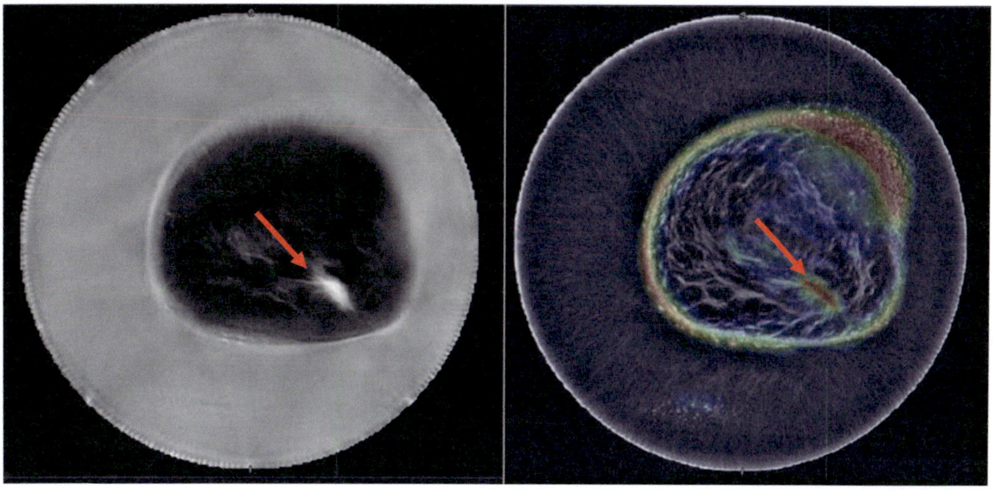

(a)

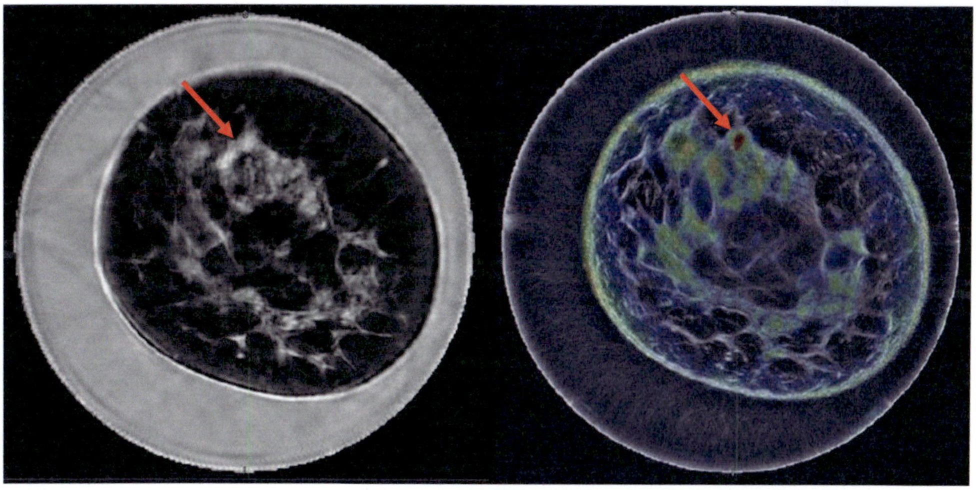

(b)

Figure 5: (a) Scar tissue. Left: SS; Right: Stiffness. (b)Benign finding – probable inspissated cyst. Left: SS; Right: Stiffness. (Red arrows indicate masses).

References

[1] Brem, R. F., Tabár, L., Duffy, S. W., Inciardi, M. F., Guingrich, J. A., Hashimoto, B. E., ... & Miller, D. P. (2014). Assessing improvement in detection of breast cancer with three-dimensional automated breast US in women with dense breast tissue: The SomoInsight Study. Radiology.

[2] Duric N, Littrup P., Li C., Roy O., Schmidt S., Seamans J., Wallen A. and Bei-Knight L.: Whole breast tissue characterization with ultrasound tomography, Proc. SPIE 9419, Medical Imaging, 94190G (2015).

[3] Carson PL, Meyer CR, Scherzinger AL, Oughton TV. Breast imaging in coronal planes with simultaneous pulse echo and transmission ultrasound. Science 1981, Dec 4;214(4525):1141-3.

[4] Andre MP, Janee HS, Martin PJ, Otto GP, Spivey BA, Palmer DA, "High-speed data acquisition in a diffraction tomography system employing large-scale toroidal arrays," International Journal of Imaging Systems and Technology 1997; Vol. 8, Issue 1:137-147.

[5] Johnson SA, Borup DT, Wiskin JW, Natterer F, Wuebbling F, Zhang Y, Olsen C. Apparatus and Method for Imaging with Wavefields using Inverse Scattering Techniques. United States Patent 6,005,916 (1999).

[6] Marmarelis VZ, Kim T, Shehada RE. Proceedings of the SPIE: Medical Imaging; Ultrasonic Imaging and Signal Processing 2003, Paper 5035-6.

[7] Liu D-L, Waag RC. "Propagation and backpropagation for ultrasonic wavefront design," IEEE Trans. on Ultras.

[8] Ferro. and Freq. Contr. 1997;44(1):1-13.

[9] Gemmeke, H and Ruiter, N. “3D ultrasound computer tomography for medical imaging”. Nuclear instruments and methods in Physics Research Section A: Accelerators, Spectrometers, Detectors and Associated Equipment, vol. 580, no. 2, pp 1057-1065, 2007.

[10] Nicole V. Ruiter, Georg Göbel, Lutz Berger, Michael Zapf and Hartmut Gemmeke, "Realization of an optimized 3D USCT", Proc. SPIE 7968, 796805 (2011)

[11] Duric N, Littrup P, Poulo L, Babkin A, Pevzner R, Holsapple E, Rama O, Glide C. Detection of Breast Cancer With Ultrasound Tomography: First Results with the Computerized Ultrasound Risk Evaluation (C.U.R.E) Prototype. Medical Physics Feb 2007; Vol 34 (2), pp. 773-785.

[12] Glide-Hurst C, Duric N, Littrup P. Volumetric breast density evaluation from ultrasound tomography images. Med Phys. 2008; Vol. 35, Issue 9, pp. 3988-3997.

[13] S. Schmidt, Z. Huang, N. Duric, C. Li and O. Roy. “Modification of Kirchhoff migration with variable sound speed and attenuation for acoustic imaging of media and application to tomographic imaging of the breast:. Med. Phys. 38, 998 (2011).

[14] C. Li, N. Duric, P. Littrup, L. Huang. In vivo Breast Sound-Speed Imaging with Ultrasound Tomography.Ultrasound in Medicine & Biology, Volume 35, Issue 10, Pages 1615-1628. 2009.

[15] Ranger B, Littrup P, Duric N, Chandiwala-Mody P, Li C, Schmidt S and Lupinacci J. Breast ultrasound tomography versus magnetic resonance imaging for clinical display of anatomy and tumor rendering: Preliminary results. AJR Am J Roentgenol Jan 2012; 198(1):233-9.

[16] Duric, N. et al. Ultrasound Tomography Systems for Medical Imaging, in Emerging Imaging in Medical Diagnosis and Therapy. 2012. Taylor &Francis, Editors: Mark A. Anastasio; Patrick La Riviere. CRC Press.

[17] Duric, N., Boyd, N., Littrup, P., Sak, M., Myc, L., Li, C., ... & Albrecht, T. (2013). Breast density measurements with ultrasound tomography: A comparison with film and digital mammography. Medical physics, 40, 013501

[18] Duric, Neb, Peter Littrup, Cuiping Li, Olivier Roy, Steven Schmidt, Xiaoyang Cheng, John Seamans, Andrea Wallen, and Lisa Bey-Knight. "Breast imaging with SoftVue: initial clinical evaluation." In SPIE Medical Imaging, pp. 90400V-90400V. International Society for Optics and Photonics, 2014.

[19] http://pubs.rsna.org/doi/pdf/10.1148/rg.305095144

Postprocessing workflow of 3D USCT: bridging the gap to the clinic

T. Hopp, M. Zapf, H. Gemmeke, and N.V. Ruiter

Karlsruhe Institute of Technology, Institute for Data Processing and Electronics, Karlsruhe, Germany
E-mail: torsten.hopp@kit.edu

Abstract

As first USCT systems are approaching clinical application, it is an essential task to prepare the reconstructed images for intuitive diagnosis and conform to clinical standards. We describe our post-processing workflow consisting of automated breast segmentation, image fusion, DICOM export and the methods to transfer images to the clinic. The segmentation was tested with 14 images resulting in an average surface deviation of 2.7 mm from semi-automatically segmented images. Modalities were fused applying empiric thresholds for sound speed and attenuation. The exported DICOM files were checked for consistency and tested with open source and commercial DICOM viewers. A teleradiology connection to University Medicine Mannheim was established based on the DICOM e-mail concept. We consider segmentation and image fusion as essential steps for intuitive diagnosis. Using medical standards like DICOM and PACS allows convenient integration into clinical workflows.

Keywords: Image processing, Segmentation, Image fusion, DICOM

1 Introduction

First Ultrasound tomography (USCT) systems are approaching clinical application, e.g. [1, 2]. At Karlsruhe Institute of Technology (KIT) we are developing the world's first full 3D USCT systems, which we are currently testing in clinical trials [3]. Bridging the gap from a purely research system to a clinically applicable system, not only requires the system aspects like fast data acquisition and fast image reconstruction, but also the clinical workflow related aspects in order to prepare the images for intuitive diagnosis, to conform with clinical standards and to seamlessly integrate the new modality into the clinical workflow.

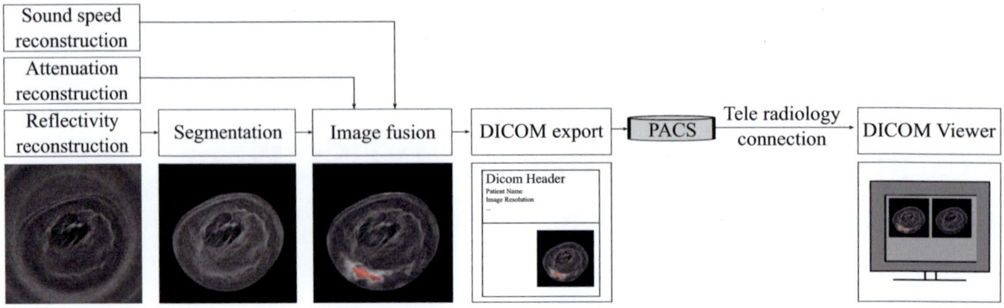

Figure 1: Postprocessing workflow of the KIT 3D USCT.

In this paper we describe our post-processing workflow (Figure 1) for USCT images which consists of the following processing steps:

1. Automated segmentation of the breast from the background in order to remove the water background and artifacts outside the breast like aperture reflections.
2. Fusion of the three imaging modalities (reflectivity, sound speed, attenuation) to enable intuitive diagnosis at a glance.
3. Export of the image data into DICOM format to conform with clinical standards.
4. Transfer of image data to the clinic.

2 Methods

2.1 KIT 3D USCT

The KIT 3D USCT consists of a semi-ellipsoidal aperture with a diameter of 26 cm and a depth of 16 cm. The surface of the aperture is equipped with 628 dedicated ultrasound emitters and 1413 receivers which are grouped into 157 transducer array systems (TAS). Approximately spherical waves are emitted by a single ultrasound transducer at a center frequency of 2.5 MHz (approximately 50% bandwidth) while all other receivers acquire the reflected and transmitted signals. Repeating the measurement process for all sender-receiver-combinations results in approximately 890,000 signals, so-called Amplitdue scans (A-scans). Rotational and translational motion of the aperture create further virtual transducer positions to increase the amount of A-scans further. Approximately 10 million A-scans are currently acquired during patient imaging in our clinical studies for one breast volume. From the acquired signal data, transmission volumes are reconstructed using a ray-based algebraic reconstruction technique (ART) [4, 5] and reflection images are reconstructed using Synthetic Aperture Focusing Technique (SAFT) [3].

2.2 Breast segmentation

Though huge datasets with up to 10 million A-scans and 40GB raw data per breast are acquired, the aperture is still sparse. Due to the sparseness, reflection images typically suffer from grating lobe artifacts, i.e. the water surrounding the breast is not imaged as homogeneous background. For diagnosis and further processing like image registration, volume measurement, etc., segmentation of the breast from the background is essential.

The segmentation problem to be solved is the detection of the breast edge, which appears bright in the reflectivity images due to the change in acoustical impedance between water and skin. We developed an automated breast segmentation [6] based on three-dimensional active contours.

Active contours can be described as an energy minimization problem (equation 1) according to *Kass et al.* [7] as follows:

$$E(t_k) = w_{int} \int_0^1 E_{int}(x(s,t_k))\,ds + w_{ext} \int_0^1 E_{ext}(x(s,t_k)) \rightarrow \min \tag{1}$$

where $x(s,t_k)$ describes a parametric curve depending on the spatial parameter s and time point t_k, and w_{int} respectively w_{ext} represent weighting factors for the internal energy E_{int} and the external energy E_{ext}. The internal energy describes the smoothness of the parametric curve's geometric shape by introducing an inner tension using the first and second order derivatives. The external energy estimates the proximity of the parametric curve to edges in the image by computing the image gradient at the position of the parametric curve. The minimization problem is tackled by an iterative deformation of the parametric curve based on an Euler-Lagrange modeling [6].

In our formulation we use gradient vector flow (GVF) [8] for computation of the external energy in order to enhance the capture range of contours in the images. As SAFT images depict changes in the impedance we expect high image intensity values at the boundary of the breast, which the method should detect. Consequently we code the intensity information as additional external energy term. Moreover, the 3D USCT aperture characteristics cause a spatially varying contrast of tissue boundaries compared to the water background. Therefore an additional weighting factor is introduced, which depends on the spatial position of the parametric curve. It is determined by the region of interest (ROI) of the 3D USCT, which was previously defined and optimized to produce the optimal illumination, contrast and resolution [9]. The semi-ellipsoidal ROI of the current 3D USCT prototype has dimensions of $10 \times 10 \times 10$cm. The ROI is modeled by a representation of the ROI in a Gaussian filtered image, which additionally delivers weights on the external force for the parametric curve.

The initial parametric curve has a major influence on the active contour algorithm. For 3D USCT the initial parametric curve is discretized to a three dimensional surface polygon mesh.

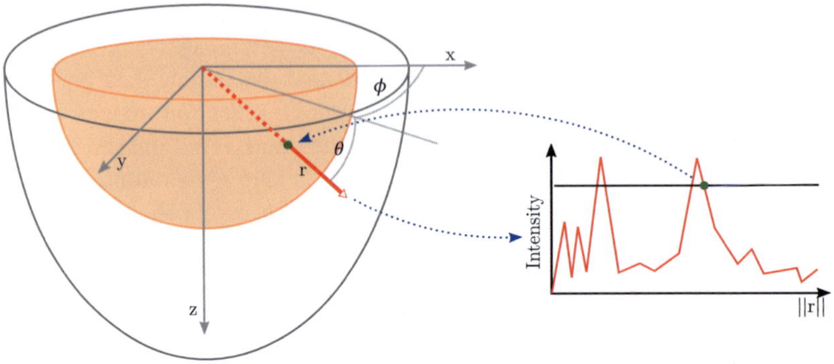

Figure 2: Ray-based detection of the breast surface for initialization of the active contour approach: Along a ray $\vec{r}$ from the center of the USCT aperture intensities are interpolated, resulting in an intensity against radius plot (right). To determine the breast surface reflection, the last occurring intensity peak above a threshold, which is defined by the average intensity of the background, is detected.

Each surface node is generated by a ray based approach as depicted in Figure 2. Image intensities along a ray $\vec{r}$ with elevation angle θ and azimuth angle ϕ and starting at the center of the USCT (red arrow in Figure 2 left) are interpolated from the volume image. Assuming an approximately hemispherical breast shape, the ray thereby intersects the breast boundary approximately normal to the surface. Furthermore assuming that there are no major scattering objects outside the breast, the breast surface is estimated by determining the outermost intensity peak along the ray using a threshold (Figure 2 right). The threshold is chosen by the average intensity of the water background $\bar{I}_{water}$ multiplied with an empirical factor s, which is iteratively decreased from $s = 1.5$ until an intensity value along the ray (I_{ray}) is above the threshold t, i.e. $I_{ray} > t$ with $t = \bar{I}_{water} \cdot s$. The final initial parametric curve is then generated using a polynomial fit to remove outliers from the threshold based surface detection. The purpose is to provide a good first estimate of the position, size and the rough shape of the breast.

The initial parametric curve is iteratively deformed. The iterative process is stopped at a maximum number of iterations, or if the average motion of the parametric curve is smaller than a given tolerance level. The final contour is then used to create a binary segmentation mask which is zero for voxels outside the closed contour. By multiplying the binary segmentation mask voxel-vise with the reconstructed images, the water background can be removed in all three modalities (sound speed, attenuation, reflectivity) as they are imaged in one data acquisition step.

2.3 Image fusion

To facilitate diagnosis we apply an image fusion in order to combine the diagnostic information from all modalities in a single image. The basic idea is to combine high resolution reflectivity images with the quantitative sound speed and attenuation maps. We perform the fusion of two images (sound speed and reflectivity, attenuation and reflectivity) as well as the fusion of all

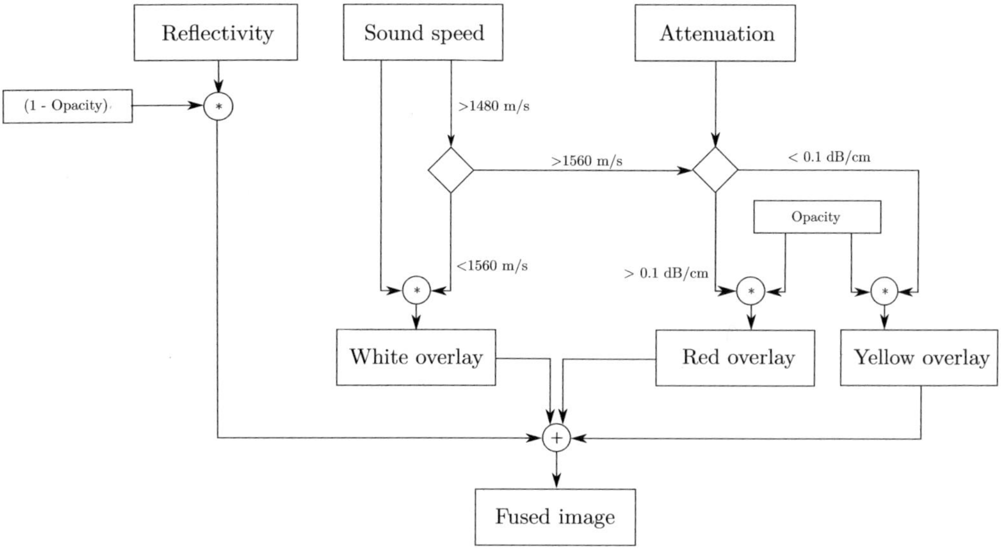

Figure 3: Workflow of the three-modality image fusion, which combines reflectivity with sound speed and attenuation information.

three images. For pair-wise fusion the reflectivity image is rendered as a gray scale background with additional adaption of the contrast by a gray scale windowing. The sound speed map is color-coded in a range between 1300 m/s (blue) to 1600 m/s (dark red). In the same fashion the attenuation map is color-coded in a range between 0 dB/cm (blue) to 1.5 dB/cm (dark red).

To combine all three modalities, several approaches have been proposed, e.g. [10, 11]. Based on our empiric experience with collaborating radiologists we decided to adapt the image fusion developed by *Ranger et al.* [10]. In this method the reflectivity is rendered as gray scale background. An empiric window of sound speed values is used to mask areas with fibroglandular structures and render them overlaid as a cloud like white structure on the reflectivity background. We adapted the method by weighting the opacity of the overlay with the actual sound speed value, i.e. higher sound speeds in the fibroglandular sound speed value window are rendered with less transparency than low sound speed values. Furthermore the method uses a second threshold for the sound speed and a threshold for the attenuation map to mask out a lesion. The attenuation threshold serves as basis to distinguish a benign from a malignant mass. Areas with high sound speeds and high attenuation are therefore rendered as red overlay on the reflectivity background to mark malign lesions, while areas with high sound speed and low attenuation are rendered in yellow to mark benign lesions (Figure 3).

We adapted the thresholds of this method empirically: A sound speed window 1480 m/s to 1560 m/s is used to mask the area of fibroglandular tissue, areas with sound speeds higher than 1560 m/s and attenuation higher than 0.1 dB/cm are considered as malign masses, areas with sound speed higher than 1560 m/s and attenuation lower than 0.1 dB/cm are considered as benign masses.

2.4 Export to DICOM

All segmented and fused images are thereafter exported into the DICOM format, which is a standard for storing and transmitting medical images [12]. DICOM provides a container format which encapsulates the image data together with metadata in a single file. The so-called header holds information about the patient, the image acquisition and image reconstruction. In the KIT 3D USCT case we automatically create the DICOM header by extracting metadata from the data acquisition process (e.g. acquisition date and time, patient position) and the image reconstruction process (e.g. pixel spacing, modality type, windowing levels). The volume dataset is split into slices according to a user selected slicing direction (coronal, transversal, sagittal). Each slice is exported to a single DICOM file without data compression. In case of fused images, the photometric interpretation header tag is set to RGB and the RGB values are exported accordingly.

DICOM uses Information Object Definitions (IOD) to define a standard set of header tags required for certain imaging modalities to conform with the standard. As currently no IOD for USCT images is defined in the DICOM standard, we apply the CT IOD and fill header tags with pseudo values if needed.

The DICOM files are created using the MATLAB image processing toolbox. To evaluate the conformity with the DICOM standard, the exported files are checked with the DICOM validator software "dciodvfy" by *D.A. Clunie* [13]. Visual inspection of the images is carried out using the DICOM viewer RadiAnt [14].

2.5 Data transfer to the clinic

As the image reconstruction for our 3D USCT prototype is in our current clinical study performed on a multi-GPU system at KIT, resulting images need to be transferred to the clinic in order to evaluate the diagnostic information in a concordance study in comparison to MRI. For this purpose we apply the established teleradiology transfer of the clinic. For our current clinical study, the transfer method is based on DICOM e-mails [15]. The architecture of the data exchange infrastructure is depicted in Figure 4. v

After DICOM export the files are automatically send to a local Picture Archiving and Communication System (PACS) using the DICOM Toolkit (DCMTK). We use an installation of the public domain Conquest DICOM software [17] as PACS. From the PACS a data transfer can be triggered. On transfer request the DKON3 software provided by University Medicine Mannheim encrypts the DICOM files using Pretty Good Privacy (PGP), attaches them to an e-mail and sends the e-mail via a mail server to the destination mail server [15]. On the receiver site the e-mail attachments are decrypted and images are sent to the clinic PACS, from which they can be accessed from DICOM viewer workstations.

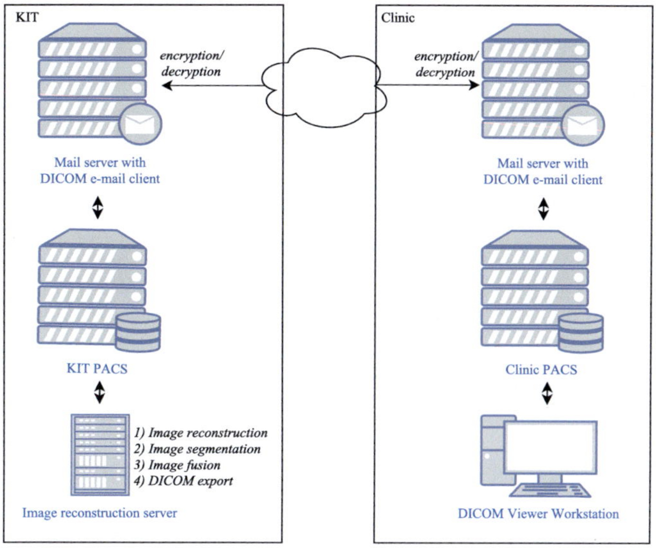

Figure 4: Architecture of the DICOM infrastructure for data transfer to the clinic. At KIT images are reconstructed, segmented, fused and exported to DICOM in a reconstruction server, which send the images to a local PACS. To transfer the data to the clinic, encrypted DICOM e-mails are sent to the destination where they are decrypted and images are transferred to the clinic PACS.

3 Results

The breast segmentation was tested with 14 images from 9 patients. Images were reconstructed with an isotropic pixel resolution of $(0.74\,mm)^3$. A semi-automated segmentation based on edge detection, manual corrections and three-dimensional surface fitting as described in our earlier publication [18] served as ground truth for evaluation. The deviation of both segmented breast surfaces was determined by calculating the mean three-dimensional Euclidean distance of the surface nodes of the active contour to the closest surface voxels of the semi-automated segmentation and vice versa. Both measurements were averaged to get the final deviation metric. Applying our model-based initialization and the traditional active contour approach with GVF but without including USCT aperture characteristics, the average of mean surface distance was 3.2 mm (standard deviation $\pm 1.3\,mm$). By including the USCT aperture characteristics the average of mean surface distances was $2.7\,mm$ ($\pm 1.1\,mm$). These experiments were conducted with a constant initial parameter set.

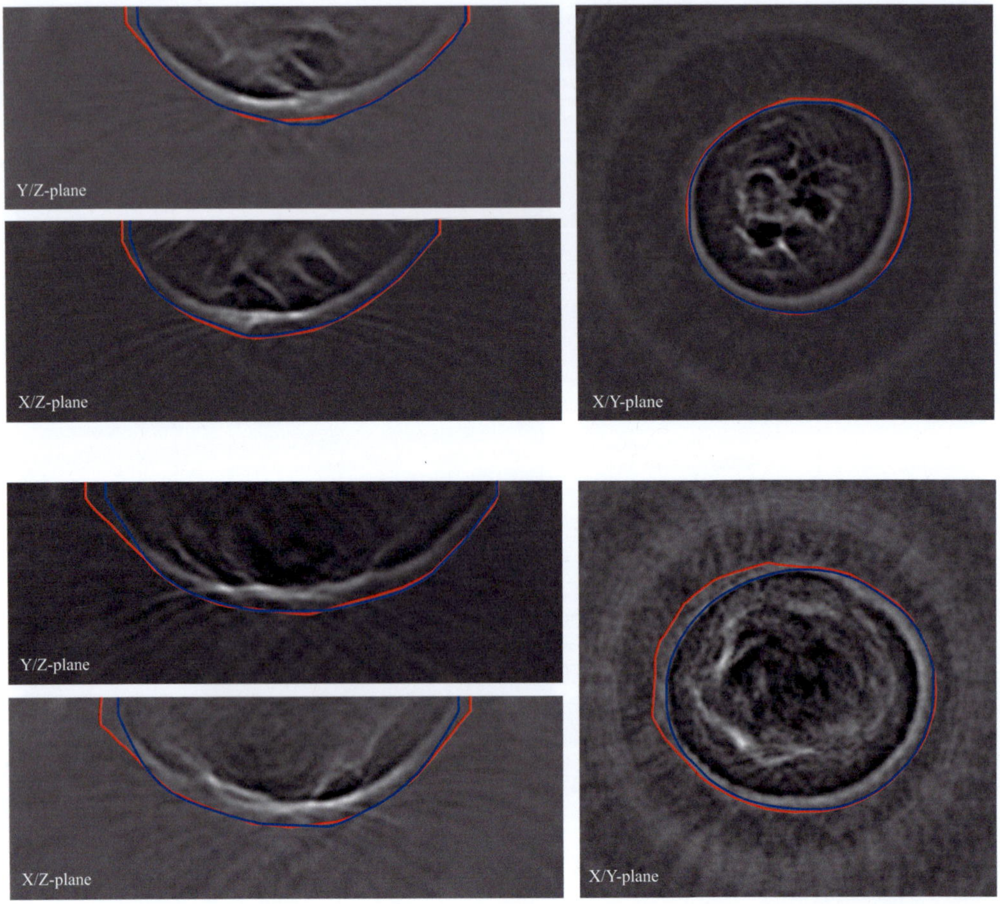

Figure 5: Segmentation result of a patient volume. The blue outline shows the semi-automated segmentation which serves as ground truth for evaluation, the red outline shows the result of the fully automated segmentation. Top images: patient volume reconstructed from signals at ten aperture positions with an average surface deviation of $0.9\,mm$. Bottom images: patient volume reconstructed from signal at four aperture positions with an average surface deviation of $1.5\,mm$

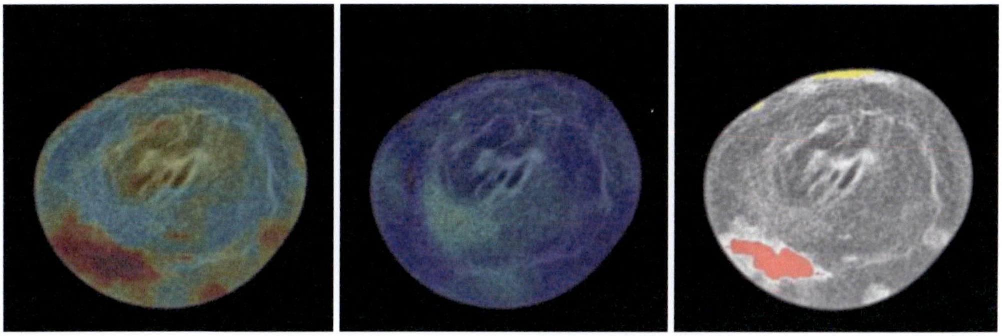

Figure 6: Results for the image fusion methods, from left to right: combination of reflectivity and sound speed, combination of reflectivity and attenuation, combination of all three modalities.

Figures 5 shows segmentation results with patient data. The largest segmentation errors could be observed close to the top of the USCT aperture (Figure 5, top in each image on the left), where the contrast of the breast against the background is decreased significantly due to the aperture geometry. It appeared that varying the threshold for the contour initialization had a major influence on the results. To demonstrate the influence, we changed the threshold parameter once to a different empiric constant for all datasets and manually selected for each dataset the more accurate segmentation. Thereby the average surface distance further decreased to $2.2\,mm$ ($\pm\,1.3\,mm$).

After image fusion with the method described above (Figure 6), the images of our first clinical study with 10 patients were successfully exported to DICOM. The DICOM validation successfully tested the header attributes against the requirements of the IOD, the encoding of data elements, the data element value representation against the DICOM data dictionary and the consistency of attributes.

The PACS installation was tested successfully by automatically transferring the exported DICOM files via DCMTK. The PACS currently holds the anonymized image data of the 10 patients imaged in our first clinical study as well as image data of phantoms imaged with KIT 3D USCT. It is constantly growing by adding the image data of our ongoing second clinical study. The PACS can be accessed at KIT with any DICOM viewer after obtaining appropriate authorization. A visual representation of an exemplary DICOM viewer connected to the local PACS system is given in Figure 7. The images are correctly represented and can be viewed side-by-side with according MRI images. The dialog in Figure 7 (right) shows the attached metadata in the DICOM header.

A teleradiology connection to University Medicine Mannheim was established based on the DICOM e-mail concept and successfully tested by transferring images from KIT to the University Medicine Mannheim and vice versa.

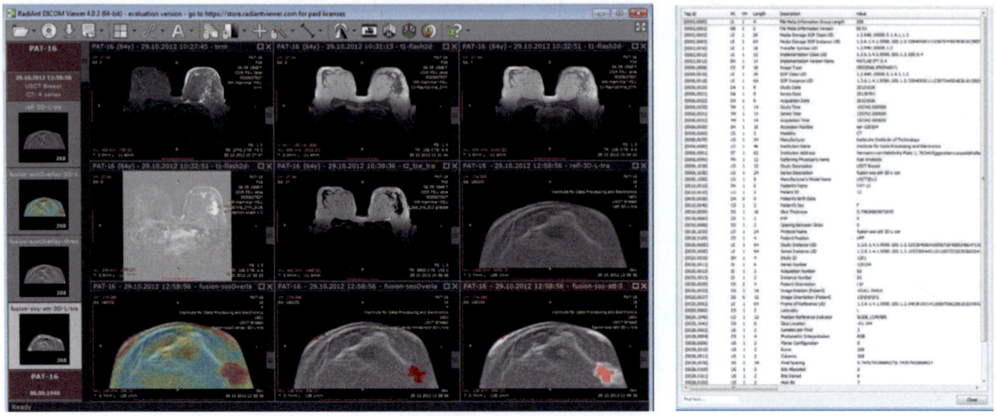

Figure 7: Visual inspection of the exported DICOM files using the RadiAnt DICOM viewer. Left: side-by-side view of USCT images with MR images of the same patient. Right: screenshot of the DICOM header dialog, which provides the attached metadata for a USCT image.

4 Discussion and conclusion

We successfully established a fully automated post-processing workflow to bring 3D USCT closer to clinical application. We consider segmentation and image fusion as an essential steps for intuitive diagnosis which is focused to the most relevant clinical information.

The accuracy achieved with our fully automated segmentation is comparable to a semi-automated segmentation with an average surface deviation of $2.7\,mm$. Based on the successful application to patient data we believe that the segmentation is robust against clinical variability of the imaging process and different anatomies of the breast. To proof this we are planning to extend the evaluation to a larger patient cohort, which will be recruited during our ongoing clinical study.

Using medical standards like DICOM and PACS will allow an easy integration into clinical workflows. By applying the validation software we ensure that the exported DICOM files follow the DICOM standard as close as possible. Yet due to the lack of an appropriate IOD, some header tags have to be filled with pseudo values. This might cause confusion with some DICOM viewer software if the DICOM header is not properly interpreted. In future we propose to extend the DICOM standard by a dedicated IOD fulfilling the metadata requirements of USCT.

In conclusion we believe that the presented work provides essential steps to integrate USCT into clinical workflows, and to establish the imaging method for clinical applicability.

References

[1] N. Duric, P. Littrup, P. Chandiwala-Mody, C. Li, S. Schmidt, L. Myc, O. Rama, L. Bey-Knight, J. Lupinacci, B. Ranger, A. Szczepanski, E. West: In-vivo imaging results with ultrasound tomography: Report on an ongoing study at the Karmanos Cancer Institute. Proc. SPIE Medical Imaging 7629 (2010), 76290M

[2] J. Wiskin, D. Borup, S. Johnson, M. Berggren, D. Robinson, J. Smith, J. Chen, Y. Parisky, J. Klock: Inverse Scattering and Refraction Corrected Reflection for Breast Cancer Imaging Proc. SPIE Medical Imaging 7629 (2010) 76290K

[3] N. Ruiter, M. Zapf, R. Dapp, T. Hopp, W. Kaiser, H. Gemmeke: First Results of Clinical Study with 3D Ultrasound Computer Tomography. Proc. IEEE Ultrasonics Symposium (2013), 651654

[4] R. Dapp, M. Zapf, N. V. Ruiter: Geometry-independent speed of sound reconstruction for 3D USCT using apriori information. Proc. IEEE Ultrasonics Symposium (2011), 14031406

[5] R. Dapp, H. Gemmeke, N. V. Ruiter: Attenuation reconstruction for 3D Ultrasound Computer Tomography. Proc. 19th International Conference on Systems, Signals and Image Processing (IWSSIP) (2012), 484487

[6] T. Hopp, W. You, M. Zapf, W.Y. Tan, H. Gemmeke, N.V. Ruiter: Automated breast segmentation in ultrasound computer tomography SAFT images, Proc. SPIE Medical Imaging 10139 (2017), 101390G

[7] M. Kass, A. Witkin, D. Terzopoulos: Snakes: Active contour models. International Journal of Computer Vision, 1(4), (1988), 321331

[8] C. Xu, J.L. Prince: Snakes, Shapes, and Gradient Vector Flow. IEEE Transactions on Image Processing, 7(3), (1998), 359369

[9] G.F. Schwarzenberg, M. Zapf, N.V. Ruiter: Aperture Optimization for 3D Ultrasound Computer Tomography. Proc. IEEE Ultrasonics Symposium (2007), 1820-1823

[10] B. Ranger, P. Littrup, N. Duric, P. Chandiwala-Mody, C. Li, S. Schmidt, J. Lupinacci: Breast ultrasound tomography versus MRI for clinical display of anatomy and tumor rendering: preliminary results. American Journal of Roentgenology, 198(1) (2012), 233239

[11] T. Hopp, M. Zapf, E. Kretzek, J. Henrich, A. Tukalo, H. Gemmeke, C. Kaiser, J. Knaudt, N.V. Ruiter: 3D Ultrasound Computer Tomography: Update from a clinical study. Proc. SPIE Medical Imaging 9790 (2017), 97909

[12] NEMA PS3 / ISO 12052, Digital Imaging and Communications in Medicine (DICOM) Standard, National Electrical Manufacturers Association, Rosslyn, VA, USA (available free at http://medical.nema.org/)

[13] D.A. Clunie: DICOM Validator - dciodvfy, available online at http://www.dclunie.com/dicom3tools/dciodvfy.html

[14] Medixant: RadiAnt DICOM Viewer, available online at https://www.radiantviewer.com/

[15] G. Weisser, U. Engelmann, S. Ruggiero, A. Runa, A. Schrter, S. Baur, M. Walz: Teleradiology applications with DICOM-e-mail. European Radiology 17 (2007), 1331-1340.

[16] The OFFIS computer science institute: DCMTK - DICOM Toolkit, available online at http://dicom.offis.de/dcmtk.php.en
[17] M. van Kerk, L. Zijp: Conquest DICOM software. Netherlands Cancer Institute. available online at https://ingenium.home.xs4all.nl/dicom.html.
[18] T. Hopp, M. Zapf, N.V. Ruiter: Segmentation of 3D Ultrasound Computer Tomography Reflection Images using Edge Detection and Surface Fitting, Proc. SPIE Medical Imaging 9040 (2014), 904066

Tissue Characterization With Ultrasound Tomography Machine Learning

G. Sandhu[1], P. Littrup[1,2,3], M. Sak[1], C. Li[1], and N. Duric[1,2]

[1]*Delphinus Medical Technologies Inc., Novi, United States*
E-mail: gsandhu@delphinusmt.com
[2]*Wayne State University, Detroit, United States*
[3]*Ascension Crittenton Hospital, Rochester, United States*

Abstract

Ultrasound tomography generates several different imaging stacks. This includes reflection, sound speed, and attenuation images. The images visualize different acoustic parameters which are useful for assessing different types of breast diseases or tissues. Typically, a radiologist views the images to determine a diagnosis for a patient. However, a learning algorithm can be trained to predict diagnoses based on the features contained within the image. Thus, we present a method to extract features from an ultrasound tomography image and label them. The extracted features with the associated label of benign or malignant are fed to a machine learning algorithm which trains a classifier model (the agent). Extracted features from an unlabeled image are then labeled according to the agent. In particular, the differences in tissue acoustic parameters and lesion heterogeneity within the tumor and its surrounding peritumoral region have great diagnostic potential. Ultimately, a radiologist has to work quickly, thus we will also demonstrate that machine learning tools can be used quickly on clinically relevant time scales.

Keywords: Ultrasound Tomography, Radiomics, Machine Learning, Supervised Learning, Feature Extraction

1 Introduction

Breast cancer is one of the leading causes of cancer mortality among women [1, 2]. Early detection of breast disease can lead to a reduction in the mortality rate [3]. However, problems exist with the sensitivity and specificity of mammography which is the current gold standard for breast cancer screening [4]. These problems are substantial within the subset of young women with dense breasts who are at an increased risk for cancer development [5]. Conventional hand-held ultrasound (HHUS) has proven to be a valuable adjunct to mammography [6, 7, 8]. HHUS aids in the detection of cancers in dense breasts and helps differentiate between malignant and benign masses by qualitatively assessing lesion morphology and thus increasing the specificity of diagnostic breast imaging. This leads to reduced anxiety, stress, and physical trauma associated with the biopsy procedure. Problems also exist for HHUS. It is highly operator dependent and difficulties exist for the reproducibility of examinations. It typically only utilizes the basic principles of pulse-echo reflection sonography which cannot use the information contained within the transmitted ultrasound (US) signal. The added cost to the healthcare system as a result of false-positives is also a problem [9, 10].

Ultrasound tomography (UST) might provide a remedy to the deficiencies of HHUS and mammography. Many research groups have investigated the use of reflection and transmission UST [11, 12, 13, 14, 15, 16, 17, 18]. In contrast to mammography, UST does not use ionizing radiation or compression. When compared to HHUS, UST is considerably less operator dependent, has more reproducibility of the data acquisition process, and can utilize both reflection and transmission information. UST can utilize reflection signals to create tomographic B-mode images of the breast [19]. The transmitted portion of an US signal contains information about the sound speed and attenuation properties of the insonified medium [20, 21, 22, 23, 24, 25]. These properties can aid in the differentiation of fat, fibroglandular tissues, benign masses, and malignant cancer [20, 21, 22, 23, 24, 25, 26, 27, 28, 29]. The UST device used for this study and its ring array has been described in our previous work [30, 31].

The goal of developing a UST device is for its eventual application in a clinical setting. There, a radiologist will review the images of a scanned patient and make a diagnosis based on what is seen. In particular, radiologists use their experience and training to make a decision on the presence of any focal imaging abnormality. However, their decision are not always correct, and a possible method to boost their classification ability could utilize radiomic features and classification using supervised machine learning techniques [32, 33, 34, 35, 36, 37, 38, 39, 40]. We will focus on assessing breast tissue acoustic parameters and heterogeneity of a breast mass while comparing its tumoral and peritumoral (i.e. surrounding a tumor) regions. For example, in Figure 1, we see an example of the visualization of an invasive ductal carcinoma breast cancer using UST sound speed, reflection, and attenuation images. A magnification of the region surrounding the tumor at 11 o'clock helps define its irregular margins and spiculation. Note the differences in the acoustic parameters and tissue heterogeneity between the tumoral and peritumoral areas. The goal of this paper is to use machine learning techniques to properly classify lesions as benign or malignant based on the differences between these areas. Doing so could improve the classification ability of experienced radiologists as well as boosting novice radiologists so that they perform with increased ability.

In the following sections, we will outline the machine learning method which includes dataset generation for the tumor/peritumoral regions, feature extraction, feature selection, supervised learning, and evaluation metrics. We will show how using different features subsets which correspond to methods which can or can not be done on clinically relevant time scales affect the classification accuracy. We will conclude with our conclusions on the efficacy of the method and future work.

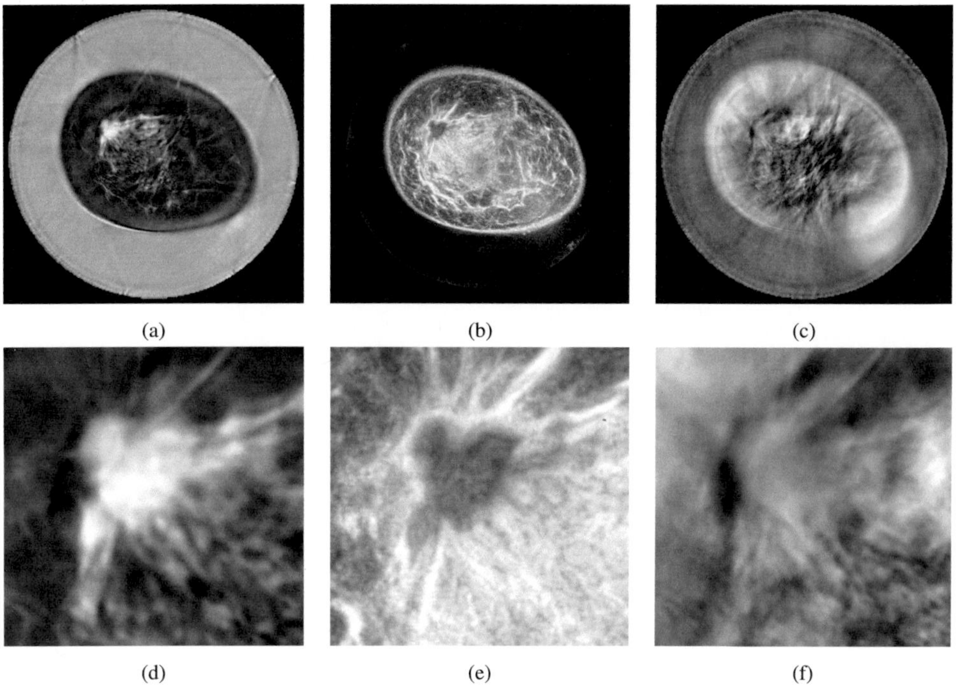

Figure 1: Ultrasound tomography images of an invasive ductal carcinoma in the 10:00 position of a breast with scattered parenchymal density. Note tumor location on the interface between fibroglanduar and adipose tissue (IFGA). In contradistinction to benign masses, magnifications views show heterogeneity extending beyond the cancer and into the surrounding peritumoral regions. (a) Sound speed; (b) Reflection; (c) Attenuation; (d) Magnification of Sound Speed; (e) Magnification of Reflection; Magnification of Attenuation.

2 Materials and Method

Tissue characterization of UST images using machine learning techniques requires a series of steps. First, a data set of images must be created which contain examples of different types of tissues and masses. A trained radiologist must then locate and segment the tissue of interest by generating a binary region-of-interest (ROI) mask. Features are then extracted from the ROI. Using feature selection techniques, the most relevant features are then fed to a machine learning classifier model. The trained algorithm can then be fed features from an unknown tissue sample to predict a label for the sample.

2.1 Region of Interest Generation

ROIs are identified within each image which encapsulate a particular tissue or mass. ROI creation is demonstrated in Figure 2. An example of a sound speed image with a well-circumscribed bilobed fibroadenoma in the peripheral 8:00 position is seen in Figure 2a. A mask is drawn around the mass (Figure 2a) to a generate a binary mask as seen in Figures 2b and 2c. The ROI can be expanded to assess features within the surroundings peritumoral region as shown in Figures 2d and 2e. Note, that instead of using a detailed ROI as shown in Figure 2, an elliptical ROI encompassing the lesion could also be created or morphed from the original ROI. For the purposes of this study, we used a data set containing 161 (93 benign and 68 malignant) samples of lesions which includes 38 cysts, 55 fibroadenomas, and 68 cancers.

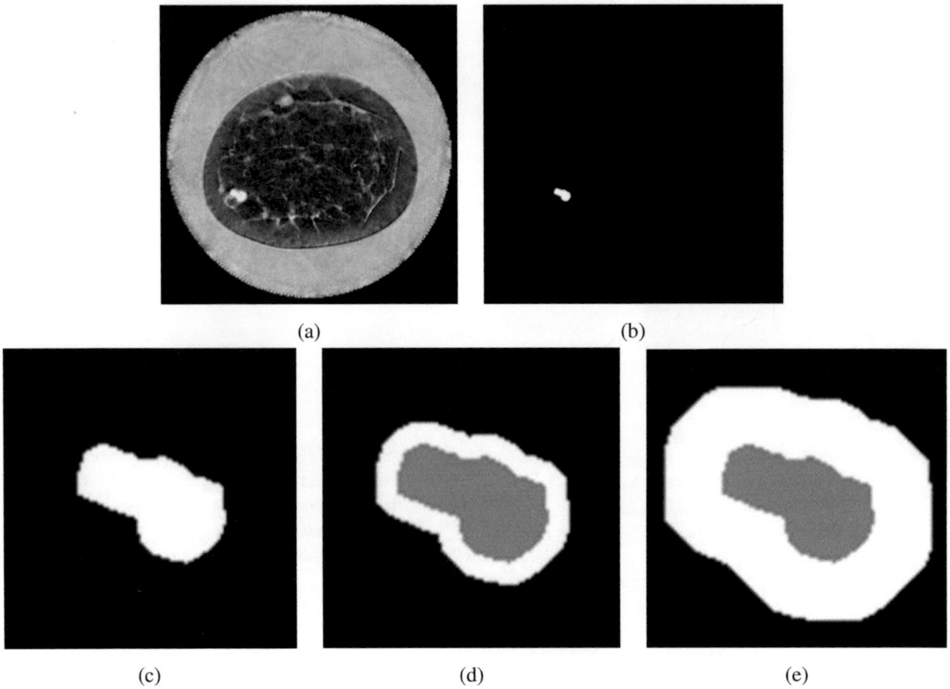

Figure 2: Region-of-Interest (ROI) creation. (a) Sound speed image with a well-circumscribed bilobed fibroadenoma in the peripheral 8:00 position; (b) ROI; (c) Magnification of ROI; (d) ROI with small a peritumoral region. (e) ROI with a larger peritumoral region.

2.2 Feature Extraction

Once an ROI is generated, it can be applied to the various imaging modalities to extract features [41]. Some examples of features include various order statistic assessments of the acoustic parameters or assessments of the texture of the tissue. This includes order statistics such as mean, standard deviation, skewness, etc. Quantitative morphological information can also be obtained from the tumor ROI. Texture metrics include 1st order histogram statistics, 2nd order Gray Level Co-Occurrence Matrix (GLCM) features, as well higher order methods such

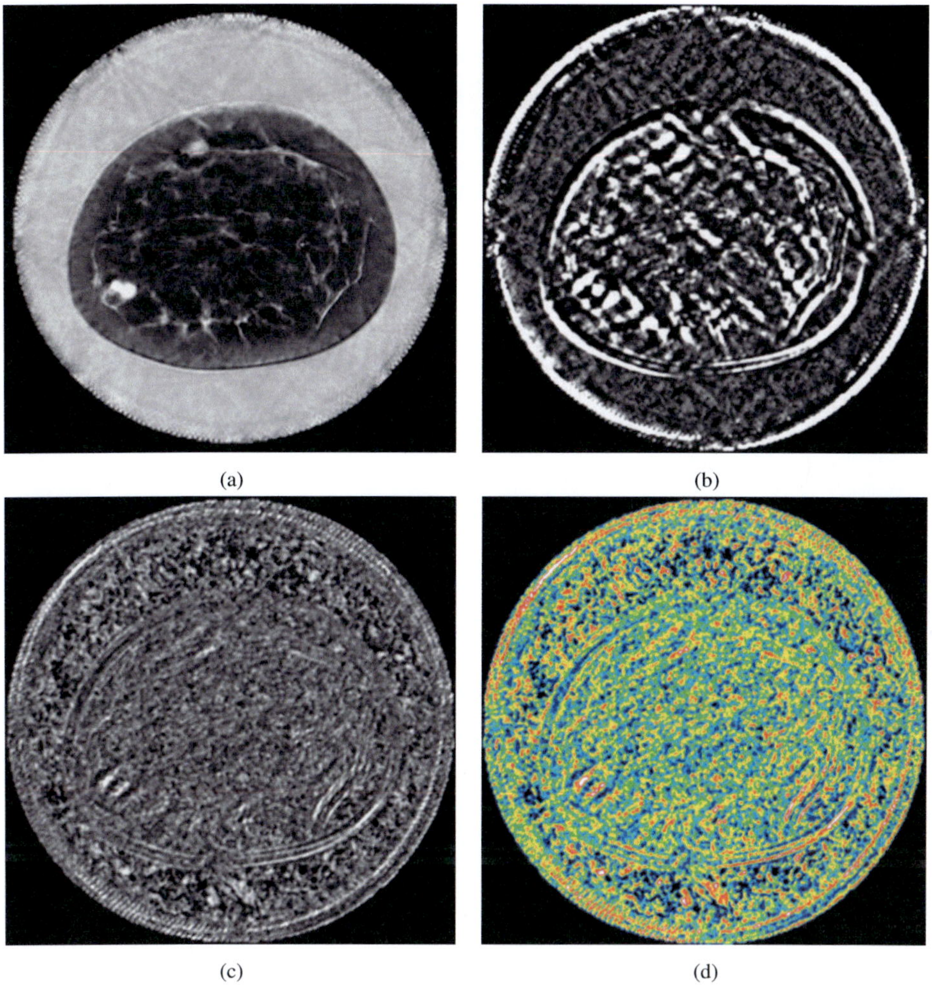

Figure 3: Examples of higher order textural features of the Law's maps. (a) Sound speed image; (b) EE map; (c) ESSE map; (d) ESSE map 4-bit color.

as texture maps. An example of some of Law's texture maps are seen in Figure 3. Additional features can be extracted from permutations of how the images were contrasted, the differences between the features within the tumor and peritumoral regions, and the imaging type.

In addition to the features that are extracted from the images, a radiologist could also provide a score that assesses the degree of malignancy. This is crucial as all *a priori* information that can be provided boosts the classification accuracy of a machine learning algorithm [42]. Thus, we have created our own single BI-RADs-like criterion which assesses the degree of heterogeneity in tumor morphology. This score, called the Mass Boundary (MB) score rates a

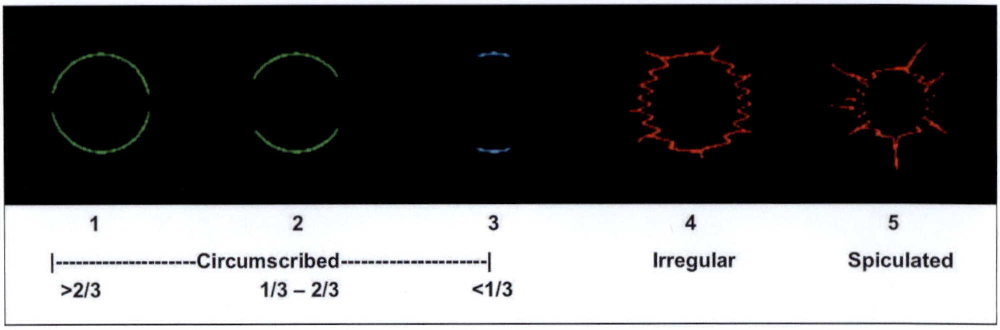

Figure 4: Examples of using the mass boundary score. A lower score reflects more well-defined lesions with circumscribed margins while a higher score reflects more spiculated lesions.

tumor on a scale of 1 to 5. A low value reflects a well circumscribed lesion with well-defined margins while a higher score reflects an irregular or spiculated lesion with ill-defined margins extending into the peritumoral region. An example of this is seen in Figure 4. If greater than 2/3 of the lesion is circumscribed, then a score of 1 is given. If this perimeter is between 1/3 and 2/3, a score of 2 is given. If less than 1/3 of the lesion is circumscribed, then a score of 3 is given. If the lesion is quite irregular, a score of 4 is given. Likewise, if distinct speculations are seen, a score of 5 is given. Therefore, the MB score differs somewhat from an overall BI-RADs score in that the MB score classifies only the tumor/peritumoral morphology and is not meant to convey clinical decision of 12-month follow-up (BI-RADs 1 and 2), 6-month follow-up (BI-RADs 3), or recommendation for biopsy (BI-RADs 4 and 5). Indeed, the MB score likely represents a smoother transition of cancer probability rather than the sharp inflection in probability from $<2\%$ with BI-RADs 3 to approximately 10-50% with BI-RADs 4.

2.3 Feature Selection

Given that multiple imaging modalities are used, that we use both the tumor and peritumoral regions, the various contrast choices that can be made, and other permutations, the number of features we obtain quickly explodes to be much greater than the number of patient samples we have. In order to mitigate this dimensionality curse, we must prune the number of features [43]. Some methods to accomplish this include simulated annealing, genetic algorithms, forward selection, backward elimination, and decision tree pruning. We used decision tree pruning to reduce the dimensionality of the hypothesis space. Subsets of features were fed to a decision tree classifier. The top nodes of the trees were aggregated. This allowed reduction in the number of features while keeping features with the greatest information gain.

To demonstrate that machine learning techniques can be used on clinically relevant time scales, we partitioned our features into subcategories. These categories include all acoustic parameter and textural features obtained using a detailed hand-drawn ROI (R), the same features but with a coarse elliptical ROI (RE), quantitative morphological features obtained from the detailed hand-drawn ROI (M), and the mass boundary (MB) score.

2.4 Supervised Learning

Given a vector of features $\vec{x}$ and a label y, the goal of supervised machine learning is to train a classifier model f such that $f(\vec{x}) = y$. In particular, the function f is taught to predict labels by being fed a training set S of features and labels: $S = \{(\vec{x}_1, y_1), (\vec{x}_2, y_2), \ldots, (\vec{x}_N, y_N)\}$. In this manner, the classifier model f does the best job it can on obtaining the proper label. However, the classifier model can be overfitted such that it gives the proper label for each sample. Thus, a true test of the ability of a classifier model to generalize a data set would lie on its performance on a testing data set.

We tested several classifier models including decision trees, nearest neighbor classifiers, neural networks, support vector machines, and boosted decision stumps [44, 45, 46, 47, 48, 49, 50]. Hyperparameter training was done across reasonable parameters until the greatest classification accuracy was obtained. We evaluated both the Weka and scikit-learn machine learning libraries [51, 52].

2.5 Evaluation Metrics

The efficacy of our feature extraction and machine learning method was evaluated by using the sensitivity (SEN), specificity (SPF), and positive predictive value (PPV) of our classifiers. Note that these definitions of SEN, SPF, and PPV are not what they might typically mean for detecting lesions in medical images. Instead, the radiologist has already found the lesion and contoured it. It is the job of the classifier to label the region as benign or malignant. The classifier's SEN, SPF, and PPV thus reflects the ability to properly label the region as benign or malignant. To reduce over-fitting and have a classifier model which generalizes well, it is important to test the classifier on a separate testing set. However, for our testing, the data was not explicitly partitioned into a training and testing set. Instead, a stratified shuffle split cross-validation approach was used. Also, we do not cite the raw SEN, SPF, and PPV values. Instead, we cite the improvement over randomly guessing the classification to better estimate eventual clinical utility.

3 Results

In this section, we will show improvements in SEN, SPF, and PPV over random guessing when using certain subsets of features. The results are seen in Table 1.

Feature Category	SEN	SPF	PPV
R	27.9%	25.1%	34.8%
RE	23.6%	20.8%	29.4%
R + M	31.0%	28.3%	38.9%
R + MB	35.4%	38.0%	51.5%
RE + MB	32.5%	39.1%	52.9%

Table 1: The improvements in sensitivity (SEN), specificity (SPF), and positive predicative value (PPV) over random guessing when using certain categories of features. See Section 2.3 for the definitions of R, RE, M, and MB.

4 Discussion and Conclusions

From Table 1, it is seen that using only acoustic parameters and textural information from the UST images generates better classification accuracy over random guessing. This is true when using either the detailed ROI (R) or the elliptical ROI (RE). However, the detailed ROI provides better improvements compared to the elliptical ROI. In addition, if we use a detailed ROI in conjunction with quantitative morphological information obtained from the ROI (R + M), then the classification accuracy improves with respect to not using the morphological information (R). If instead of the quantitative information, we insert additional information from the radiologists in the form of the MB score, the classification accuracy improves further (R + MB). However, since the radiologists assessment of the MB score is such a highly filtering feature, we obtain similar classification accuracy if using an elliptical ROI (RE + MB). Thus, the performance of the detailed ROI and elliptical ROI is comparable (R + MB vs. RE + MB). Since we see vast improvements in classification accuracy over random guessing, we would surmise that machine learning tools will allow a radiologist to boost their ability to assess lesion malignancy. Since the elliptical ROI in conjunction with the MB score performs just as well as the detailed ROI, a radiologist should be able to use machine learning tools on clinically relevant time scales where every click or movement of a mouse is aggregated in terms of clinical cost.

For our future work, we will incorporate a much larger patient data pool. This should improve the classification accuracy which can be seen by developing learning curves from toy datasets such as those available on the UCI repository [53]. When developing learning curves, one uses increasing fractions of the total data to develop their classifier models. It is typically seen for many problems that the classification accuracy improves as we incorporate more training samples. However, it does eventually saturate. Based on the sample size used in this paper, we should be far away from this saturation point.

References

[1] C. DeSantis, J. Ma, L. Bryan, and A. Jemal. Breast cancer statistics, 2013. *CA: a cancer journal for clinicians*, 64(1):52–62, 2014.

[2] A. Jemal, F. Bray, M. M. Center, J. Ferlay, E. Ward, and D. Forman. Global cancer statistics. *CA: a cancer journal for clinicians*, 61(2):69–90, 2011.

[3] A. M. Leitch, G. D. Dodd, M. Costanza, M. Linver, P. Pressman, L. McGinnis, and R. A. Smith. American cancer society guidelines for the early detection of breast cancer: update 1997. *CA: A cancer Journal for Clinicians*, 47(3):150–153, 1997.

[4] P. C. Gøtzsche and O. Olsen. Is screening for breast cancer with mammography justifiable? *The Lancet*, 355(9198):129–134, 2000.

[5] N. Arora, T. A. King, L. M. Jacks, M. M. Stempel, S. Patil, E. Morris, and M. Morrow. Impact of breast density on the presenting features of malignancy. *Annals of surgical oncology*, 17(3):211–218, 2010.

[6] W. A. Berg, J. D. Blume, J. B. Cormack, E. B. Mendelson, D. Lehrer, M. Böhm-Vélez, E. D. Pisano, R. A. Jong, W. P. Evans, M. J. Morton, et al. Combined screening with ultrasound and mammography vs mammography alone in women at elevated risk of breast cancer. *Jama*, 299(18):2151–2163, 2008.

[7] T. M. Kolb, J. Lichy, and J. H. Newhouse. Comparison of the performance of screening mammography, physical examination, and breast us and evaluation of factors that influence them: an analysis of 27,825 patient evaluations. *Radiology*, 225(1):165–175, 2002.

[8] A. T. Stavros, D. Thickman, C. L. Rapp, M. A. Dennis, S. H. Parker, and G. A. Sisney. Solid breast nodules: use of sonography to distinguish between benign and malignant lesions. *Radiology*, 196(1):123–134, 1995.

[9] B. L. Sprague, N. K. Stout, C. Schechter, N. T. Van Ravesteyn, M. Cevik, O. Alagoz, C. I. Lee, J. J. Van Den Broek, D. L. Miglioretti, J. S. Mandelblatt, et al. Benefits, harms, and cost-effectiveness of supplemental ultrasonography screening for women with dense breastssupplemental ultrasonography screening for women with dense breasts. *Annals of internal medicine*, 162(3):157–166, 2015.

[10] J. H. Youk and E.-K. Kim. Supplementary screening sonography in mammographically dense breast: pros and cons. *Korean journal of radiology*, 11(6):589–593, 2010.

[11] M. P. André, H. S. Janée, P. J. Martin, G. P. Otto, B. A. Spivey, and D. A. Palmer. High-speed data acquisition in a diffraction tomography system employing large-scale toroidal arrays. *International Journal of Imaging Systems and Technology*, 8(1):137–147, 1997.

[12] S. A. Johnson, D. T. Borup, J. W. Wiskin, F. Natterer, F. Wubeling, Y. Zhang, and S. C. Olsen. Apparatus and method for imaging with wavefields using inverse scattering techniques, December 21 1999. US Patent 6,005,916.

[13] P. L. Carson, C. R. Meyer, A. L. Scherzinger, and T. V. Oughton. Breast imaging in coronal planes with simultaneous pulse echo and transmission ultrasound. *Science*, 214(4525):1141–1143, 1981.

[14] N. Duric, P. Littrup, A. Babkin, D. Chambers, S. Azevedo, A. Kalinin, R. Pevzner, M. Tokarev, E. Holsapple, O. Rama, et al. Development of ultrasound tomography for breast imaging: Technical assessment. *Medical Physics*, 32(5):1375–1386, 2005.

[15] D.-L. Liu and R. C. Waag. Propagation and backpropagation for ultrasonic wavefront design. *IEEE transactions on ultrasonics, ferroelectrics, and frequency control*, 44(1):1–13, 1997.

[16] V. Z. Marmarelis, T.-S. Kim, and R. E. Shehada. High resolution ultrasonic transmission tomography. In *Proc SPIE Med Imaging*, volume 5035, pages 33–40, 2003.

[17] N. V. Ruiter, G. Göbel, L. Berger, M. Zapf, and H. Gemmeke. Realization of an optimized 3d usct. In *Proc. SPIE*, volume 7968, page 796805, 2011.

[18] J. F. Greenleaf, S. Johnson, R. C. Bahn, and B. Rajagopalan. Quantitative cross-sectional imaging of ultrasound parameters. In *Ultrason Symp Proc*. IEEE, 1800.

[19] S. Schmidt, N. Duric, C. Li, O. Roy, and Z.-F. Huang. Modification of kirchhoff migration with variable sound speed and attenuation for acoustic imaging of media and application to tomographic imaging of the breast. *Medical physics*, 38(2):998–1007, 2011.

[20] C. Li, N. Duric, and L. Huang. Comparison of ultrasound attenuation tomography methods for breast imaging. *Ultrasonic Imaging and Signal Processing], McAleavey, SA and Dhooge, J., eds., Proc. SPIE*, 6920:692015–1, 2008.

[21] C. Li, N. Duric, and L. Huang. Clinical breast imaging using sound-speed reconstructions of ultrasound tomography data. *Ultrasonic Imaging and Signal Processing], McAleavey, SA and Dhooge, J., eds., Proc. SPIE*, 6920:692009–1, 2008.

[22] C. Li, N. Duric, P. Littrup, and L. Huang. In vivo breast sound-speed imaging with ultrasound tomography. *Ultrasound in medicine & biology*, 35(10):1615–1628, 2009.

[23] G. Sandhu, C. Li, O. Roy, S. Schmidt, and N. Duric. Frequency domain ultrasound waveform tomography: breast imaging using a ring transducer. *Physics in medicine and biology*, 60(14):5381, 2015.

[24] G. Y. Sandhu, C. Li, O. Roy, S. Schmidt, and N. Duric. High-resolution quantitative whole-breast ultrasound: in vivo application using frequency-domain waveform tomography. In *Proc. SPIE*, volume 9419, page 94190D, 2015.

[25] G. Y. S. Sandhu, C. Li, O. Roy, E. West, K. Montgomery, M. Boone, and N. Duric. Frequency-domain ultrasound waveform tomography breast attenuation imaging. In *Medical Imaging 2016: Ultrasonic Imaging and Tomography*, volume 9790, page 97900C. International Society for Optics and Photonics, 2016.

[26] F. A. Duck. *Physical properties of tissues: a comprehensive reference book*. Academic press, 2013.

[27] P. Edmonds, C. Mortensen, J. Hill, S. Holland, J. Jensen, P. Schattner, A. Valdes, R. Lee, and F. Marzoni. Ultrasound tissue characterization of breast biopsy specimens. *Ultrasonic imaging*, 13(2):162–185, 1991.

[28] S. Goss, R. Johnston, and F. Dunn. Comprehensive compilation of empirical ultrasonic properties of mammalian tissues. *The Journal of the Acoustical Society of America*, 64(2):423–457, 1978.

[29] N. F. Boyd, L. J. Martin, M. Bronskill, M. J. Yaffe, N. Duric, and S. Minkin. Breast tissue composition and susceptibility to breast cancer. *Journal of the National Cancer Institute*, 102(16):1224–1237, 2010.

[30] N. Duric, P. Littrup, S. Schmidt, C. Li, O. Roy, L. Bey-Knight, R. Janer, D. Kunz, X. Chen, J. Goll, et al. Breast imaging with the softvue imaging system: First results. In *Proc. SPIE*, volume 8675, page 86750K, 2013.

[31] O. Roy, S. Schmidt, C. Li, V. Allada, E. West, D. Kunz, and N. Duric. Breast imaging using ultrasound tomography: From clinical requirements to system design. In *Ultrasonics Symposium (IUS), 2013 IEEE International*, pages 1174–1177. IEEE, 2013.

[32] B. Ranger, P. J. Littrup, N. Duric, P. Chandiwala-Mody, C. Li, S. Schmidt, and J. Lupinacci. Breast ultrasound tomography versus mri for clinical display of anatomy and tumor rendering: preliminary results. *American Journal of Roentgenology*, 198(1):233–239, 2012.

[33] E. Honda, R. Nakayama, H. Koyama, and A. Yamashita. Computer-aided diagnosis scheme for distinguishing between benign and malignant masses in breast dce-mri. *Journal of digital imaging*, 29(3):388–393, 2016.

[34] F. Davnall, C. S. Yip, G. Ljungqvist, M. Selmi, F. Ng, B. Sanghera, B. Ganeshan, K. A. Miles, G. J. Cook, and V. Goh. Assessment of tumor heterogeneity: an emerging imaging tool for clinical practice? *Insights into imaging*, 3(6):573–589, 2012.

[35] E. J. Sutton, J. H. Oh, B. Z. Dashevsky, H. Veeraraghavan, A. P. Apte, S. B. Thakur, J. O. Deasy, and E. A. Morris. Breast cancer subtype intertumor heterogeneity: Mri-based features predict results of a genomic assay. *Journal of Magnetic Resonance Imaging*, 42(5):1398–1406, 2015.

[36] B. Malik, J. Klock, J. Wiskin, and M. Lenox. Objective breast tissue image classification using quantitative transmission ultrasound tomography. *Scientific reports*, 6:38857, 2016.

[37] H. Li, Y. Zhu, E. S. Burnside, E. Huang, K. Drukker, K. A. Hoadley, C. Fan, S. D. Conzen, M. Zuley, J. M. Net, et al. Quantitative mri radiomics in the prediction of molecular classifications of breast cancer subtypes in the tcga/tcia data set. *NPJ breast cancer*, 2, 2016.

[38] H. Li, Y. Zhu, E. S. Burnside, K. Drukker, K. A. Hoadley, C. Fan, S. D. Conzen, G. J. Whitman, E. J. Sutton, J. M. Net, et al. Mr imaging radiomics signatures for predicting the risk of breast cancer recurrence as given by research versions of mammaprint, oncotype dx, and pam50 gene assays. *Radiology*, 281(2):382–391, 2016.

[39] R. J. Gillies, P. E. Kinahan, and H. Hricak. Radiomics: images are more than pictures, they are data. *Radiology*, 278(2):563–577, 2015.

[40] W. N. Street, W. H. Wolberg, and O. L. Mangasarian. Nuclear feature extraction for breast tumor diagnosis. In *IS&T/SPIE's Symposium on Electronic Imaging: Science and Technology*, pages 861–870. International Society for Optics and Photonics, 1993.

[41] R. Jain, R. Kasturi, and B. G. Schunck. *Machine vision*, volume 5. McGraw-Hill New York, 1995.

[42] Y.-C. Ho and D. L. Pepyne. Simple explanation of the no-free-lunch theorem and its implications. *Journal of optimization theory and applications*, 115(3):549–570, 2002.

[43] A. L. Blum and P. Langley. Selection of relevant features and examples in machine learning. *Artificial intelligence*, 97(1):245–271, 1997.

[44] J. R. Quinlan. *C4. 5: programs for machine learning*. Elsevier, 2014.

[45] L. Breiman, J. H. Friedman, R. A. Olshen, and C. J. Stone. Classification and regression trees. wadsworth & brooks. *Monterey, CA*, 1984.

[46] P. Indyk and R. Motwani. Approximate nearest neighbors: towards removing the curse of dimensionality. In *Proceedings of the thirtieth annual ACM symposium on Theory of computing*, pages 604–613. ACM, 1998.

[47] R. Hecht-Nielsen et al. Theory of the backpropagation neural network. *Neural Networks*, 1(Supplement-1):445–448, 1988.

[48] C. J. Burges. A tutorial on support vector machines for pattern recognition. *Data mining and knowledge discovery*, 2(2):121–167, 1998.

[49] R. E. Schapire. The boosting approach to machine learning: An overview. In *Nonlinear estimation and classification*, pages 149–171. Springer, 2003.

[50] T. M. Mitchell et al. Machine learning. WCB, 1997.

[51] M. Hall, E. Frank, G. Holmes, B. Pfahringer, P. Reutemann, and I. H. Witten. The weka data mining software: an update. *ACM SIGKDD explorations newsletter*, 11(1):10–18, 2009.

[52] F. Pedregosa, G. Varoquaux, A. Gramfort, V. Michel, B. Thirion, O. Grisel, M. Blondel, P. Prettenhofer, R. Weiss, V. Dubourg, J. Vanderplas, A. Passos, D. Cournapeau, M. Brucher, M. Perrot, and E. Duchesnay. Scikit-learn: Machine learning in Python. *Journal of Machine Learning Research*, 12:2825–2830, 2011.

[53] M. Lichman. UCI machine learning repository, 2013.

Challenges and Applications of Registering 3D Ultrasound Computer Tomography with Conventional Breast Imaging Techniques

P. Cotic Smole[1], N.V. Ruiter[1], N. Duric[2], and T. Hopp[1]

[1] *Karlsruhe Institute of Technology, Institute for Data Processing and Electronics, Karlsruhe, Germany*
E-mail: patricia.smole@kit.edu, torsten.hopp@kit.edu
[2] *Barbara Ann Karmanos Cancer Institute, Department of Oncology, Detroit, USA*

Abstract

To evaluate the diagnostic value of Ultrasound Computer Tomography (USCT), the imaging results have to be correlated with conventional breast imaging techniques. This is challenging due to different patient positioning in the modalities with nonlinear deformations of the breast tissue. We have developed a patient-specific image registration method, which simulates different breast positionings in both X-ray mammography and Magnetic Resonance Imaging (MRI) through biomechanical modelling. An average registration error below 5 and 17 mm for MRI to USCT and USCT to mammography registration, respectively, allowed us to evaluate the diagnostic performance of USCT. It was shown that regions of high sound speed corresponded well with the tumour position indicated from the MRI contrast kinetic map. Moreover, the quantitative analysis of sound speed and attenuation values with respect to the segmented mammograms revealed that sound speed gives a better distinction between breast tissue, whereas their combined information further improves the classification. Although the results are based on a preliminary study, the promising outcome points that the registration could assist radiologists in comparing the USCT with both MRI and X-ray mammography.

Keywords: Breast image registration, Ultrasound computer tomography, X-ray mammography, Magnetic resonance imaging, Multimodal diagnosis

1 Introduction

3D Ultrasound Computer Tomography (USCT) is a promising imaging method for breast cancer diagnosis that is currently undergoing first evaluations in clinical trials [1, 2, 3]. The method aims to provide high resolution 3D images of the undeformed breast by using ultrasonic waves, thereby enabling patient-friendly conditions. For image acquisition, more than two thousands ultrasound transducers surround the breast in a water bath. The transducers emit unfocussed ultrasound waves and record the reflected and transmitted signals that are generated upon interaction of the wave with the breast tissue. A single image acquisition allows the reconstruction of three tissue characteristics: reflectivity, sound speed and attenuation. While reflectivity images visualize the tissue boundaries, sound speed and attenuation images provide quantitative tissue characterization [4].

In the current development state, it is essential to correlate USCT images to conventional imaging modalities to evaluate its diagnostic value and further improve the data acquisition and image reconstruction process. Besides the screening modality X-ray mammography, magnetic resonance imaging (MRI) is frequently used for early breast cancer diagnosis. To directly compare USCT with both modalities, the challenge is to overcome the substantial differences in patient positioning and breast deformation in order to provide a spatial correspondence between images. Another obstacle is the different dimensionality of images (3D USCT vs. 2D mammograms).

In this paper, we present a patient-specific image registration method that estimates the spatial transformation between images, governed by the differences between imaging modalities. Patient-positioning conditions and breast deformations are simulated by employing biomechanical modelling and an X-ray like projection of the USCT volume is used to enable a comparison with 2D mammograms. We give a review of its recent developments, present the first evaluation results of USCT's diagnostic value and raise open challenges.

2 Methods

The aim of the registration approach is to spatially align the breast shape observed in one modality (source image) as good as possible with the shape observed in the compared modality (target image). With a biomechanically-based registration we aim in modelling the different conditions in patient-positioning and breast deformation of imaging modalities:

- USCT: breast in prone position, immersed in water;
- X-ray mammography: breast in upright position, compressed between parallel plates;
- MRI: breast in prone position, placed within MRI breast coils.

Hence, the following loading conditions are simulated for the registration of MRI to USCT respectively USCT to X-ray mammography:

- MRI to USCT: the buoyancy effect is simulated on the MRI volume to estimate the approximate gravity-free state of the breast observed in USCT;

- USCT to X-ray mammography: the breast compression is simulated on the USCT volume to mimic the mammographic compression.

In the following, a detail description of the breast image registration workflow is presented.

2.1 Breast image registration

The registration approach is based on the biomechanical modelling used in the registration of MRI with X-ray mammography [5]. The model is generated from the MRI volume (MRI-USCT registration) respectively USCT volume (USCT-mammography registration). To estimate the breast stiffness distribution for MRI to USCT registration, the MRI volume is segmented into background, fatty and glandular breast tissues using unsupervised fuzzy c-means algorithm [6] and Level-Set-Evolution [7]. Young's moduli of fatty (E_{fat}) and glandular tissue (E_{gland}) are initially applied constant for all patients and are subsequently updated by a patient-specific parameter optimization. Initial E_{fat} and E_{gland} are in the range of experimental values in literature [8]: $E_{fat} = 900\,\text{Pa}$ and $E_{gland} = 1200\,\text{Pa}$. The segmented MRI volume is further cropped at the sternum in anteroposterior direction to take into account only the relevant part of the breast for the registration with USCT.

For USCT to X-ray mammography registration, a patient-specific stiffness distribution model is constructed from the preprocessed USCT sound speed image that provides a voxel-based model. The motivation for using a voxel-based stiffness distribution is two fold. First, automated segmentation of breast tissue types in USCT images is challenging and not yet developed. Second, due to the physical relationship between the sound speed and elastic properties of tissue, the Young's modulus E can be estimated for each voxel from the sound speed map.

The geometry of the segmented MRI volume respectively USCT sound speed image is generated by a volumetric meshing algorithm [9] using 4-node tetrahedrons. A hyperelastic neo-hookean material model is used. The neo-hookean material constants are computed based on the relationship between the Young's modulus and the shear and bulk modulus as described in e.g. Bower [10]. A Poisson ratio close to 0.5 assumes the breast tissue to be nearly incompressible.

For both MRI to USCT and USCT to X-ray mammography registration, the simulation of different loading conditions is implemented using the commercial Finite Element Methods (FEM) software ABAQUS [11]. For MRI to USCT registration, the buoyancy effect is simulated by applying a body load $F = \rho V g$, where ρ refers to the density of water, V to the volume of the water displaced by the breast and g is the gravitational acceleration factor in anteroposterior direction. In the case of USCT to X-ray mammography registration, the mammographic compression of the breast is modelled by a displacement-driven movement of two parallel plates in the craniocaudal direction until a compression thickness retrieved from the mammogram's metadata is achieved. The deformation of the breast is governed by a contact definition between the plates and the breast. During both simulation strategies, the posterior-most nodes are kept in position to model the fixation of the breast at the chest wall. For the comparison of the USCT volume with the 2D mammograms, a maximum intensity projection is additionally derived from the deformed USCT volume.

The presented registration process is based on several preprocessing parameters that govern the biomechanical model creation and simulation. To adapt the process to patient-specific conditions, we allow the optimization of the most influencing patient-specific parameters with respect to maximizing the image similarity between the deformed source image and target image. We focused on optimizing the following parameters: the rotation around the anteroposterior direction that accounts for any relative rotation and tilting of the patient between both modalities (MRI-USCT, USCT-X ray mammography), the cropping position of the MRI volume in anteroposterior direction (MRI-USCT), the Young's moduli of fatty and glandular tissue (MRI-USCT). The image similarity is calculated based on the surface agreement between the deformed MRI volume and the USCT volume, respectively gradient correlation between the projection of the deformed USCT volume and the 2D mammogram. The optimization is implemented using the simulated annealing algorithm [12] with a stopping condition of 100 iterations.

In addition to the biomechanically-based registration, both registration approaches underwent an additional surface-based registration that directly matches the volume surface of the source to the target image, thereby enabling direct comparison of imaging modalities. In the case of USCT to X-ray mammography registration, the 3D profile of the breast was approximated by a semi-ellipsoidal shape, where the projection of the breast boundary was extracted from the mammogram and the height matched the compression thickness given from the mammogram's meta data. The use of this second registration step aimed to overcome the uncertainties and simplifications made in biomechanical modelling such as neglecting tissue structures like Cooper ligaments or neglecting breast deformations caused by the MRI breast coils.

The outcome of the registration approach is a registered breast volume of the source image that directly matches the volume in the target image. A workflow of the registration approach is schematically depicted in figure 1 for the example of USCT to X-ray mammography registration. A detail description of the whole registration is beyond the scope of this paper and can be found in [13, 14].

2.2 Evaluation method

To evaluate the approach for MRI to USCT registration, nine datasets from a clinical study performed at the University Hospital Jena were used, whereas USCT to X-ray mammography registration was evaluated from nine datasets acquired at the Karmanos Cancer Institute. Each consisted of volume images of the three USCT image types (reflectivity, attenuation and sound speed), as well as the corresponding T1-weighted MRI volume respectively craniocaudal mammogram. The registration accuracy was measured based on landmarks such as lesions, predominant connective tissue structures or breast implants that could be clearly delineated in both compared modalities. The borders of the landmarks were manually annotated by using a freehand tool. In the case of USCT to X-ray mammography, the target registration error (TRE) was calculated as the 2D Euclidean distance between the centre positions of the annotation in the projection of the deformed USCT volume and mammogram, whereas the average closest distance between pairs of annotation points in the deformed USCT volume and the MRI volume served for calculating the 3D TRE for USCT to MRI registration. Note that the different calculation approach of TRE arises as both studies were performed independently.

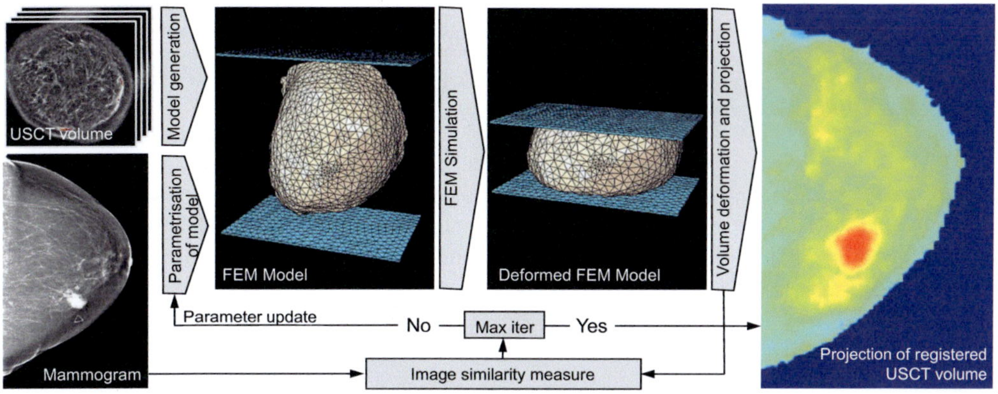

Figure 1: Schematic workflow presentation of the biomechanically-based image registration of USCT with X-ray mammography.

3 Results

3.1 Registration accuracy

For the analysed preliminary datasets, the presented registration approach showed to improve the registration accuracy by more than a factor of two compared to rigid alignment of the volumes at their centres of mass (table 1). As evident from the table, the mean TRE for USCT to X-ray mammography is more than three times larger than the TRE reached for MRI to USCT registration (16.2 mm vs. 4.7 mm) and has a much larger variance (9.0 mm vs. 1.7 mm). On one hand, this could be explained by the fact that the compression simulation induces much larger nonlinear deformations of the soft breast tissue compared to the buoyancy simulation and is as such more sensitive to uncertainties and simplifications in the breast modelling. On the other hand, differences in TRE could also arise as both registration strategies did not employ a common calculation approach for TRE.

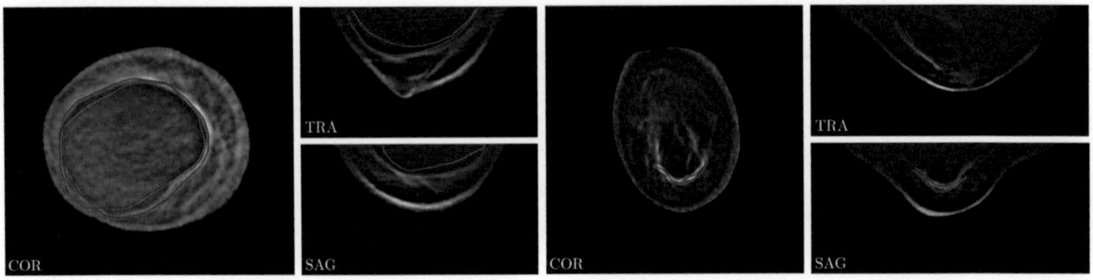

(a) Patient with a breast implant (b) Healthy patient

Figure 2: Resulting images of two patients for MRI to USCT registration. An overlap of the registered MRI annotation (red) and USCT annotation (blue) on the coronal (COR), sagittal (SAG) and transversal (TRA) USCT reflectivity slices. (a) A patient with a breast implant, (b) a healthy patient showing a high intensity connective tissue structure. Figures acquired from [14].

Figure 2 shows the resulting images of two patients for MRI to USCT registration, where the registered MRI annotation contour (red) is overlapped together with the USCT annotation contour (blue) on the USCT reflectivity image. The presented cases refer to a patient with a breast implant (figure 2a) and a healthy patient with a clearly visible connective tissue structure (figure 2b). In both cases, the annotations are well overlapping and can be delineated in the same slice in both modalities. The average TRE for these cases was 3.6 mm and 1.9 mm respectively.

3.2 Evaluation of USCT diagnostic value with MRI

In comparing USCT with MRI, we focused in assessing the diagnostic value of USCT for tumour detection by qualitative evaluation of USCT sound speed images with respect to the MRI contrast kinetic. The MRI contrast kinetic is a commonly used method to visualize tumours in contrast enhanced MRI and is based on monitoring the contrast agent uptake and washout over time through so called parametric maps, in which the three time point (3TP) method [15] is applied. The image intensity is evaluated at three time points: before, shortly after and approximately 6 to 7 minutes after the contrast agent was applied. For each voxel, both the contrast agent uptake between the first and second time point, as well as the wash out between the second and third time point are categorized into three intensity classes each. The washout categories are color-coded in red, green and blue and are together with the uptake-related brightness categories overlaid on the native MRI.

Biomechanical registration	$\mu_{\text{TRE}} \pm \sigma_{\text{TRE}}$	$TRE_{\text{Reg}}/\text{TRE}_{\text{Rigid}}$
MRI-USCT	4.7 ± 1.7 mm	2.2
USCT-Mammography	16.2 ± 9.0 mm	2.5

Table 1: Summary of mean target registration error (μ_{TRE}), standard deviation (σ_{TRE}) and ratio between mean TRE obtained from biomechanical image registration and mean TRE obtained from mere rigid alignment of volumes ($TRE_{\text{Reg}}/\text{TRE}_{\text{Rigid}}$).

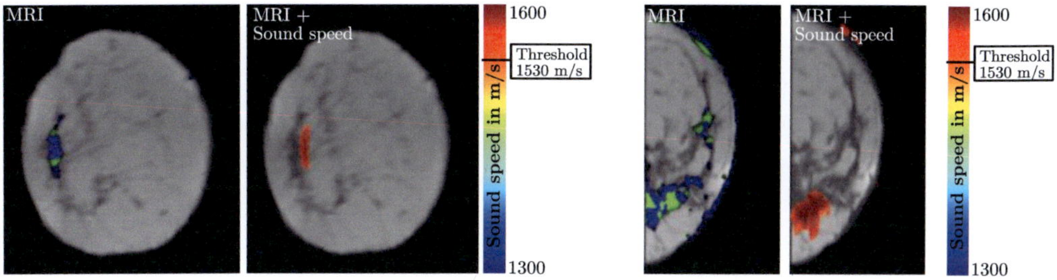

Figure 3: Comparison of registered native MRI with color-coded contrast kinetic analysis by the 3TP method (left subimage for each patient) and fused image from registered native MRI background and color-coded thresholded USCT sound speed (right subimage for each patient) for two patients (left and right image). Regions of high sound speed (red) correspond well with the tumour position in MRI indicated from the contrast kinetic as strong contrast agent uptake and a persistent respectively strong washout (green and blue). Figures acquired from [14].

A qualitative comparison of USCT and MRI for tumour detection is shown in figure 3 for two patients in terms of image fusion. Here, the USCT sound speed is presented as color-coded overlay on the MRI native grey-scale background in comparison to the MRI contrast kinetic analysis. From the fused images from USCT sound speed and native MRI, an area of high sound speed can be detected at approximately the same position, where the high contrast agent uptake and persistent respectively strong washout in the MRI refers to a detected tumour. This qualitative comparison of both modalities depicts that the registration is accurate enough for performing image fusion and that USCT sound speed may have a comparable diagnostic value for tumour detection as MRI contrast kinetic analysis.

3.3 Evaluation of USCT diagnostic value with X-ray mammography

Besides qualitatively evaluating the diagnostic value of USCT sound speed for the detection of tumours, the interest is to analyse whether a quantitative characterization of different tissue types is possible based on both the attenuation and sound speed values. We performed this analysis based on the registered USCT and X-ray mammography images. As a ground truth for the different tissue types, the mammogram was segmented into fatty, glandular and tumorous tissue using interactive thresholding and morphological closing, whereas the lesion was manually annotated. By comparing the projections of the registered sound speed and attenuation images to the mammogram, the segmentation served as a tissue mask to evaluate the average sound speed and attenuation values in fatty, glandular and tumorous tissue for each of the patients. To evaluate how well the average sound speed and attenuation values can separate different tissue types, a classification was further performed using a linear support vector machine (SVM) algorithm [16]. We used both the average sound speed and attenuation values obtained for each patient as features for a 3-class problem aiming in separating fatty, glandular and tumorous tissue. In a repeating process for all combinations of training-test-partitions, eight patient datasets were used in the training, whereas one dataset remained for testing.

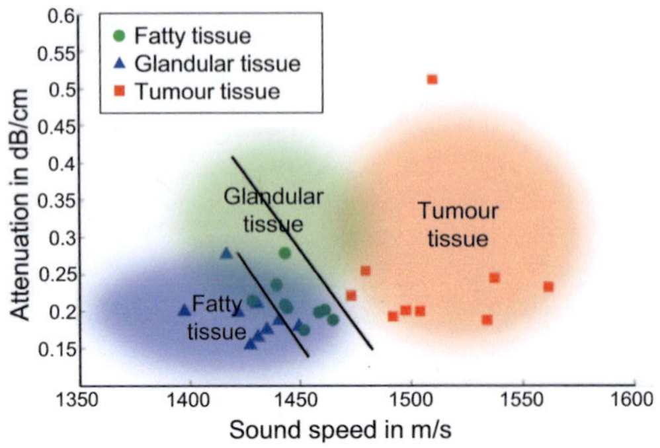

Figure 4: A scatter plot of average sound speed and attenuation values for fatty, glandular and tumorous tissue types for each patient in combination with the two tissue separation lines as obtained from SVM for the 3-class problem. The three transparent color clouds show approximately the expected tissue classification as obtained from Greenleaf et al. [4].

Figure 4 shows a scatter plot of average sound speed and attenuation values for fatty, glandular and tumorous tissue types for each patient in combination with the tissue separation lines as obtained from SVM for the 3-class problem. The training and test errors were 13% respectively 15%. As evident from the figure, the high error appeared due to hard separation between fatty and glandular tissue. That was also supported by a 2-class problem, where both the training and testing error were 0% in separating the fatty and glandular part from the tumorous part.

To present the fused information of both mammograms and projections of USCT sound speed, figure 5 presents an example where the tissue-characteristic sound speed is shown as a color-coded overlay on the grey-scale mammogram background. The different tissue regions in the sound speed image are separated based on the SVM classification output.

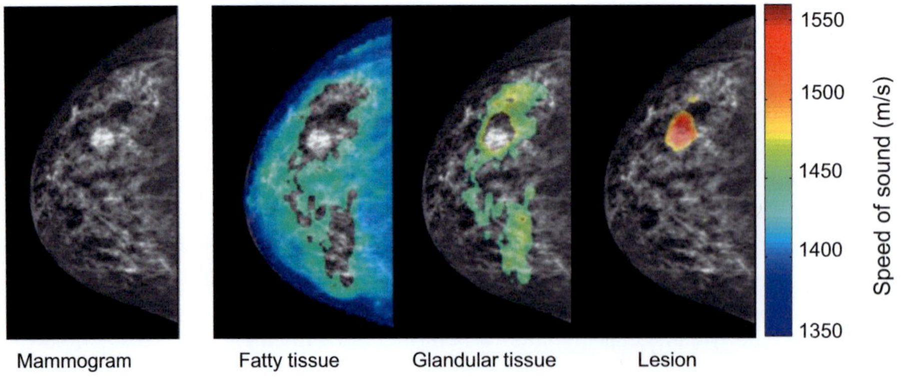

Figure 5: Image fusion of USCT sound speed projection and mammography. A color-coded overlay of tissue-specific sound speed values is shown on the grey-scale mammogram background. The different tissue regions in the sound speed image are separated based on the SVM classification.

4 Summary and Conclusion

We have developed and implemented a fully automated biomechanically-based image registration approach that matches the USCT reflectivity, sound speed and attenuation images with both MRI and X-ray mammography. By optimizing a set of the most influencing parameters, we enable a patient-specific registration. The evaluation with a preliminary dataset showed that the registration approach improves the registration accuracy by more than a factor of two in comparison to rigid alignment of the volumes at their centres of the mass. The average achieved target registration error for USCT to MRI matching was smaller than 5 mm, whereas an average accuracy of 16.2 mm was reached for USCT to X-ray mammography.

The achieved registration accuracy enabled us to evaluate the diagnostic performance of USCT with respect to both modalities. In visually comparing the USCT sound speed image to the registered MRI contrast kinetic map that depicts lesions, areas of high sound speed appeared to match approximately the same lesion region as detected from the contrast kinetic map. Moreover, quantitative evaluation of the average sound speed and attenuation values for different tissue types revealed that automatic classification of fatty, glandular and tumorous tissue may be possible and is more accurate when both image modalities are taken into account.

The presented method and its evaluation showed promising results in registering and fusing information from USCT with two different modalities with significant differences in patient positioning and breast deformation. Although the results were derived from a preliminary dataset, the approach clearly depicts that a direct correlation of tissue structures from different modalities may be possible. Therefore, it is likely to help assisting radiologists in the time consuming and challenging multimodal diagnosis of USCT data.

The presented biomechanical model was subjected to several uncertainties and simplifications in the modelling, which were overcome with a second surface-based registration. In order to omit this step, we plan to further extend the model by simulating tissue structures like Cooper ligaments, the breast-muscle interface, as well as pre-deformations of the breast caused by the MRI breast coils. In addition, we plan to investigate several registration strategies, such as the accuracy achieved in registering MRI to USCT in comparison to USCT to MRI, as well as the effect of the three-modal registration compared to the two-modal. Finally, additional approaches to evaluate the quantitative information of USCT images will be tackled.

References

[1] N.V. Ruiter, M. Zapf, R. Dapp, T. Hopp, W.A Kaiser, H. Gemmeke: First results of a clinical study with 3D ultrasound computer tomography. In: Ultrasonics Symposium (IUS), 2013 IEEE International, 651-654.

[2] N. Duric, P. Littrup: Clinical breast imaging with ultrasound tomography: A description of the SoftVue system. The Journal of the Acoustical Society of America 135(4) (2014) 2155.

[3] T. Hopp, M. Zapf, E. Kretzek, J. Henrich, A. Tukalo, H. Gemmeke, C. Kaiser, J. Knaudt, N.V. Ruiter: 3D ultrasound computer tomography: update from a clinical study. In: SPIE Medical Imaging 2016. Proc. of SPIE Vol. 9790, 97900A.

[4] J.F. Greenleaf, R.C. Bahn: Clinical imaging with transmissive ultrasonic computerized tomography. IEEE Trans Biomed Imaging 28(2) (1981) 177-185.

[5] T. Hopp, M. Dietzel, P.A. Baltzer, P. Kreisel, W.A. Kaiser, H. Gemmeke, N.V. Ruiter: Automatic multimodal 2D/3D breast image registration using biomechnical FEM models and intensity-based optimization. Medical Image Analysis 17 (2013) 209-218.

[6] J.C. Bezdek: Pattern Recognition with Fuzzy Objective Function Algorithms, Kluwer Academic Publishers, Norwell, MA, USA (1981).

[7] C. Li, R. Huang, Z. Ding, J. Gatenby, D. Metaxas, J. Gore: A Level Set Method for Image Segmentation in the Presence of Intensity Inhomogeneities With Application to MRI. IEEE Transactions on Image Processing 20(7) (2011) 2007-2016.

[8] T.J. Carter, C. Tanner, D.J. Hawkes: Determining material properties of the breast for image-guided surgery. In: Proc. SPIE Medical Imaging 7261 (2009) 726124.

[9] Q. Fang, D. Boas: Tetrahedral mesh generation from volumetric binary and grayscale images. In: IEEE International Symposium on Biomedical Imaging: From Nano to Macro 2009 (2009) 1142-1145.

[10] A. Bower: Applied Mechanics of Solids, Taylor and Francis (2011).

[11] Dassault Systems Simulia Corp, ABAQUS Analysis User's Manual (2014).

[12] S. Kirkpatrick, C.D. Gelatt, M.P. Vecchi: Optimization by Simulated Annealing. Science 220(4598) (1983) 671-680.

[13] T. Hopp, N. Duric, N.V. Ruiter: Image fusion of Ultrasound Computer Tomography volumes with X-ray mammograms using a biomechanical model based 2D/3D registration. Computerized Medical Imaging and Graphics 40 (2015) 170-181.

[14] T. Hopp, R. Dapp, M. Zapf, E. Kretzek, H. Gemmeke, N.V. Ruiter: Registration of 3D Ultrasound computer Tomography and MRI for evaluation of tissue correspondences. In: SPIE Medical Imaging 2015. Proc. of SPIE Vol. 9419, 94190Q-1.

[15] E.A. Hauth, C. Stockamp, S. Maderwald, A. Mhler, R. Kimming, H. Jaeger, J. Barkhausen, M. Forsting: Evaluation of the three-time point method for diagnosis of breast lesions in contrast-enhanced MR mammography. Clinical Imaging 30(3) (2006) 160-165.

[16] N. Cristianini, J. Shawe-Taylor: An introduction to Support Vector Machines and other kernel-based learning methods. New York, NY, USA: Cambridge University Press 2000.

A simple method for measurement of acoustic properties from cancerous lung tissue and its implementation into the clinical workflow

Frank Wolfram, Thomas G Lesser

SRH Walkdklinikum Gera, Dept. of Thoracic and Vascular Surgery, Gera, Germany
E-mail: Frank.Wolfram@SRH.de

Abstract

During USCT examination, tissue morphology, as well as acoustic properties such as speed of sound is extracted. Data based upon malignant tissue is limited, so is its reliability as a prognostic factor indicating a malignant or benign nature. It's hard to obtain tumour tissue because of their pathological use for staging. Therefore, this work will present a simple method of acoustic properties measurement and its implementation in a clinical workflow.
A broadband – dual immersion technique was used to determine speed of sound and attenuation of malignant and benign Lung Cancer. Tumours were resected during surgery containing Adeno-, Squamous Carcinoma and Benign as well as metastatic tissue from breast and colon carcinoma. Measurements were performed after resection before fixation and histological staining. A clinical workflow was implemented that didn't interfere with the pathological procedures. Additionally, a literature study was performed to compare the determined properties with published data.
All cancer types had higher speed of sound (1560–1670 m/s) than water. The speed of sound was higher in malignant tissue than in benign. Impedance was highest for squamous carcinoma (1.88 MRayl). Attenuation varied between 0,31 – 0,8 dB/cm/MHz and showed no significant difference between the histological subtypes. The proposed measurement technique could be implemented into the surgical - pathological workflow without disturb-ance of the histological management.
There exists comprehensive literature for acoustic properties from parenchymal, but a limited one for cancerous tissue. Measurements revealed that malignant tissue has higher speed of sound than benign tissue and might therefore be a valuable parameter for tissue classification in USCT. More work is demanded in order to determine acoustic properties from mammary tumours of different histological subtypes.

Keywords: tissue properties, speed of sound, attenuation

1 Introduction

USCT is used for 3D holography to analyse anatomic structures. But tomography acquires additional information such as pulse arrival time and amplitude which are related speed of sound and attenuation [1]. These parameters can be used for tissue characterization.

In this work the determination of acoustic properties from cancerous lung tissue was presented. It has been early investigated that Lung in ventilated condition is a total acoustic absorber independent of inflation status and frequency range. Lung ultrasound is clinical only used to detect pleural processes and exclude pneumothorax [2]. But our approach is based on replacing air content in one lung wing section with saline and therefore generating acoustic access. This is called One Lung Flooding and generates gas free lung saline tissue compound where lung tumours are sonographic visual [3]. In order to understand the interaction of acoustic waves in lung, the acoustic properties of lung cancer tissue needed to be determined [4].

Lung cancer entities comprise adeno as well as squamous carcinoma. Such histological subtypes are also present for breast cancer, the outcome of those measurements might be of interest for ultrasound tomography.

The main literatures of published acoustic properties have investigated parenchymal tissue of almost all organs including bone and blood as seen in Table 1. But properties from cancerous tissue are investigated only from a few organs such as from prostate, breast, liver and uterus. It needs to be noticed that there is a high variability of measurement conditions found in the publications. So tissue fixations with saline and formaldehyde, temperature range from room to 37°C and a wide frequency range (1- 450 MHz) have been found as well as different methods (transmission, ultrasound microscopy). It is difficult to compare the results and find confidence in their reliability. One reason for such circumstance might be the fact that cancerous tissue plays an important role in the surgical quality process. Therefore this work will present a simple method for determining acoustic properties and how to implement this in the clinical workflow.

Tissue	Speed of sound [m/s]	Attenuation [dB/cm/MHz]	Literature
Kidney	1570	0,5	Gross et al. 1978
Skin	1537	0,2408	Gross et al. 1978
Liver	1530-1600	0,4 - 0,6	Johnston et. al. 1979 Bamber et al, 1981
Muscle / Myocardium	1590-1620	0,94	Marsh, 2016/ Saijo et. al. 1997
Spleen	1520-1580	0,4	Johnston et. al. 2014
Tendon	1750	3	Gross et al. 1978
Uterus	1615	0,3	Keshavarzi et. al. 2001
Prostate	1614	1,8	Tanoue, 2012
Breast fatty tissue	1422		Li et. al. 2009 / Duck ,1990
Breast parenchyma	1487 1504	0,96	Li et. al. 2009 Hanani et. al. 2014
Fibroglandular tissue	1514	0,774	Li et. al. 2009
cancerous			
Uterine myoma	1610	0,33	Keshavarzi et. al. 2001
Prostate malign.	1585-1660	1,42	Tanoue 2012
Breast malign.	1548	-	Li et. al. 2009
Breast benign.	1531 1584	- 0,7	Li et. al. 2009 Duck, 1990

Table 1: Summary of literature determining acoustic properties from parenchymal and cancerous tissue

2 Methods

2.1 Measurement Setup

The experimental Setup contain a temperature (35°C) controlled tank of degased isotonic saline with two identical immersion ultrasound transducer (Smart Material, Dresden, Germany). A through transmission broadband technique was used to determine acoustic parameter speed of sound and attenuation. Cancer tissue was fixed centrally between them, while the total distance of transducers was set to 20 mm. These customized broadband transducers with 3 mm active diameter cover an acoustic 10 dB Bandwidth between 1 MHz and 5 MHz. The transmitter is connected with a function generator (33126A, Agilent Technologies Inc., Santa Clara, CA, USA) pulsing 30 Vpp positive flank with repetition rate of 10 Hz. The data's from receiver are stored by Digital Oscilloscope (54622D, Agilent Technologies Inc., Santa Clara, CA, USA) with sample rate of 100 Ms/s. A trigger line was used for synchronisation. Signal noise was removed by averaging 16 times the receive pulse before transmitted to PC.

The density of cancerous tissue was determined with calibrated Pyknometer (Brand, Wertheim, Germany). Weight of cancerous tissue and pyknometer with water and tissue was measured by EMB 200-2 (Kern&Sohn, Balingen, Germany).

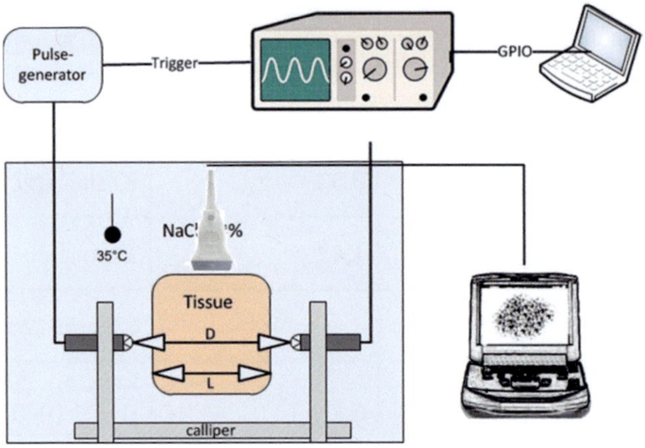

Figure 2: Schematic measurement setup with dual immersion transducers. D- distance between transducers, L thickness of tissue

Data processing:

Speed of sound should be calculated first regarding Eq. 1 with c_0 [1520 m/s] corresponding to speed of sound in water at 35°C. τ is the time delay between the arrival time of the saline and tissue pulse. It can be automatic estimated by using a cross correlation function, where the maximum of the correlation function represents the propagation delay τ.

Acoustic Impedance (Z [MRayls]) was calculated by multiplication of density and speed of sound (Eq.2). The density of tissue (Eq.3) was estimated using a pyknometer, which requires tree individual measurements of weight, from the tissue, the pyknometer with tissue saline filled and with saline only [5].

The pulse waveform was captured in degased saline Y0(t) and with cancer tissue Y(t) of thickness L. Acoustic attenuation versus frequency was calculated by logarithmic dividing the spectrum of Y and Y0 (Eq. 4). The amplitude spectrum is estimated by FFT transformation to be $S_{tissue}(f)$ and $S_{water}(f)$. Additionally, a reflection coefficient r is used to estimate the intensity loss on the crossing from saline into and out of tissue (Eq. 5). The equitation not takes scatter losses into account, which can cause overestimation of attenuation when not using r.

The attenuation course is interpolated using a simple exponential function. Most of tissues have a typical frequency dependence where n is around 1,2 (Eq. 6).

Important to notice is that the correction factor of attenuation can be calculated just after the density measurement.

$$c = c_0 \cdot \frac{L}{\tau \cdot c_0 + L} \qquad ; \tau = \arg\max_t (Y * Y_0) \tag{1}$$

$$\mathrm{Z} = c \cdot \rho_{tissue} \tag{2}$$

$$\rho_{tissue} = \frac{\mathrm{m_{tissue}}}{\mathrm{m_{tissue}} + \mathrm{m}_{\mathrm{H}_2O} - \mathrm{m_{pycno}}} \cdot \rho_{\mathrm{H_2O}} \tag{3}$$

$$\alpha(f) = \frac{1}{L} \cdot 20 \log_{10} \left(\frac{S_{water}(f)}{S_{tissue}(f)} \right) r \tag{4}$$

$$r = \frac{p_r}{p_e} = \left| \frac{Z_1 - Z_0}{Z_0 + Z_1} \right| \tag{5}$$

$$\alpha(f) = A \left[\frac{dB}{cm\ MHz}\right] f^n \; ; \; n = 0{,}9 - 1{,}5 \tag{6}$$

2.2 Clinical Workflow

It can be assumed that the tissue resected during surgery is not of any use and most of it will be thrown away. But it plays an important role in the clinical workflow. Usually all the resected tissue is send straight to pathology. Beside the cytological examination the pathologists performs often detailed histology and in particular biomarker and immunological staining which are performed from external labs. Additionally the pathologist analyses the resection margins which requires the entire resected organ including the tumour. All this information is reported to the tumour board which makes treatment decisions based on those results. Most important aspect is the assessment of surgical intervention, was it a completeness of (R0) tumour resection. The biomarker analysis defines adjuvant systemic treatment. In summary the process loop between surgery and pathology is closed, and here our measurement is placed in between with all its own needs, regarding fixation, transport logistics and timing issues (Fig. 2).

In order to manage its implementation into the workflow, pre-defined conditions were agreed. Prior to surgery the cancer cytology should defined by biopsy. Surgery is scheduled early morning so that it can make sure that the tissue arrives on the same day in pathology. Finally the surgeon documents the incisions and changes done to the tissue. All the tissue not needed for acoustic measurement goes straight to pathology and just as little as needed for measurement can be picked up from surgery immediately during surgery. From surgery to measurement the tissue is immerged in saline and then after measurement fixated in formaldehyde before transportation to pathology.

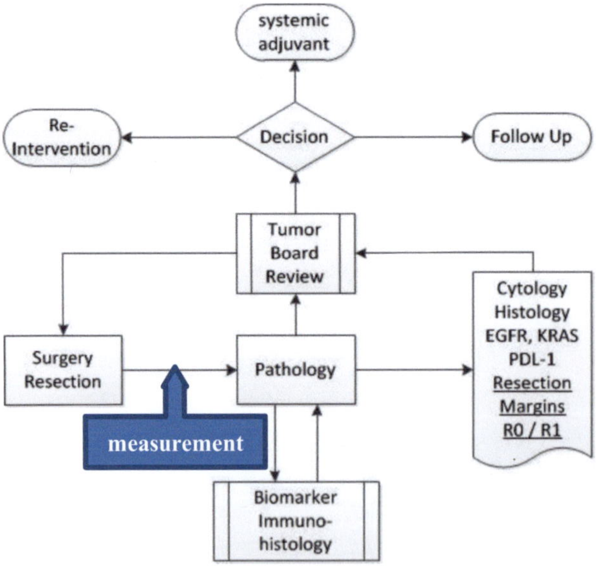

Figure 2: Clinical workflow between surgery pathology and tumour board.

3 Results

The measurement with its tissue sampling directly from surgery could be implemented into the clinical workflow without disturbance of the pathological yield for staging and resection qualification. Speed of sound from primary lung cancer is in range of 1580-1640 ms, the same values showed lung metastases from breast (IDC) and colon (CRC). The benign lung tumour showed lower speed of sound of only 1500 m/s. The corresponding impedances of NSCLC (Non-Small Cell Lung Cancer) is 1,75 MRayl where the squamous carcinoma showed highest value of 1,88 MRayl. Impedance from metastases was identical to NSCLC. Attenuation from metastases and lung cancer tissue are similar (0,42 -0,5 dB/cm/MHz). Only the benign lung tumour show almost twice as high value of 0,8. The frequency dependence of attenuation was in the range of 1,1-1,4.

Gewebe	$c[1000\, m/s]$	Z [MRayl]	$A[dB/cm\,MHz]$	n	R^2
Lung Tumor					
NSCLC	1,60	1,75	0,42	1,2	0,93
ADC	1,58± 0,03	1,76± 0,11	0,45	1,2	0,95
SQC	1,64± 0,12	1,88± 0,10	0,43	1,4	0,97
Benign	1,50	1,60	0,80	1,1	0,9
Metastases					
IDC	1,60	1,75	0,50	1,15	0,93
CRC	1,62	1,80	0,45	1,1	0,9

Table 2: Summary of measured speed of sound and attenuation from lung cancer tissue and pulmonary metastases.

4 Discussion & Outlook

As mentioned in the introduction, there has been no interest in acoustic properties of lung cancer tissue because of their unavailability for ultrasound in ventilated lung therefore no reference data exists. But recently a publication presented speed of sound and attenuation measured in single cells using ultrasound microscopy including lung cancer cells [6]. The speed of sound of single lung cancer cells is in the range of 1600-1700 m/s as measured with boot methods. In addition our attenuation measurement revealed an attenuation of 0,45 dB/cmMHz for malignant tissue which is equal to the mean of the cell lines.

A comparison of published data from parenchymal and cancerous breast tissue with the measured one can lead to the assumption that attenuation and speed of sound might be valuable parameters for tissue differentiation regarding its malignant or benign nature. Speed of sound in cancerous tissue might be higher than 1550 m/s while attenuation lower than 0,5 dB/cm/MHz.

What should be done in the future?

A comprehensive and proved data source is needed in order to extract diagnostic information from speed of sound and attenuation images. Therefore properties from cancerous tissue should be investigated intensively including their subtypes as well as necrotic tissue. It would be favorable using specialized USCT for tissue samples measurement instead of a dual transmission technique as presented. This would give a 2D or even 3D image where changes and tissue specific transitions can be monitored.

This work suffers also from several limitations.

The presented workflow is very complex. This might be caused due the highly malignant nature of lung cancer. There was no statistical analysis performed due to a low number of samples in particular for breast metastatic tissue.

References

[1] Ozmen N, Dapp R, Zapf M, Gemmeke H, Ruiter N, van Dongen K. Comparing different ultrasound imaging methods for breast cancer detection. In: IEEE Trans Ultrason Ferroelectr Freq Control; 2015. p. 637-46.

[2] Reissig A, Kroegel C. Transthoracic sonography of diffuse parenchymal lung disease: the role of comet tail artifacts. J Ultrasound Med. 2003;22(2):173-180.

[3] Lesser T, Schubert H, Bischoff S, Wolfram F. Lung flooding enables efficient lung sonography and tumour imaging in human ex vivo and porcine in vivo lung cancer models. European Journal of Medical Research. 2013;18(23).

[4] Wolfram F, Reichenbach J, Lesser T. An ex vivo human lung model for ultrasound guided HIFU therapy using lung flooding. Ultrasound in Med & Biol. 2013;40(3):496-503.

[5] DiResta M, Lee J, Lau N, Ali F, Galicich J, Arbit E. Measurement of brain tissue density using pycnometry. Acta Neurochir. 1990;51:34-36.

[6] Miura K, Yamamoto S. A scanning acoustic microscope discriminates cancer cells in fluid. Sci Rep. 2015;19(5).

The New Generation of the KIT 3D USCT

H. Gemmeke, L. Berger, T. Hopp, M. Zapf, W. Tan, R. Blanco, R. Leys, I. Peric, and N. Ruiter

Karlsruhe Institute of Technology, Karlsruhe, Germany
E-mail: hartmut.gemmeke@kit.edu

Abstract

The first clinical studies with our current prototype, 3D USCT II, enabled us to identify the necessary improvements for transition of our method to clinical practice. The main goals are to improve the contrast of reflection and transmission tomography, and to optimize the coverage of the imaged breast by a new geometry of the transducer distribution. Furthermore, for cost-effective industrial mass production, a self-calibration method allows us to relax the precision of the positioning of the transducers to 0.1 mm. The readout of the transducer arrays is now carried out by an ASIC, developed for a more cost-effective design. The coupling of the measuring device to the patient was optimized to cover the full size of the breast up to the pectoral muscles. Finally, the data acquisition and readout time were reduced to 1.5 minutes each by new micro-TCA electronics and larger FPGAs.

Keywords: breast cancer, medical imaging, reflection tomography, transmission tomography

1 Introduction

Our 3D Ultrasound Computer Tomography system for breast imaging [1] is shown in Fig. 1. It consists of a patient bed with an embedded ellipsoidal measuring device covered by 2041 transducers contained in 157 transducer arrays (TAS) [2]. The ellipsoidal aperture has a diameter of 26 cm and a depth of 18 cm. The coupling medium is water at body temperature. Using 10 million A-scans, which describe the pressure over time, we could reconstruct 3D reflectivity images of the breast with sub-millimeter resolution using synthetic aperture technique [3]. The speed-of-sound and attenuation were reconstructed from the same raw data set by a straight ray based algebraic reconstruction technique [4]. The necessary fast data acquisition (DAQ) electronics was adapted from our development for the cosmic ray experiment AUGER [5].

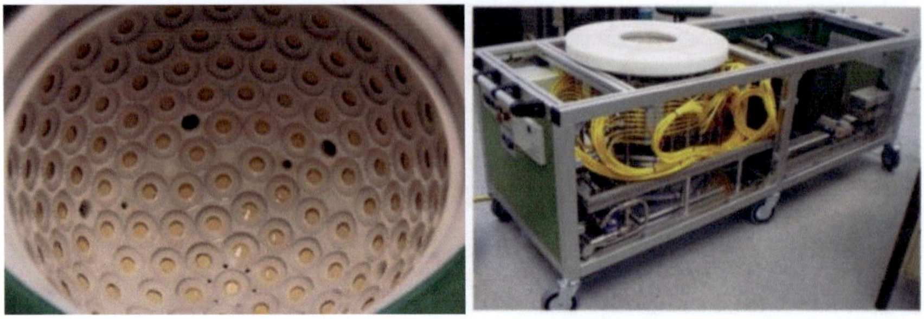

Figure 1: KIT 3D USCT with look in the inner structure (left) and transducer aperture (right).

At the University Hospital Jena we carried out a pilot study with the prototype, 3D USCT II, which enabled us to identify the necessary improvements for transition of our method to clinical practice. The main goals are:

1. Improvement of the contrast in reflection and transmission tomography by a new geometry of the transducer distribution. A uniform random distribution of transducers may minimize the artifacts of the sparse aperture and maximize the contrast in the reconstructed images.
2. The interface of the measuring device to the patient should be optimized to cover the full size of the breast up to the pectoral muscles.
3. A further aim was to enlarge the aperture for better immersion of large breasts into the device.
4. Finally, the DAQ and readout time should be reduced by a new electronic.

The strategy of development, the steps of optimization of geometry, their improvements to reflection and transmission tomography and the produced measuring device are described in the following sections. Furthermore, the new frontend ASIC for driving and receiving the ultrasound signals and the new data acquisition electronics are introduced and finally the so far obtained results discussed.

2 Strategy of Development

To lower the risk in the overall development we carry out the implementation in two steps. Starting from the current measuring system 3D USCT II with 157 TAS with 4 emitters and 9 receivers each, we test the production technology of a new transducer array system [6].

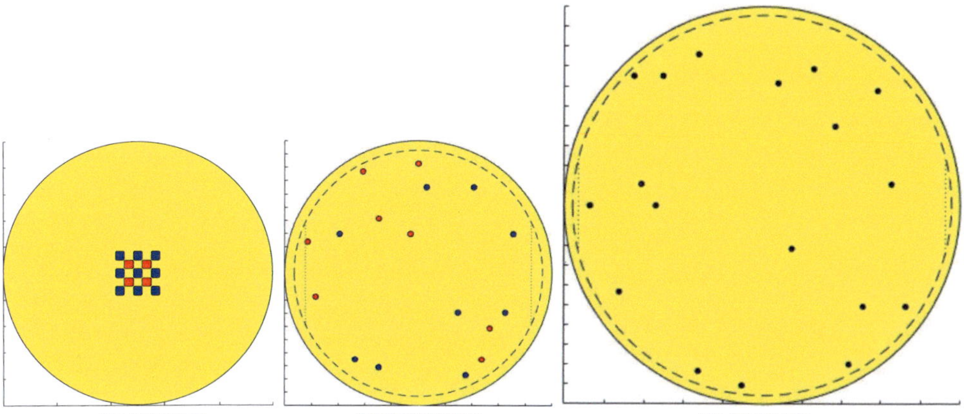

Figure 2: Distribution of transducer at 3D USCT II, II.5 and III displayed in the same scale. Red describes the emitter and blue the receivers. Whereas the TAS of USCT II and II.5 have the same diameter of 28 mm, the TAS of 3D USCT III has a diameter of 43 mm and its transducer (black) are operated omnidirectional.

The three types of TAS for 3D USCT II, II.5 and III are shown in Fig. 2. Due to the omnidirectional characteristic of the transducers in 3D USCT III, the obtained number of A-scans per used transducers quadruplicate and the number of aperture positions (AP) could be reduced by the same scale. For a sufficient contrast and resolution about 1e7 A-scans are required. Whereas for 1e7 A-scans with 3D USCT II 10 APs are necessary, this number is reduced for 3D USCT II.5 to 5 APs and for 3D USCT III to 2 APs, thereby reducing the time-consuming aperture movements and minimizing the DAQ time from 6 to 4 and 2 minutes respectively.

The size of the aperture with 26 cm is to small to cover breasts of 20 cm diameter with limited opening angles of the transducers and to achieve a constant point-spread-function over the size of the breasts. Especially the boyancy in the water enlarges the horizontal diameters for fatty breasts. Based on simulations we choose an diameter of 36 cm for 3D USCT III.

3 Optimal Geometry of Measuring System

For a globally uniform distribution of transducer on the surface of the measuring device the TAS have to be spaced as tightly as possible, i.e. the area of the surface not covered by TAS has to be as small as possible. The aim was to increase the density of coverage with transducer arrays from 75% in 3D USCT II to 80% in 3D USCT III.

3.1 Minimize holes in coverage

Covering a sphere or ellipsoid with circles is an old unsolved mathematical problem, named Thomson's problem [7]. Numerically it may be approximated by minimizing the energy of Coulomb charges on the surface of the measuring device. In the case of a half-sphere or semi-ellipsoid an effective method is to fill the surface row by row starting from the bottom. This method of optimization of TAS distribution was described in a patent application [8]. It starts with a fixed size of the measuring device and varies the size and number of TAS per row, places them as dense as possible and ascends to the next row. For fine tuning, the radius of the measuring device is varied until the predetermined number of TAS is reached and the efficiency of coverage is maximized.

3.2 Global uniform random distribution of transducers

We optimized possible transducer distributions using Monte Carlo simulations in respect to contrast, coverage of the region of interest (hemisphere of 20 cm diameter), and minimization of artifacts. For a cost-effective industrial mass production, the TAS design should be identical for each TAS. To achieve a global uniform random distribution of the transducers and avoiding constant angle differences between the transducers, the TAS can be rotated randomly. Scoring the uniform randomness, the surface was subdivided into equal areas and the frequency distribution of the hits in these areas by the position of the transducers was analyzed by a chi-square test similarly to the test of uniform random number generators [9].

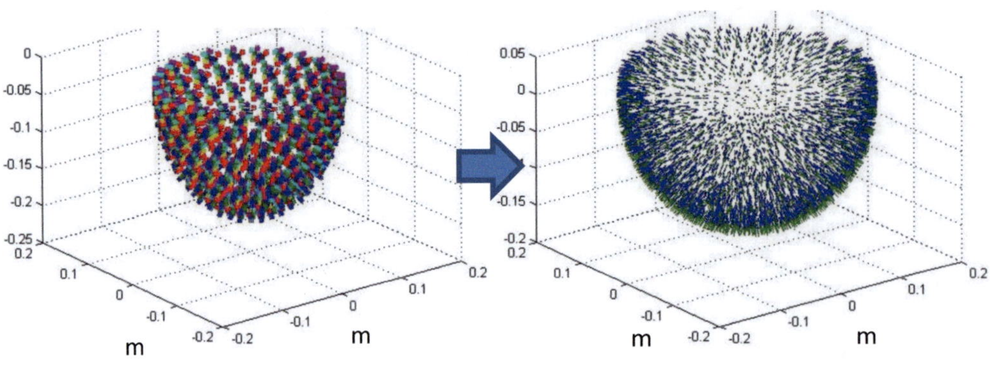

Figure 3: Transducer distribution in USCT II (left) with 12 APs and USCT III (right) with 2 APs.

The improvement in the distribution of transducers from 3D USCT II to 3D USCT III can be easily seen in Fig. 3. For one aperture position, a more uniform distribution without using the non-omnidirectional character of the transducer in 3D USCT II was obtained. To achieve a fair comparison, we use in both simulations the same number of A-scans.

4 Results

4.1 Contrast improvement in reflection tomography

Due to speed-of-sound correction we were able to achieve sub-wavelength resolution for reflection tomography with phantoms. Scattering and refraction does not significantly decrease resolution in the used frequency range of 2.5 MHz [10]. Yet, the contrast in reflection tomography is limited as we apply sparse array imaging. The artifacts, i.e. grating lobes, arise due to regular sampling at two orders of magnitude below the Nyquist limit, see Fig. 4 left, obtained with 900 000 A-scans or 1 AP with 3D USCT II. The artifacts can be reduced by a uniform random distribution of the transducers, see Fig. 4 right. By selection of 900 000 A-scans out of 10 APs with a uniform distribution of emitter and receiver, the grating lobes are greatly reduced. The same improvement we observed after increasing the number of APs to 22 [11]. Similar effects were observed at 2D sparse arrays [12].

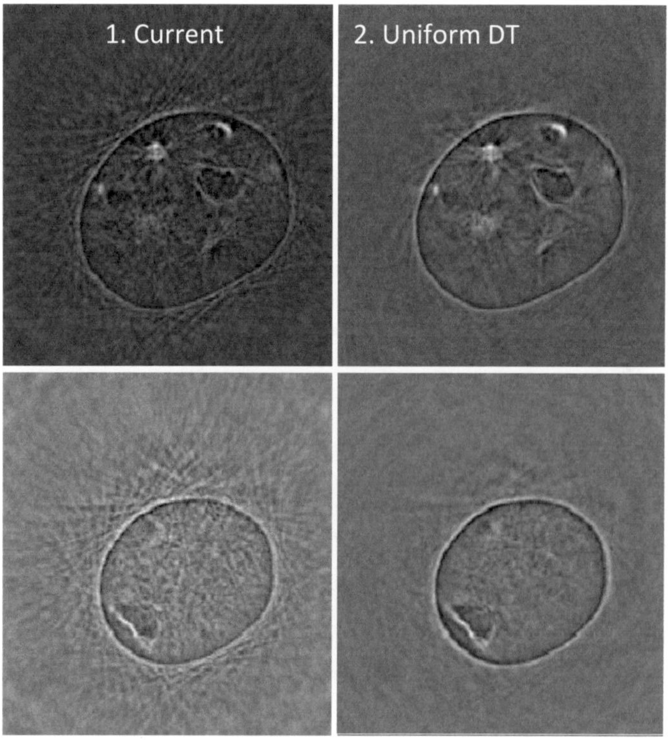

Figure 4: Increasing contrast in reflection tomography from left to right by a more uniform distribution of transducers (DT). The number of A-scans is in both cases the same.

4.2 Improvement of transmission tomography

We tested the improvements on transmission tomography by a straight ray simulation for 3D USCT II and II.5 including the characteristics and distribution of the transducers and added noise. The simulated phantom (with a gradient of c = 1460 to 1500 m/s) is embedded in water (c = 1530 m/s) and contains eight lesions with a diameter of 5 to 12 mm testing the resolution, and seven lesions with a diameter of 10 mm and c = 1475 to 1560 m/s testing the contrast. The results are shown in Fig. 5. The reconstructed image with the 3D USCT II setup in Fig. 5b does not clearly depict the outline of the phantom for 1AP, but gives a more reasonable result at 16 AP in Fig. 5c. A reconstruction, Fig. 5d, with a 15° larger opening angle, ±35°, solves this problem, but still the contrast is low. Less clustering of the transducers results in a visibility of most test lesions in Fig. 5e still at 1 AP.

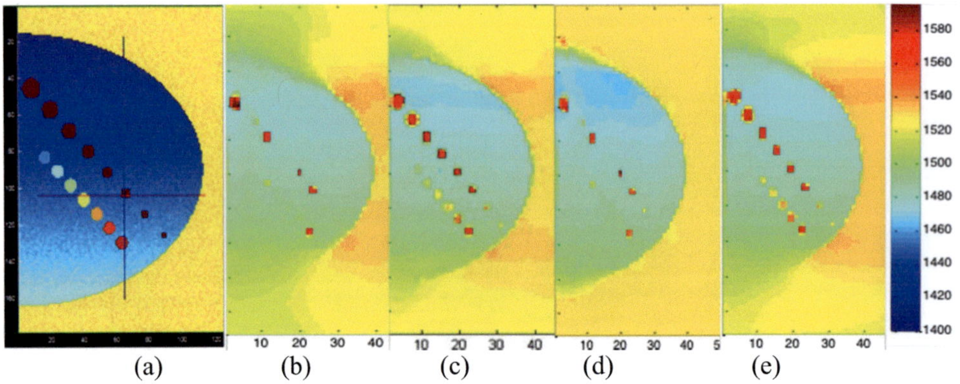

Figure 5: 3D simulation of a phantom (a) and reconstruction for 3D USCT II with different transducer distributions and parameters. 3D USCT II with 1 AP (b) and 16 AP (c), about 15° larger opening angles 1 AP (d) and 1 AP but uniform transducer distribution (e).

4.3 Final new aperture

Following these simulations, we choose for 3D USCT III a larger opening angle for the transducers and an enlarged aperture with a diameter of 36 cm (3D USCT II has 26 cm). By these changes we enlarge the field of view and depth of field from a diameter of 10 cm to 15 cm and 20 cm in version II.5 and III, respectively.

Due to the design, which allows vertical displacements of the measuring device, we lost in USCT 3D II 25 mm of the measuring range to the pectoralis, see Fig. 6 (right). By a new construction for 3D USCT III with a membrane (Fig. 6 left) we allow the same stroke of about 20 mm but reduce the losses to 5 mm. A small dead zone is acceptable, because tissue out of plane can also be reconstructed due to refraction and forward scattering.

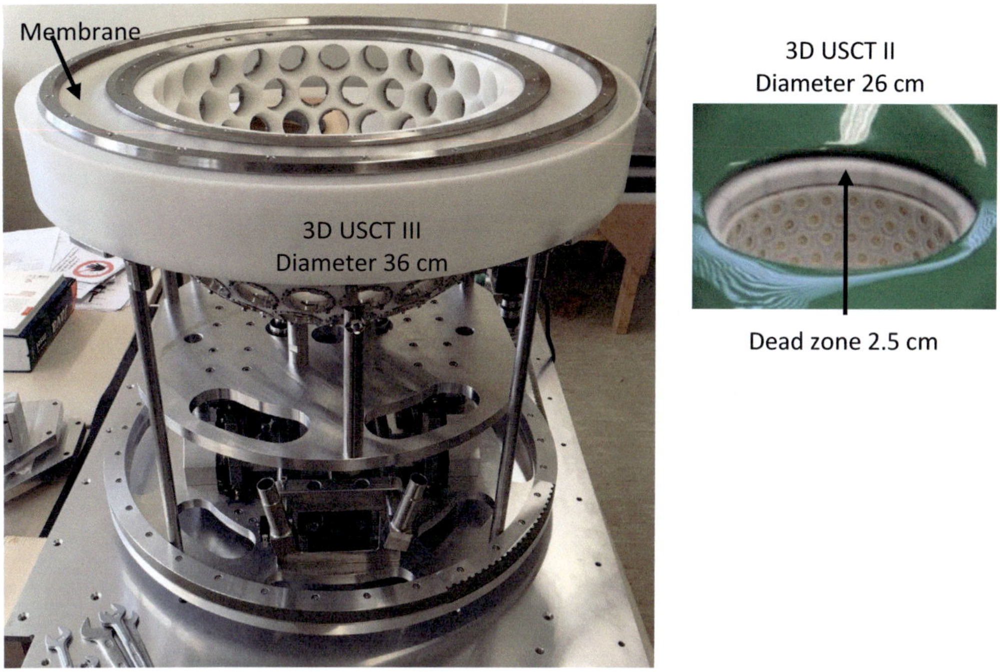

Figure 6: Hemispherical measuring device of 3D USCT III with 128 TAS (left) and the same for 3D USCT II with 157 TAS (right).

Furthermore, the transducers can be mounted under distinct different rotation angles and thus allows a better approximation of the uniform random distribution of transducers. Using all these provisions the simulations predicted relative improvements as described in Tab 1.

Ratio of new to current aperture			
Transmission-		Reflection-Tomography	
Resolution	2.0	Variability PSF	3.0
Contrast	3.0	Contrast	6.8
Visibility	2.3	Illumination	2.0

Table 1: Relative comparison of the quality of 3D USCT II and expected quality of 3D USCT III as extracted from simulations described in chapter 4.1 and 4.2.

4.4 New calibration method

The mechanical parts for the measuring device are machined with a precision of 20 microns to ensure positioning of the transducers with this accuracy. That is not a precision, which is standard for industrial mass production. Therefore, we developed a method to calibrate the position of transducers [13]. To test the method, we measured a sphere of stainless steel of diameter 50 mm, see Fig. 7a, which was fabricated with a precision of 50 µm. First results of the calibration measurement Fig 7b, c showed, that we can reconstruct the position of the transducers to 0.1 mm, if their initial position is within 1mm of the intended position. Furthermore, the individual delays of the electronical channels are corrected. This makes us more independent from the limitations of industrial mass production and reduces the costs.

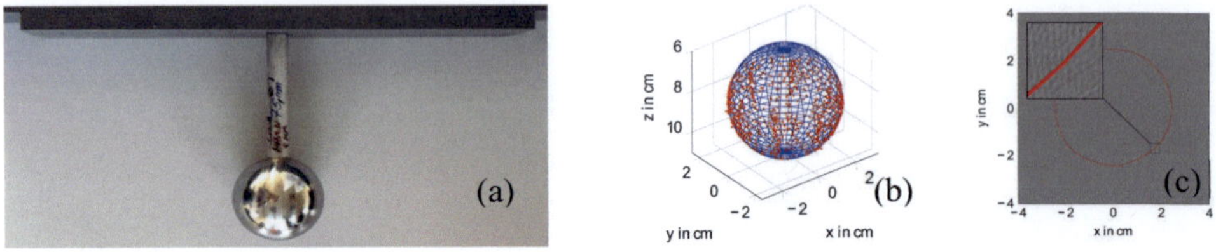

Figure 7: (a) Sphere of 50 mm stainless steel for calibration of our 3D USCTs, (b) first reconstruction of the sphere and (c) by a factor 5 enlarged zone at the surface showing the precision of result.

5 Fast readout electronics

5.1 Integrated TAS electronics via an ASIC

To reduce the costs for the transducer arrays we designed an ASIC, see Fig. 8, which can readout and drive 9 transducers with up to 100 Vpp. The applied technology was AMS 350 nm HVCMOS. By this design, transducers can be operated. One selectable HV amplifier drives the emitter channel, see Fig. 9. The nine receiver preamplifiers are multiplexed to three readout channels. The 3 dB bandwidth of the 3-stage preamplifier is 3 MHz around a middle frequency of 2.5 MHz. The gain can be programmed between 40 and 720. The noise related to the input is ~4 μV, the crosstalk -30 dB.

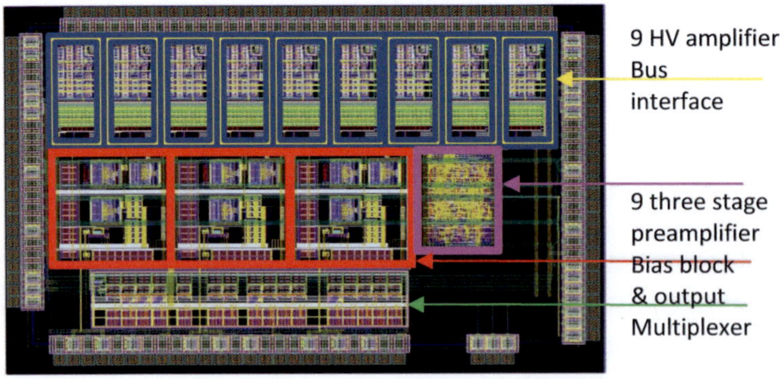

Figure 8: Layout of the ASIC. At the upper side of the ASIC the nine HV amplifier channels could be recognized, well separated to reduce the cross coupling. Below these HV stages are in 3 blocks 3 three stage preamplifier. Bus interface and output multiplexer complete these functions.

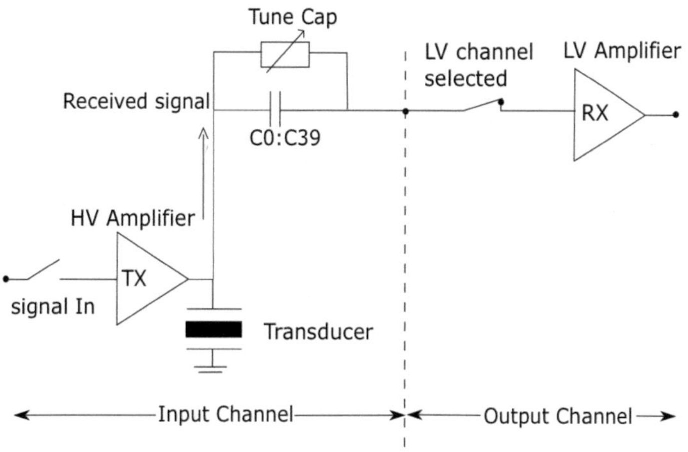

Figure 9: Simplified schematic of the ASIC consisting of high voltage (HV) amplifier and preamplifier (LV).

5.2 Performance increase by a new DAQ hardware

The large number of A-scans (10^7) was obtained in 3D USCT II by 10 motion-steps of the aperture. The DAQ speed for USCT 2.5 was increased by two changes. Firstly, we use a stronger motor for faster movements reducing the DAQ time from 8 to 6 minutes. The use of each transducer as emitter and receiver increases the number of emitters per aperture position and A-scans by a factor two. 3D USCT III will have a factor 1.6 more transducers (128 TAS with 18 transducers each) and therefore will need only two aperture positions to obtain the same number of A-scans as before. The new electronics will reduce the DAQ-time further by a factor of 2 to 2 minutes. Also, the probability for patient movement will be reduced by this factor 5 shorter measuring time.

Our micro-TCA system (Fig. 10) developed in a collaboration with DESY [14] contains a Kintex 7 FPGA from Xilinx which is large enough to do signal preprocessing. That reduces the necessary time of signal processing by nearly two orders of magnitudes by the massive parallel processing in the FPGA. A fast PCI-Express linked to a serial ATA disk reduces the readout time from 15 to 1.5 minutes. The use of a new generation of GPUs accelerate the reconstruction by more than half an hour, so that the total DAQ and reconstruction time shrinks from roughly 2 hours to less than a quarter of an hour, see Tab. 2.

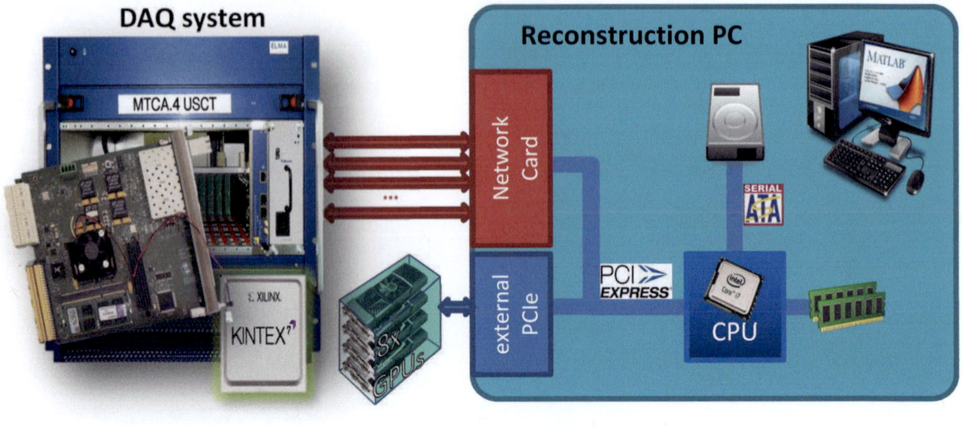

Figure 10: DAQ system and reconstruction PC. The DAQ system is based on a micro TCA system equipped with a Xilinx Kintex 7 FPGA. The reconstruction PC has as support 8 GTX Titan GPUs.

	DAQ	Signal preprocessing	Readout time	TOFI-SAFT	Total
3D USCT II	6 min	Matlab: 55 min	15 min	8 GTX 590: 41min	117 min
3D USCT III	2 min	12 Kintex 7: 2.5 s	1.5 min	8 GTX Titan: 9 min	12.5 min

Table 2: Comparison of 3D USCT II and III in respect to DAQ, signal preprocessing, read out and reconstruction time.

6 Discussion and Conclusion

So far, all known demands of 3D ultrasound tomography are fulfilled to achieve all three modalities reflection-, speed of sound, and attenuation tomography with high image quality.
Most of the parts of the new system are ready for assembly. The measuring aperture was enlarged to 36 cm, see Fig. 5, to cover a semi-spherical volume of interest with a diameter of 20 cm. The distribution of transducers over the aperture's surface is homogeneous and random to allow statistical sampling of the volume. The simulations promise an increase of contrast for the reflection tomography of a factor 6 and significant more contrast and visibility for transmission tomography. Especially by the new construction of the lifting mechanism the measuring device can be moved within 5 mm directly to the breast cage. The data acquisition time for 10^7 A-scans will be 2 minutes and the readout will be performed within 1.5 minutes. The ASIC has a bandwidth of 3 MHz and allows reconstruction also at frequencies as low as 0.75 MHz. The total imaging time including DAQ and image processing will shrink from about 2h to 13 minutes.

References

[1] N.V. Ruiter, M. Zapf, R. Dapp, T. Hopp, W.A. Kaiser, H. Gemmeke, "First results of a clinical study with 3D Ultrasound computer tomography", IEEE Ultrasonics Symp., 2013.

[2] P. D. Dragnev, D. A. Legg, and D. W. Townsend, "Discrete logarithmic energy on the sphere". Pacific J. Math. 207 (2002), no. 2, 345–358.

[3] H. Gemmeke, T. Hopp, M. Zapf, C. Kaiser, N.V. Ruiter, "3D ultrasound computer tomography: Hardware setup, reconstruction methods and first clinical results", Nuclear Instr. and Methods in Physics Research, A873 (2017) 59-65.

[4] H. Gemmeke, R. Dapp, T. Hopp, M. Zapf, N.V. Ruiter, "An Improved 3D Ultrasound Computer Tomography System", IEEE Ultrasonics Symposium (IUS), (2014) 1009.

[5] A. Kopmann, T. Bergmann, H. Gemmeke et al.: "FPGA-based DAQ system for multi-channel detectors," *Proc. IEEE NSS,* (2008), Dresden.

[6] M.Zapf, P. Pfistner, C.I. Liberman, "Dice-and-fill single element octagon transducers for next generation 3D USCT", Proceeding of International Workshop on Medical Ultrasound Tomography, 2017, in press.

[7] Henry Cohn and Abhinav Kumar, "Universally optimal distribution of points on spheres", J. Amer. Math. Soc. 20 (2007), no. 1, pp. 99-148.

[8] Patent PCT/EP2015/000369, WO 2015/124301 A1.

[9] Donald E. Knuth, Seminumerical Algorithms, volume 2 of The Art of Computer Programming. Addison-Wesley, 1969.

[10] M. Hardt, "Distributed Simulations for 3D ultrasound computer tomography," PHD-thesis KIT 2012, pp.68-84, AV Akademieverlag Saarbrücken, Germany, ISBN: 978-3-8381-3476-5.

[11] N.V. Ruiter, M. Zapf, T. Hopp, H. Gemmeke, "Experimental evaluation of noise generated by grating lobes for a sparse 3D ultrasound computer tomography system," Proc. SPIE Medical Imaging 2013: Ultrasonic Imaging, Tomography, and Therapy, 2013.

[12] B. Diarra, M. Robini, P. Tortoli C. Cachard, H. Liebgott, "Design of optimal 2D nongrid sparse arrays for medical ultrasound", IEEE Trans Biomed Eng. 2013, 60(11):3093-102.

[13] W. Y. Tan, T. Steiner, N.V. Ruiter, "Upper Bound of Accuracy for Self-Calibration of an 3D Ultrasound Tomography System without Ground Truth", Proceeding of International Workshop on Medical Ultrasound Tomography, 2017, in press.

[14] P. Kaever, M. Balzer, A. Kopmann, M. Zimmer and H. Rongen, The Common Data Acquisition Platform in the Helmholtz Association", Journal of Instrumentation, Volume 12, April 2017.

Comparison of two ray tracing methods for sound speed imaging

Xiaoyue Fang, Yun Wu, Mingyue Ding, Ming Yuchi

Department of Biomedical Engineering, School of Life Science and Technology, Key Laboratory of Molecular Biophysics of the Ministry of Education , Medical Ultrasound Laboratory, Huazhong University of Science and Technology, Wuhan, Hubei, China
E-Mail: m.yuchi@hust.edu.cn

Abstract

Ultrasound computed tomography (USCT) is a promising technology for early breast cancer detection. Sound speed imaging in USCT is a kind of functional imaging mode which can provide valuable information for differentiating normal tissue and tumor. One of the key problems of sound speed reconstruction is ray tracing. Common ray tracing methods include shortest path method, finite difference method, interpolation method and so on. This paper compares the sensitivity and the accuracy of the finite difference method and the linear interpolation method, came to the conclusion that the sensitivity of the linear interpolation is higher, while the accuracy of the finite difference method is higher probably resulting from the "expanding wavefront" scheme used.

Keywords: Ultrasound computed tomography, Sound speed reconstruction, Ray tracing, Finite difference, Linear interpolation

1 Introduction

Breast cancer is the most common cancer for women worldwide. Ultrasound computed tomography (USCT) is a promising technology for early breast cancer detection [1-4]. Sound speed imaging in USCT is performed by reconstructing the velocity distribution of the breast tissue [5-6]. One of the key problems of sound speed reconstruction is ray tracing. The ray tracing result directly determines the reconstruction sensitivity and accuracy. Common ray tracing methods include shortest path method [7], finite difference method [8-9], interpolation method [10] and so on.

Here, the finite difference method and the linear interpolation method are compared, including the travel times calculated in receiver location and the first-arrival time diagram, which reveal the sensitivity and accuracy of the two methods.

2 Material and Methods

2.1 Finite difference method

Vidale (1988) presented a method that could obtain the first arrival travel times by a finite-difference solution of the eikonal equation [8],

$$\left(\frac{\partial T}{\partial x}\right)^2 + \left(\frac{\partial T}{\partial z}\right)^2 = s(x,z)^2 , \tag{1}$$

where T(x, z) is the first arrival time for seismic energy propagating from a point source through a medium with a slowness distribution of s(x, z).

Vidale proposed the following scheme to solve equation (1):

For a source located at point A, in Fig. 1, the arrival times at the four points B_1, B_2, B_3, and B_4 can be computed by taking the product of the distance h and the average slowness between points A and B_i

$$T_{B_i} = h\frac{(s_{B_i}+s_A)}{2} , \tag{2}$$

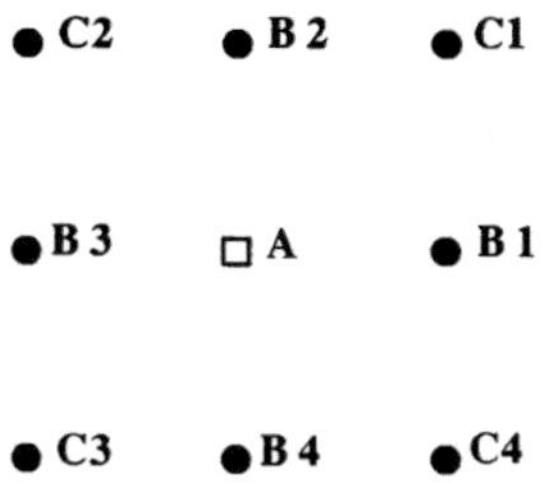

Figure 1: Finite-difference mesh centered about source point A, where arrival times at B_i and C_i for i = 1, 2, 3, 4 are to be calculated [9].

Then the arrival times at C_i at the four corner points can be computed with the following formulas:

$$T_{C_i} = T_A + \sqrt{2(h\bar{s}_i)^2 - (T_{B_{i+1}} - T_{B_i})^2}, \tag{3}$$

$$\overline{s_i} = \frac{1}{4}(s_A + s_{C_i} + s_{B_i} + s_{B_{i+1}}) \,, \tag{4}$$

where $T_A=0$, since it is the origin time of the source.

The procedures for computing travel times can be found in [9].

2.2 Linear interpolation method

Asakawa (1993) presented a linear interpolation method [10], which considered a ray path crossing segment AB on a certain cell boundary and reaching point D on the opposite side of the boundary as shown in Fig. 2. The method tries to calculate the ray crossing point C and the travel time T_D at point D, given that the travel times T_A and T_B are known at points A and B, respectively.

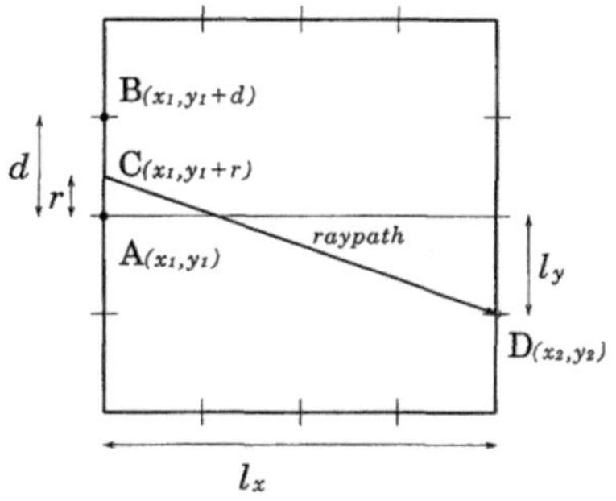

Figure 2: Geometrical representation of a ray path crossing a cell with equally spaced grid points on the cell boundaries [10].

After some manipulations, the travel time T_D and the distance r are given by

$$T_D = T_A + \Delta T \frac{l_y}{d} + \frac{l_x}{d}\sqrt{S^2 d^2 - \Delta T^2}, \tag{5}$$

$$r = \frac{\Delta T l_x}{\sqrt{S^2 d^2 - \Delta T^2}} - l_y, \tag{6}$$

where $\Delta T = T_A - T_B$.

The constraint of the linearity assumption over the segment AB are

$$S^2 d^2 \frac{{l_y}^2}{{l_x}^2 + {l_y}^2} \leq (\Delta T)^2 \leq S^2 d^2 \frac{(l_y + d)^2}{{l_x}^2 + (l_y + d)^2} \tag{7}$$

The procedures for computing travel times can be found in [10].

2.3 Data acquisition

We used the software pzflex to simulate acoustic-wave propagation in a numerical phantom. A ring array with 72 elements was used (Fig. 3). The diameter of the ring array was 40mm. When one element transmitted a signal, all other elements received signals. A numerical phantom of four circles with different sound speed value were placed inside the ring array and immersed in water. The phantom is introduced in Table 1.

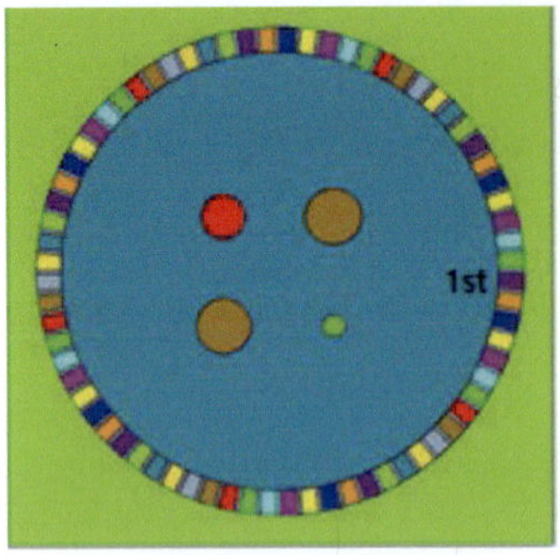

Figure 3: Illustration of a ring array and a numerical phantom immersed in water. "1st" indicates the first transducer element.

Position of circle center/color	Diameter(mm)	Material/Speed(m/s)
(5,5)/yellow	5	Nylon/2600
(-5,5)/red	4	Breast/1510
(-5,-5)/yellow	5	Nylon/2600
(5,-5)/green	2	Liver tumor/1579
--/blue	--	Water/1495

Table 1: Parameters of the four-circle phantom.

3 Results

3.1 First-arrival time diagram in forward process

The imaging area is divided into 321*321 grids firstly. The finite difference method and the linear interpolation method are used to calculate the first-arrival times in each grid, then ray paths are traced between transmitter-receiver pairs, the process is called forward process in sound speed reconstruction. The accuracy of first-arrival time calculated in each grid determines the sensitivity to "recognize" the target tissue.

First-arrival time diagram obtained using the two methods are illustrated in Fig. 4(a) and Fig. 4(b). The diagram represents the first-arrival time difference between the calculated value of the four-circle phantom and that of the phantom of all water when the first element transmits a signal. Both the two methods can "recognize" the two bigger circles with sound speed 2600 m/s. The interpolation method can show the third circle with sound speed value 1579 m/s more accurately. Both of these two method cannot "recognize" the forth circle with sound speed value 1510 m/s, although it is bigger than the third circle. The recognition result is listed in Table 2.

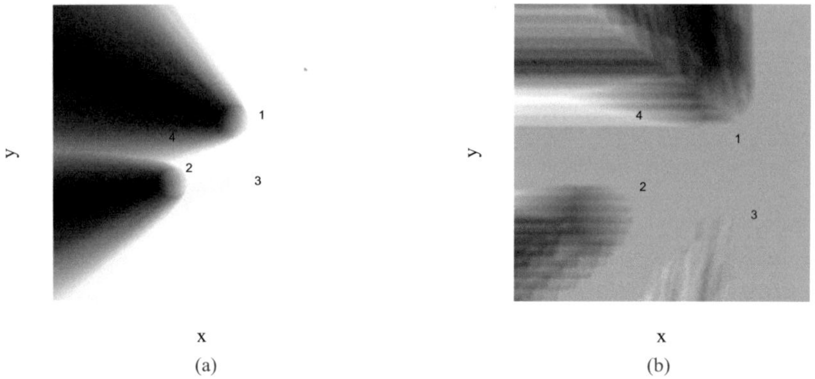

Figure 4: (a) First-arrival time diagram of the finite difference method. (b) First-arrival time diagram of the linear interpolation method.

Diameter(mm)	Material/Speed(m/s)	The finite difference method	The linear interpolation method
5	Nylon/2600	√	√
4	Breast/1510	×	×
5	Nylon/2600	√	√
2	Liver tumor/1579	×	√

Table 2: Sensitivity to "recognize" the different circle phantoms of the two methods.

3.2 Travel times calculated in receiver location

The differences of travel times calculated in receiver location in forward process and travel times detected from waveforms of receivers are the driving error to update sound speed model in inversion process. We compared the travel times in receiver position when the sound speed model is true value of the four-circle phantom with the travel times calculated in received waveforms. The less the difference of the two travel times is, the more accurate the forward process is.

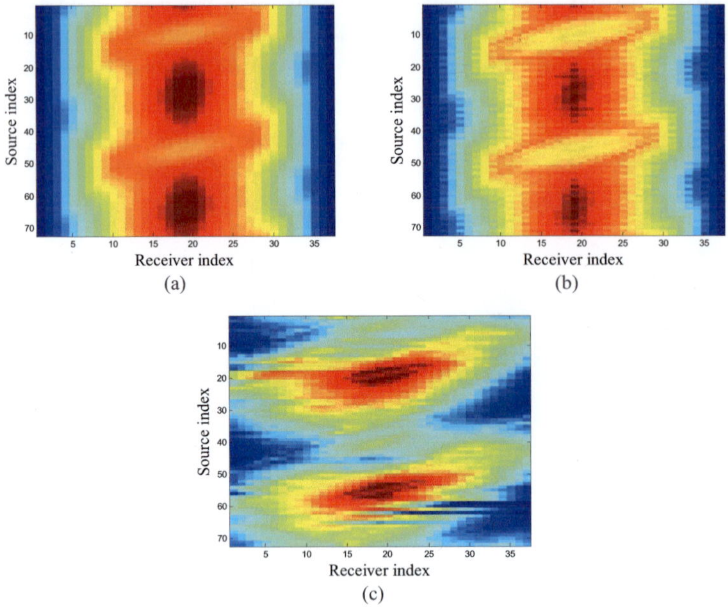

Figure 5: (a) Auto-detected travel times from waveforms generated from pzflex. (b) Travel times calculated from the finite difference method. (c)Travel times calculated from the linear interpolation method.

Firstly, we detected the travel times from the received waveforms of transducer elements within an arc of approximately 180 degrees with respect to the source transducer. Fig. 5 (a) is the standard to compare the travel times calculated from two forward process, i.e. the finite difference method in Fig.5 (b), and linear interpolation method in Fig.5 (c).

As we can see, the finite difference method's result is almost the same as the standard, however there is greater error in the interpolation method's result.

4 Discussion and Conclusion

This paper firstly generated USCT data using software pzflex. Then two ray tracing methods, i.e. the finite difference method and linear interpolation method were compared by the travel times calculated in the receiver location and the first-arrival time diagram. We found that both the two methods can "recognize" the two bigger circles with sound speed value 2600 m/s, while the interpolation method showed the circle with sound speed value 1579 m/s more accurately. Both the two methods cannot "recognize" the circle with sound speed value 1510 m/s. Travel times calculated in receiver location using finite difference method are almost the same as the standard, however there are greater error in the interpolation method's result. The comparison comes to the conclusion that the sensitivity of the linear interpolation method is higher, while the accuracy of the finite difference method is higher. Theoretically the linear interpolation method is more accurate [10], the phenomenon above probably results from the "expanding wavefront" scheme the finite difference method used, which implies the importance of the expanding scheme used.

References

[1] Wang S, Li C, Ding M and Ming Yuchi. "Frequency-shift low-pass filtering and least mean square adaptive filtering for ultrasound imaging", SPIE Medical Imaging, 9790, pp.97900P, (2016).

[2] Cuijuan Lou, Mengling Xu, Mingyue Ding, and Ming Yuchi. "Spatial smoothing coherence factor for ultrasound computed tomography", SPIE Medical Imaging, 9790, pp. 979008, (2016).

[3] Duric, N., Littrup, P., Poulo, L., Babkin, A., Pevzner, R., & Holsapple, E., et al. "Detection of breast cancer with ultrasound tomography: first results with the computed ultrasound risk evaluation (cure) prototype", Medical Physics, 34(2), pp.773-785, (2007).

[4] Neb Duric, Peter Littrup, Olivier Roy, Cuiping Li, Steve Schmidt, Xiaoyang Cheng and Roman Janer. "Clinical breast imaging with ultrasound tomography: A description of the SoftVue system", J. Acoust. Soc. Am. Papers, 135(4), pp.2155- 2155, (2014).

[5] Huang L. "Sound-speed tomography using first-arrival transmission ultrasound for a ring array", Proceedings of SPIE - The International Society for Optical Engineering, 6513, pp. 6513061-6513069, (2007).

[6] Li C, Duric N, Littrup P, et al. In vivo breast sound-speed imaging with ultrasound tomography.[J]. Ultrasound in Medicine & Biology, 2009, 35(10):1615-1628.

[7] Moser T J. Shortest path calculation of seismic rays [J]. Geophysics, 1991, 56(1):59-67.

[8] Vidale J. Finite-difference calculation of travel times [J]. Bulletin of the Seismological Society of America, 1988, 78(6):2062-2076.

[9] Qin F, Luo Y, Olsen K B, et al. Finite-difference solution of the eikonal equation along expanding wavefronts[J]. Geophysics, 1992, 57(3):478-487.

[10] Asakawa E, Kawanaka T. Seismic ray tracing using linear traveltime interpolation [J]. Geophysical Prospecting, 1993, 41(1):99-111.

Contrast resolution enhancement of Ultrasonic Computed Tomography using a wavelet-based method – Preliminary results in bone imaging

Philippe Lasaygues[1], Régine Guillermin[1], Khaled Metwally[1], Samantha Fernandez[2], Laure Balasse[2,3], Philippe Petit[4], Cécile Baron[5]

[1] *Aix Marseille Univ, CNRS, Centrale Marseille, LMA, Marseille, France*
E-mail: lasaygues@lma.cnrs-mrs.fr
[2] *Aix-Marseille Univ, CERIMED, Marseille, France*
[3] *Aix Marseille Univ, INSERM, VRCM, Marseille, France*
[4] *Dep. of Pediatric and Prenatal Radiol., "Timone" Children-Hospital, APHM, Marseille, France*
[5] *Aix Marseille Univ, CNRS, ISM, Marseille, France*

Abstract

Ultrasonic Computed Tomography (USCT) is a biological tissue imaging modality. USCT is mainly efficient in improving image resolution by eliminating noise and interferences. The strong variations in acoustic properties between soft tissues and bone generate complex signals consisting of several packets with different signatures. USCT contrast ratio is degraded. In this paper, a method to enhance USCT resolution is investigated. The method, called the "Wavelet-based Coded Excitation" (WCE) method, is based on the wavelet decomposition of the signal and on a suitable transmitted incident wave correlated with the experimental set-up, mathematically expressed using an extended form of simulated annealing. The goal of this study is to investigate the feasibility of the WCE method to enhance the Contrast-to-Noise Ratio of USCT for bone objects. Experiments are conducted with a bone phantom, and with a chicken drumstick, using a circular antenna equipped with 1MHz-transducers. Results demonstrate the capabilities and limitations of the method.

Keywords: ultrasonic tomography, resolution, coded-excitation, wavelet, bone

1 Introduction

Currently, X-ray Tomography offers significant advantages for the measurement of Bone Mineral Density (BMD). However, the limited spatial resolution of some today's devices makes an accurate measurement of cortical thickness difficult to obtain, and an assessment of cortical density almost impossible [1]. As a consequence, published data concerning cortical density should be reviewed carefully. For example, cortical density measurement limitations were confirmed in children and newborns. Significant correlations of total radius cross-sectional area, cortical area and cortical thickness with weight and height were found but with no gender differences [2]. Nevertheless, BMD remains today the "gold-standard" parameter, reporting essentially on the bone mineral contents. It is also worth noting that BMD does not describe the micro-architecture of bone, and that the ultrasonic waves are successfully used to determine other parameters than density, such as elasticity or porosity [3], [4]. X-ray (and also Magnetic Resonance Imaging-MRI) modalities are associated with different constraints and inconveniences (worse in the case of pediatric application), according to the type of examination: cost, radiation, sedation, availability, and accessibility, while Ultrasound is a non-invasive, non-irradiant, and painless modality. Ultrasound scanners are little expensive (compared to X-ray or MRI scanners) and can be used at the patient bedside. However, ultrasound has difficulty penetrating bone and, therefore, can only detect the outer surface of bony structures and not what lies within it. In current medical practice, the sub-cortical imaging is not possible, and no information on the cortical thickness and the medullar underlying tissue is available. The physical distribution of cortical bone within the measured site may influence acoustical measurements, and thus the electro-acoustical setup may not be adapted in terms of signal processing, amplification, or gain. Furthermore, the map is a bi-dimensional representation of the impedance variation between soft and hard tissues, but is not parametrical (the gray level set is not related to the value). And when a periosteal reaction occurs on adjacent bones (ribs, tibia-fibula), the resolution of echographic images may be limited, especially between the two bones. There are also limitations to the depth that sound waves can penetrate; therefore, deeper structures in larger or fatter patients may not be seen easily. For visualizing internal structure of bones or certain joints, others imaging modalities are used.

Ultrasonic Computed Tomography (USCT), a numerical two dimensional (2D) data inversion method, appears to be a possible alternative in view of the limits of medical sonography, making it possible, on one hand, to take into account the physical phenomena due to wave propagation in hard tissues, with appropriate modeling, and, on the other hand, to reach one or more significant parameters of the structure like the speed of sound or attenuation. Based on the linearization of the inverse problem of acoustic wave propagation, USCT generates cross-sectional images of biological soft tissues [5]–[7]. Difficulties occur in hard tissue imaging [7], due to the great differences between tissue impedance, and to the high echogenic index of the bone, which strongly alters the propagation of the ultrasonic waves, and generally induces low contrast resolution, and low Contrast-to-Noise Ratio (CNR). The physical phenomena associated with wave propagation make it necessary to modify the methods used for the acquisition of the ultrasonic signals. The use of low ultrasound frequencies (≤ 3MHz) provides an effective possible solution [8]. However, if the depth of the field increases, the resolution of the signals and hence that of the reconstructed images is bound to decrease. Even with low frequencies, the wave propagation process generates extremely complex acoustic signals, which are often difficult to interpret in terms of wave path, volume, guided or surface waves, and attenuation. To improve the quality of the signals, focus should be placed on signal processing such as filtering, spectrum analysis and method involving the deconvolution of the signals using a characteristic transfer function of the experimental device [9]. Deconvolution algorithms increase the bandwidth of the frequency spectrum, but they tend to be over unstable and prone to noise. Loosvelt and Lasaygues [10] developed an alternative method based on a multi-scale signal decomposition procedure, making it possible to process all the information available in terms of frequency and time. This method, called the "Wavelet-based Coded Excitation" (WCE) method, was used to determine, independently, the velocity of the ultrasonic wave and the wave path across the thickness of a 1D-parallelepiped plate. The aim of this new study is to investigate the feasibility of the WCE method as a means of CNR enhancement of bone imaging. In this two-dimensional case, the wavelet decomposition alone does not suffice to optimize the signal processing, and the incident wave reaching the object also should match the wavelets' mathematical properties. We thus propose a solution to achieve this goal, based on a zone-by-zone simulated annealing algorithm. Then, we show the usefulness of the WCE method through experimental results on a human bone (without soft tissues) mimicking phantom, and on an *ex vivo* chicken drumstick (without skin).

2 Material and method

2.1 USCT statements

By now, basic USCT principles have been clearly established in the case of weakly varying media such as low-contrast structures, i.e., almost homogeneous media [5], [6], [11]. A constant reference medium can therefore be chosen and approximations will be made over an unperturbed background. The scattering problem can be linearized by using the first-order Born approximation, and if the Green's function of the unperturbed problem (the background) is known, the forward problem can be solved with the Lippmann-Schwinger integral equation. A method to solve this inverse problem will consist in performing a far field asymptotic development. The USCT algorithm will yield the perturbation with respect to the reference problem. This leads to a linear relation between the object function (or contrast function) and the scattered field, particularly in the far-field (2D Fourier transform) case, which makes it possible to reconstruct the object function in almost real time, based on a sufficiently large set of scattering data. The details of the algorithm used in this work can be found in [12], [13]. In the case of hard biological tissues having larger acoustical impedances than those of the surrounding medium, the weak scattering hypothesis is not realistic. Nevertheless, if the imaging objective involves parameters such as the bone thickness, the problem can be viewed as how to identify a water-like cavity (the object) located in an elastic cylinder immersed in a water-like fluid. In this configuration, one solution consists in using the low frequency ultrasonic wave propagation scheme, because the penetration length of the wave will be greater than a high frequency scheme, and the Born approximation will still be satisfied. The background can be defined in terms of the solid part without any hole, surrounded by water, and the perturbation, i.e., the object to be reconstructed, would be the cavity. Image reconstruction can then be performed by means of an efficient back-projection method implemented using standard graphics algorithms [8].

2.2 USCT device and calibration

An USCT device prototype has been developed by our laboratory (Figure 1).

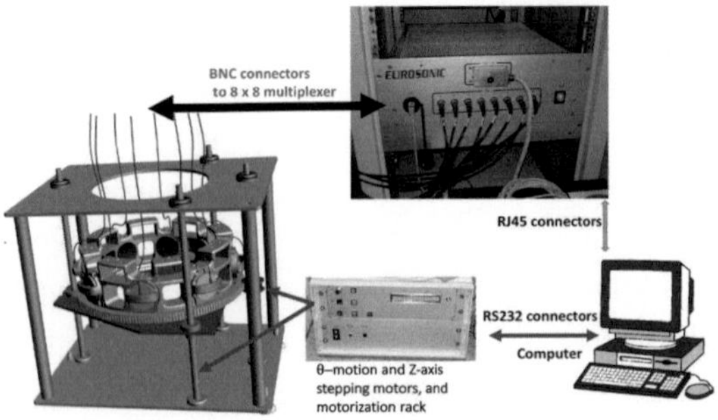

Figure 1: Photo and design drawing of the device and setup.

The device consists of a multiplexed 2D-ring antenna. The crown of the antenna has an inner radius of 150 mm and supports 8 fixed transducers distributed over 360° ($\Delta\theta = 45°$). The object to be imaged is positioned in the hypothetical geometrical center of the ring. By means of stepping motors and of an electronic motorization rack to manage the mechanical movements, the crown can turn 45° degrees in 1/100 degree increments of and move vertically for multiple image slicing (limit stroke 200mm). For a given height, it is thus possible to acquire sinograms with 64 projections (8 transmitters x 8 receivers). Then, signals from every rotation (32 in this work) are used to get a complete sinogram with 64*32 = 2048 signals, and a combination according to the angles of diffraction. Thus, we simulate an antenna comprising a greater number of emitters and receivers. The scattered pressure field is obtained by subtracting the total pressure field (measured in the presence of the object) and the incident pressure field (measured in the absence of the object). Experimentally, this consists in eliminating the data from the direct transmission between transducers facing each other with their axes aligned. The Mistras-Eurosonic™ multiplexer equipped with an 8-by-8 parallel-channel acquisition system allows the formation of arbitrary waveforms and beamforming over 8 independent channels. Transmitted and received ultrasonic radio-frequency (RF-)signals are digitized (4096 samples by signal, resolution of 12 bits, sampling frequency of 20 MHz). The power amplifier gives a variable output voltage from 10 mV to 50 mV. The 8 transducers are Imasonic™ piezo-composite transducers with a center frequency of 1 MHz, and the -6 dB bandwidth is 1.46 MHz (from 0.48 MHz to 1.95 MHz). They are equally spaced (every 45°) on the crown. Each transducer is 60 mm high and 56 mm in diameter. These transducers have a focal length of 150 mm in the Fresnel zone, a lateral aperture size of 40 mm and an axial aperture size of 30 mm. The slice thickness is 3 mm. The mean center frequency is 1.08 MHz ± 0.1 MHz. Fluctuations in the position of the transducers on the crown can give rise to time-shift variations which degrade the spatial resolution of the USCT. Here to assess these biases, a 70μm-diameter copper thread is placed in the center of the crown. For each signal, the correction process is a temporal offset between the signal and the reference signal obtained at the same angle on the thread sinogram (Point Spread Function-PSF of the device).

2.3 Pulse-mode method

The electro-acoustic device and the transducers therefore serve as a continuous, linear, stationary causal filter (Figure 2).

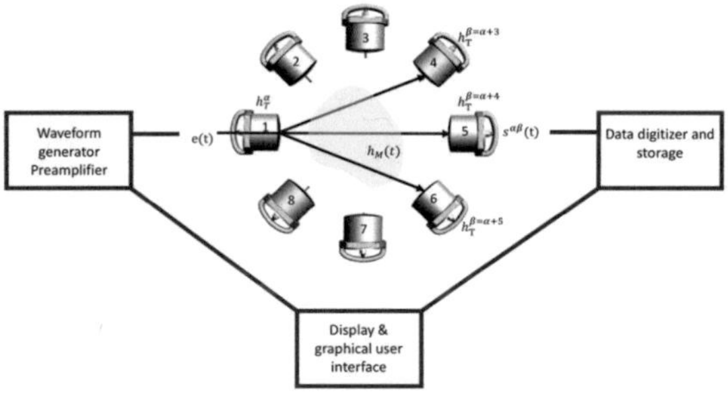

Figure 2: Electro-acoustical synoptic of the 8-parallel-channel acquisition system

The transmitted $x^{\alpha\beta}(\mathrm{t})$ and received $\mathrm{s}^{\alpha\beta}(\mathrm{t})$ signals are connected by convolution:

$$s^{\alpha\beta}(\mathrm{t}) = \mathrm{x}^{\alpha\beta}(\mathrm{t}) \otimes h_{\mathrm{M}}(\mathrm{t}) \tag{1}$$

$$\mathrm{x}^{\alpha\beta}(\mathrm{t}) = \left(h_T^{\alpha} \otimes h_{\mathrm{T}}^{\beta} \otimes \mathrm{e}\right)(\mathrm{t}) \tag{2}$$

where $\otimes$ denotes the convolution operation; e(t) is the electrical input conveyed to the transducer via the waveform generator; h_T^α and h_T^β are the responses of the electro-acoustic device including the waveform generator, multiplexer and transducers noα and noβ ($\alpha = \beta = [1,\ldots,8]$), respectively, of the circular antenna in diffraction mode; $\mathrm{h_M(t)}$ is the response of the object under investigation. At this stage, the responses of the 8 transducers are supposed identical. Here, the choice of the electrical input e(t) (independently for each pulse- or wavelet-mode method) is made on the total transmitted field in the absence of the object. The measurement is carried out in transmission between two opposite and aligned transducers ($\alpha = [1,\ldots,8]$; $\beta = \alpha + 4$). Then, in the absence of any object, the transmitted response, $h_M(t)$, in water depends on the time delay of the wave - which is proportional to the distance $d^{\alpha\beta}$ between one transmitter ($\alpha = [1,\ldots,8]$) and one receiver ($\beta = \alpha + 4$) - and on its velocity v_0. The initial output signal, $[s^{\alpha\beta}(t)]^{init}$, is therefore equal to the input signal $x^{\alpha\beta}(t)$, which is invariant by translation:

$$[s^{\alpha\beta}(t)]^{init} = x^{\alpha\beta}(t) \otimes \delta\left(t - {d^{\alpha\beta}}/{v_0}\right) = x^{\alpha\beta}(t) \tag{3}$$

Here, to obtain control experimental data, USCT is first realized using a conventional ultrasonic pulse-mode method. The electrical input signal $e(t)$ was a pulse signal, which was comparable to a Dirac delta function (in terms of the distribution), and $[s^{\alpha\beta}(t)]^{init}$ is given by

$$[s^{\alpha\beta}(t)]^{init} = \left(h_T^{\alpha} \otimes h_T^{\beta}\right)(t) \tag{4}$$

2.4 Wavelet-based coded excitation (WCE) method

Based on the orthogonal wavelet decomposition of the signal, it is possible to obtain a time versus scale diagram, giving the evolution of the frequencies with time. Like time-scale processing, wavelet decomposition lends itself very well to detecting and discriminating between signals during the data pre-processing phase as well as during the filtering step of an image reconstruction phase. If the initial received signal $x^{\alpha\beta}(t)$ is a wavelet denoted $\varphi_J(t)$, centered on the scale J ($j \in Z$) and with suitable properties for specific wavelet analysis, previously analyzed by Y. Meyer and S. Jaffard [14], [15], Eq. 1 can be written:

$$s^{\alpha\beta}(t) = \left(\varphi_J \otimes h_M\right)(t) \tag{5}$$

The coded-excitation method is thus based on a time-scale decomposition of the signal $s^{\alpha\beta}(t)$ giving the suitable coefficients $X_J^{\alpha\beta}(t)$:

$$X_J^{\alpha\beta}(t) = \langle s^{\alpha\beta}(t), \phi_j(t)\rangle = h_M(t) \otimes [\varphi_J \otimes \phi_j](t) \tag{6}$$

where ϕ_j is a wavelet centered on the scale j ($j \in \mathbb{Z}$). The properties of the wavelet decomposition, an orthogonal decomposition in this case, are such that the coefficients $X_J^{\alpha\beta}(t)$ nullify everywhere except for $j = J$ (the details of the algorithm can be found in [10]).

2.5 Acoustical modeling

As detailed in [12], reconstruction is performed using the summation of filtered back-projections" algorithm. Each pixel of the image corresponds to a coordinate of a point corresponding to a transmitter-receiver pair, that is to say, for each recorded signal. The coordinates of the point in the sinogram are the signal number (ordinate) and the time of flight (abscissa). The time of flight for each pair of transducers must be accurately measured. The working hypothesis adopted in this study is that, depending on the angle of observation, the object is comparable to a bilayer composed of two parallelepiped plates. The ultrasonic incident wave vector is perpendicular to the water/object interface. The object is taken to be homogeneous and isotropic. The first-arriving signals are assumed to be the signals from the water/bone interface and the last arriving signals are assumed to be the compressional wave propagating off the back wall. Three configurations are taken into account for this modeling: reflection (transducers α- α), back-propagation (couple of transducers α-$\alpha + 1$ and α-$\alpha + 7$), and diffraction (couple of transducers $\alpha - \alpha + 2$, $\alpha - \alpha + 3$, $\alpha - \alpha + 5$, $\alpha - \alpha + 6$). In the transmission mode, the directly transmitted wave field signals are eliminated. Only the echo mode is considered for the first and second configuration, and only the transmission mode for the third configuration. All the other phenomena (shear waves, guided waves, etc.) are insignificant or will occur too late to affect the compressional wave processes. Therefore, the received signal can be modeled as the sum of several wave packets. $h_{\mathrm{M}}(\mathrm{t})$ is comparable to a sum of Dirac delta functions.

$$s^{\alpha\beta}(\mathrm{t}) = A_1^{\alpha\beta}\varphi_{\mathrm{J}}\left(t - t_1^{\alpha\beta}\right) + A_2^{\alpha\beta}\varphi_{\mathrm{J}}\left(t - t_2^{\alpha\beta}\right) + \cdots + A_n^{\alpha\beta}\varphi_{\mathrm{J}}\left(t - t_n^{\alpha\beta}\right) \tag{7}$$

$A_n^{\alpha\beta}$ are the amplitudes of the wave packets located at $t_n^{\alpha\beta}$ between transducers noα and noβ. As indicated by Loosvelt and Lasaygues [10], $t_n^{\alpha\beta}$ can be measured by cross-correlation between the signal received $s^{\alpha\beta}(\mathrm{t})$ and a predetermined analyzing pattern. The result is the sum of the functions $X_J^{\alpha\beta}(\mathrm{t})$. The locations of times $t_n^{\alpha\beta}$ correspond to the signals from the object's inner structure.

$$\begin{aligned} X_J^{\alpha\beta}(\mathrm{t}) = {} & A_1^{\alpha\beta}\langle\varphi_{\mathrm{J}}(t - t_1^{\alpha\beta}), \phi_{\mathrm{j}}(t)\rangle + A_2^{\alpha\beta}\langle\varphi_{\mathrm{J}}(t - t_2^{\alpha\beta}), \phi_{\mathrm{j}}(t)\rangle + \cdots \\ & + A_n^{\alpha\beta}\langle\varphi_{\mathrm{J}}(t - t_n^{\alpha\beta}), \phi_{\mathrm{j}}(t)\rangle \end{aligned} \tag{8}$$

$$X_J^{\alpha\beta}(\mathrm{t}) = X_J^{\alpha\beta}(t - t_1^{\alpha\beta}) + X_J^{\alpha\beta}(t - t_2^{\alpha\beta}) + \cdots + X_J^{\alpha\beta}(t - t_n^{\alpha\beta}) \tag{9}$$

If it is possible to process the initial signal received $\mathrm{X}^{\alpha\beta}(\mathrm{t})$ in such a way that it is identical to a wavelet function, this method then yields the parameters of interest without any further filtering effects being involved. The main problem is how to digitize an initial electric input signal e(t) in order to obtain $x^{\alpha\beta}(t) = \varphi_J(t)$.

2.6 Wavelet form

In the 1D-transmission mode, Loosvelt and Lasaygues [10] previously performed direct spectral Wiener deconvolution between the wavelet $\varphi_J(t)$ and the received signal that was recorded when the electrical input signal e(t) was a Dirac delta function. In the 2D-mode measurements, although the signals mostly overlapped, considerable differences between the theoretical wavelets and those actually generated using the same algorithm and the same center frequency were observed between the transducers in diffraction mode (couple of transducers $(\alpha{-}\alpha + 2)$, $(\alpha{-}\alpha + 3)$, $(\alpha{-}\alpha + 5)$, $(\alpha{-}\alpha + 6)$). Conil et al. [16] uses a non-linear scheme and a simulated annealing algorithm [17]. The advantage of the method is that it is not necessary to know the response of the system to find a suitable input signal. This involves iteratively testing many input signals and analyzing the corresponding output signals. During the search, the probability of finding an input signal is defined as a function of the deviation between the output signal obtained and the sought signal.

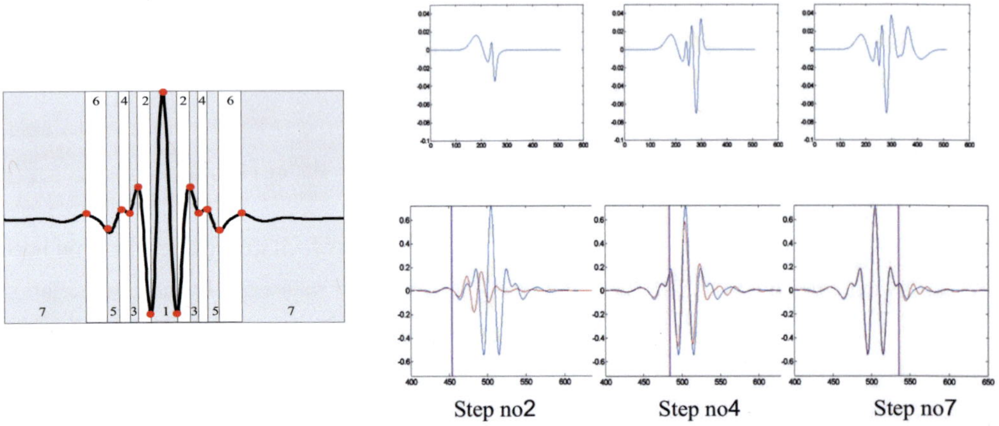

Figure 3: (left) Wavelet form (S. Jaffard function [18] with J = -4), matching zones delimited by local extrema. (right) Illustration of 3 steps of the construction of the wavelet (J = -4) by simulated annealing. (top) input signal e(t), (bottom) reconstructed signal

This probability is extended to zero; the more slowly the function tends towards zero, the better the result. Here, to limit the number of signals to be tested, which can be very important, and very time-consuming, the algorithm is adapted to the wavelet, which corresponds to the bandwidth of the 1 MHz-transducer (center frequency 0.83 MHz, bandwidth [0.42 MHz – 1.66 MHz], corresponding to J = -4) (Figure 4). This wavelet contains several local extrema (Figure 3), and the simulated annealing algorithm is applied zone by zone - the zones being delimited by local extrema. Because the wavelet is symmetrical, the number of matching zones is reduced, and the process extends iteratively from left to right of the targeted waveform (Figure 3).

The algorithm includes 8 iterations. For each step, the atoms (main functions calculating during the simulated annealing algorithm) are determined one after the other. Once all the atoms are defined, all their parameters are adjusted to obtain the best output signal.

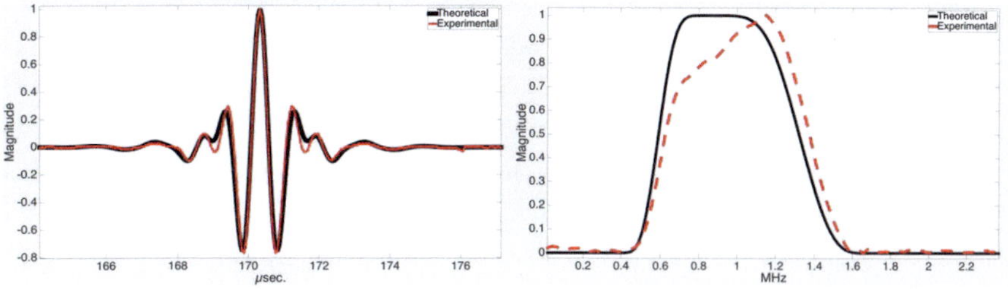

Figure 4: Time (left) and spectral (right) graph of the theoretical (black line) and the experimental (red dash line) wavelet between transmitter n°1 and receiver n°4 ($\theta = 135°$) in the absence of any object

<table>
<tr><td>A: X-ray CT</td><td>B: USCT - pulse mode</td><td>C: USCT - WCE</td></tr>
<tr><td colspan="3">Sawbones™ composite bone mimicking phantom</td></tr>
<tr><td>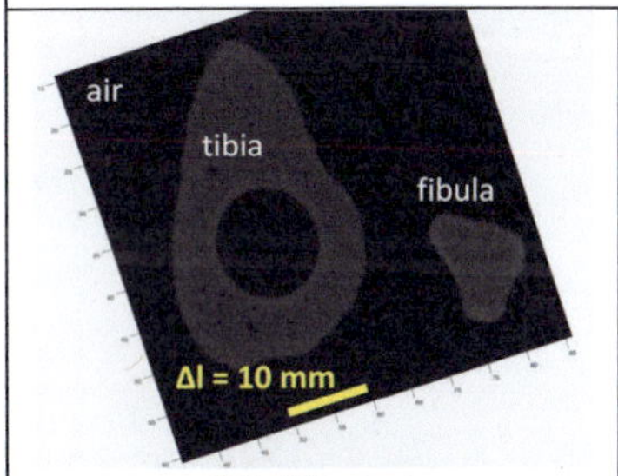
</td><td>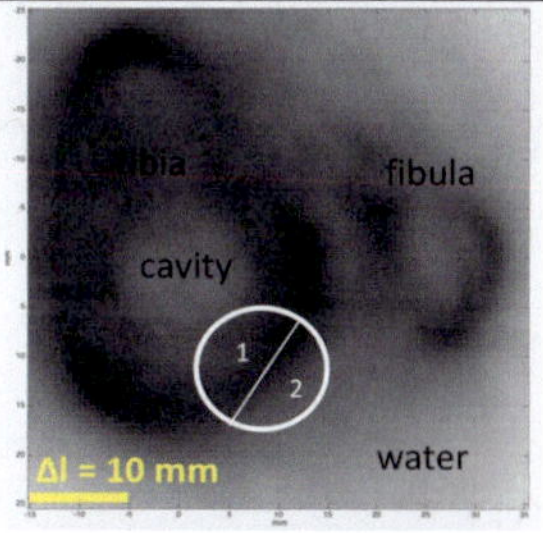
</td><td>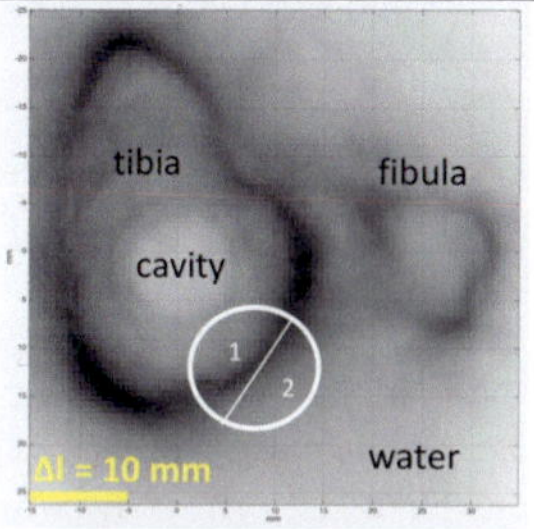
</td></tr>
<tr><td>478x478 pixels</td><td>127x127 pixels; CNR = 0.88</td><td>127x127 pixels; CNR = 1.53</td></tr>
<tr><td colspan="3">Ex vivo chicken drumstick</td></tr>
<tr><td>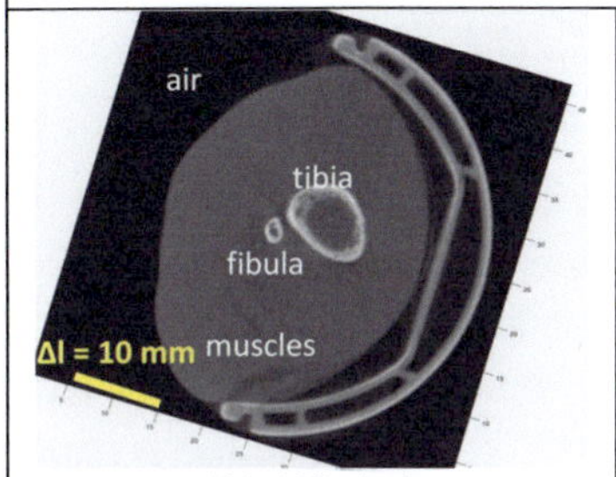
</td><td>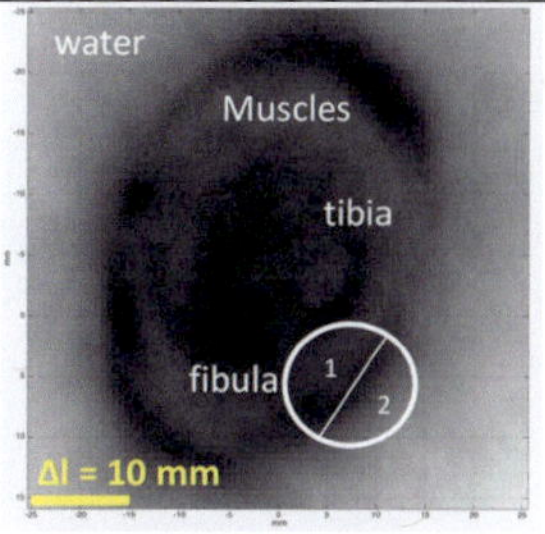
</td><td>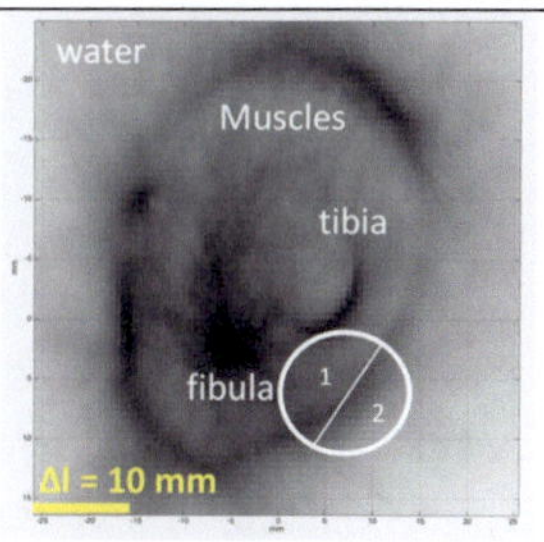
</td></tr>
<tr><td>188x188 pixels</td><td>127x127 pixels; CNR = 1.20</td><td>127x127 pixels; CNR = 1.35</td></tr>
</table>

Figure 5: X-ray CT (A), USCT using an electric pulse (B), and wavelet $\varphi_{-4}(t)$ (C), of a Sawbones™ composite bone mimicking phantom (top) and an *ex vivo* chicken drumstick without skin (bottom). The white circle represents the regions involved in Contrast-to-Noise Ratio calculation.

3 Results

Experiments were conducted to confirm the performance of the developed method. Two objects were analyzed. One human bone mimicking phantom (Sawbones™, tibia-fibula), and one *ex vivo* chicken drumstick without skin were studied. The cavity diameter of the tibia mimicking phantom was 12.5 mm, and its overall length 42 cm, and the fibula mimicking phantom had no inner cavity. The distance between bones (~ 8 mm) was measured using a caliper. The objects were set in water at room temperature prior to the experiments. The water tank temperature was 21°7 and the ultrasonic wave velocity in water was 1486 m/s. USCT images of objects were compared with X-ray computed tomography (X-ray CT) images obtained at the same cross-section levels, with a nanoScan® PET/CT preclinical imager (Mediso™, Hungary). The slice thickness for the X-ray cross-section was 1.5 mm and the number of projections was 360. Cross-sections were chosen in the cortical areas of the bones; 100 mm from the proximal epiphysis for the bone phantom; and 25 mm for the chicken drumstick. The 2D-ultrasonic tomograms were obtained from two excitation modes: the pulse excitation mode used an electric pulse as the input signal (Figure 5-B), while the WCE method used a signal corresponding to the wavelet φ_{-4} (Figure 5-C). The parameter commonly adopted to determine the quality of ultrasonic tomographic reconstructions is the Contrast-to-Noise Ratio (CNR) [19][20]. This criterion defines the contrast between two adjacent media as:

$$CNR_{1,2} = |\overline{D_1} - \overline{D_2}| \Big/ \sqrt{\sigma_1^2 + \sigma_2^2} \tag{10}$$

$\overline{D_1}$ and $\overline{D_2}$ are the mean pixel values in regions 1 and 2, and σ_1 and σ_2 are the corresponding standard deviations. Both regions contain the same number of pixels. The object (region no1) contrast is assessed in comparison with the background (region no2). As CNR increases, noise decreases and quality increases.

4 Conclusion

The resolution of images obtained by USCT is not as good as that of images obtained by X-ray Computed Tomography. It was nevertheless possible to observe qualitatively the tibia and fibula cortical shells on the USCT-images for both phantom and chicken samples. When the WCE method was applied to USCT, a 42.5% increase in contrast was observed for the phantom object. The diameter of the inner cavity was found to be in the 11-13 mm range, which is close to the actual value of 12.5 mm. The external distance between tibia and fibula was found to be in the 5-7 mm range, rather far from the actual value (8mm). For the chicken drumstick, the contrast increased by 11%. The differentiation between tibia and fibula was more difficult. The image of the tibia was not complete, and its diameter could not be measured. The image of the fibula was not well resolved, and the distance between the two bones could not be measured. By applying the WCE method, the definition of the outer and inner boundaries of each bone was obtained with a much better contrast resolution than when using the electric pulse. The boundaries of the tibia were retrieved but the quality of this reconstruction was not satisfactory; the inner structure of the tibia was not resolved. To conclude, by applying the WCE method to cortical bone USCT, boundary imaging resolution was enhanced, even though sizes were different from the actual sizes.

Acknowledgements

This research was supported by the ANR funds, under Grant No. 11-BS09-032. The authors are grateful to Eric Debieu and Vincent Long at the Laboratory of Mechanics and Acoustics, (LMA) for their help in setting up experiments. The authors also thank Eduardo Morais Carvalho at Aix-Marseille University and Gladys Leger, at Centrale Marseille for their internship work.

References

[1] P. Augat, T. Link, T. F. Lang, J. C. Lin, S. Majumdar, and H. K. Genant, "Anisotropy of the elastic modulus of trabecular bone specimens from different anatomical locations," *Med. Eng. Phys.*, vol. 20, no. 2, pp. 124–131, Mar. 1998.

[2] T. L. Binkley, R. Berry, and B. L. Specker, "Methods for measurement of pediatric bone," *Rev. Endocr. Metab. Disord.*, vol. 9, no. 2, pp. 95–106, Jun. 2008.

[3] C. Baron, M. Talmant, and P. Laugier, "Effect of porosity on effective diagonal stiffness coefficients (cii) and elastic anisotropy of cortical bone at 1MHz: A finite-difference time domain study," *J. Acoust. Soc. Am.*, vol. 122, no. 3, pp. 1810–1817, Sep. 2007.

[4] P. Laugier and G. Haïat, *Bone quantitative ultrasound.* Dordrecht; New York: Springer Science, 2011.

[5] N. V. Ruiter, T. O. Müller, R. Stotzka, and H. Gemmeke, "Evaluation of Different Approaches for Transmission Tomography in Ultrasound Computer Tomography," in *Bildverarbeitung für die Medizin 2005*, H.-P. Meinzer, H. Handels, A. Horsch, and T. Tolxdorff, Eds. Berlin/Heidelberg: Springer-Verlag, 2005, pp. 430–434.

[6] N. Duric *et al.*, "Detection of breast cancer with ultrasound tomography: First results with the Computed Ultrasound Risk Evaluation (CURE) prototype: Detection of breast cancer with ultrasound tomography," *Med. Phys.*, vol. 34, no. 2, pp. 773–785, Jan. 2007.

[7] P. Lasaygues, S. Mensah, R. Guillermin, J. Rouyer, and E. Franceschini, "Nonlinear inversion modeling for ultrasonic computed tomography: transition from soft to hard tissues imaging," in *Proceedings of SPIE*, 2012, vol. 8320, p. 832004.

[8] P. Lasaygues, "Assessing the cortical thickness of long bone shafts in children, using two-dimensional ultrasonic diffraction tomography," *Ultrasound Med. Biol.*, vol. 32, no. 8, pp. 1215–1227, Aug. 2006.

[9] P. Lasaygues, J. P. Lefebvre, and S. Mensah, "High resolution low frequency ultrasonic tomography," *Ultrason. Imaging*, vol. 19, no. 4, pp. 278–293, Oct. 1997.

[10] M. Loosvelt and P. Lasaygues, "A Wavelet-Based Processing method for simultaneously determining ultrasonic velocity and material thickness," *Ultrasonics*, vol. 51, no. 3, pp. 325–339, Apr. 2011.

[11] J.-P. Lefebvre, P. Lasaygues, and S. Mensah, "Acoustic Tomography, Ultrasonic Tomography," in *Materials and Acoustics Handbook*, M. Bruneau and C. Potel, Eds. London, UK: ISTE, 2009, pp. 887–906.

[12] P. Lasaygues, D. Tanne, S. Mensah, and J. P. Lefebvre, "Circular antenna for breast ultrasonic diffraction tomography," *Ultrason. Imaging*, vol. 24, no. 3, pp. 177–189, Jul. 2002.

[13] J. P. Lefebvre, P. Lasaygues, S. Mensah, S. Delamare, and A. Wirgin, "Born Ultrasonic Tomography: Some Limits and Improvements," in *Acoustical Imaging*, vol. 25, M. Halliwell and P. N. T. Wells, Eds. Boston: Kluwer Academic Publishers, 2002, pp. 79–86.

[14] Y. Meyer, "Orthonormal Wavelets," in *Wavelets*, J.-M. Combes, A. Grossmann, and P. Tchamitchian, Eds. Berlin, Heidelberg: Springer Berlin Heidelberg, 1989, pp. 21-37.

[15] S. Jaffard, Y. Meyer, and R. D. Ryan, *Wavelets: Tools for Science and Technology*. Society for Industrial and Applied Mathematics, 2001.

[16] F. Conil, D. Gibert, and F. Nicollin, "Nonlinear synthesis of input signals in ultrasonic experimental setups," *J. Acoust. Soc. Am.*, vol. 115, no. 1, p. 246, 2004.

[17] S. Kirkpatrick, C. D. Gelatt, and M. P. Vecchi, "Optimization by Simulated Annealing," *Science*, vol. 220, no. 4598, pp. 671–680, May 1983.

[18] S. Jaffard, "Construction of Wavelets on Open Sets," in *Wavelets*, J.-M. Combes, A. Grossmann, and P. Tchamitchian, Eds. Berlin, Heidelberg: Springer Berlin Heidelberg, 1989, pp. 247–252.

[19] R. C. Waag and R. J. Fedewa, "A ring transducer system for medical ultrasound research," *IEEE Trans. Ultrason. Ferroelectr. Freq. Control*, vol. 53, no. 10, pp. 1707–1718, Oct. 2006.

[20] J. Rouyer, S. Mensah, C. Vasseur, and P. Lasaygues, "The benefits of compression methods in acoustic coherence tomography," *Ultrason. Imaging*, vol. 37, no. 3, pp. 205–223, Jul. 2015.

Fast reflectivity imaging in 3D using SAFT

N.V. Ruiter, M. Zapf, T. Hopp, and H. Gemmeke

Karlsruhe Institute of Technology, Karlsruhe, Germany
E-mail: nicole.ruiter@kit.edu

Abstract

The computational burden for 3D Synthetic Aperture Focusing Technique (SAFT) is large as for each voxel the delay for each acquired A-scan has to be calculated, e.g. $O(N^5)$ for N^3 voxels and N^2 A-scans. For 3D reconstruction of objects which are large in terms of the wavelength, e.g. $\geq (100\ \lambda)^3$, the computation of one volume takes several days on a current multicore PC. If the 3D distribution of speed of sound is applied to correct the delays for objects with varying speed of sound the computation time increases further. This overview paper presents the implementations for 3D SAFT developed by the KIT group and discusses their computational performance.

Keywords: 3D SAFT, reflectivity imaging, GPU, acceleration

1 Introduction

The KIT's 3D USCT system [1] has a semi-ellipsoidal aperture with 628 emitters and 1413 receivers, see Figure 1. The aperture's semi-axes are 0.13 m and 0.16 m. Four emitters and nine receivers are grouped into one transducer arrays system (TAS). 157 TAS are uniformly distributed on the surface of the aperture. The device, the aperture and patient positioning are shown in Fig. 1. Approx. spherical wavefronts are generated by using a single emitter at 2.5 MHz with approx. 50% bandwidth. Rotational and translational motion of the complete sensor system, so-called aperture positions, creates further virtual positions of the ultrasound transducers. The data acquisition is carried out with an FPGA-based system, which can store up to 80 GB of A-scans.

Reflection, attenuation and speed of sound images can be reconstructed from the same raw data set. For reconstruction of reflectivity volumes, i.e. qualitative imaging of the gradient of the acoustic impedance, a 3D synthetic aperture focusing technique (3D SAFT) is applied.

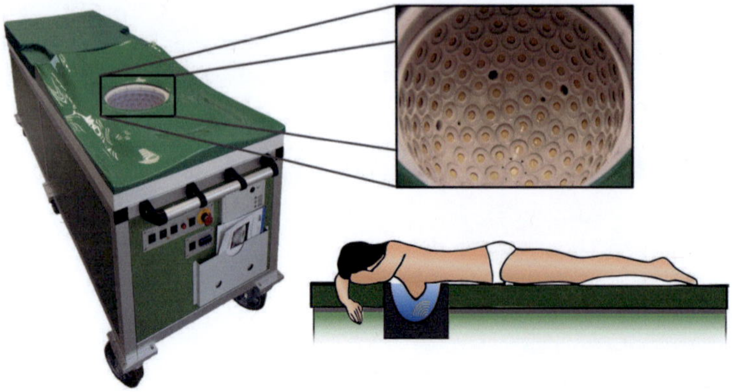

Figure 1: KIT 3D USCT with patient bed (left), transducer aperture (top right) and patient position (bottom right).

The computational burden for 3D SAFT is large as for each voxel the delay for each acquired A-scan has to be calculated, e.g. $O(N^5)$ for N^3 voxels and N^2 A-scans. For 3D reconstruction of objects which are large in terms of the wavelength, e.g. the female breast with diameters $\geq (100\ \lambda)^3$, the computation of one volume takes several days on a current multicore PC. For acceleration we developed a fast 3D SAFT implementation using multiple GPUs [2], reducing the computing time up to several minutes for a breast in resolution comparable to MRI.

Yet, for reflectivity volumes of high resolution up to $(0.5\ \lambda)^3$ speed of sound correction is necessary as the breast possesses a large range of speed of sound values [3], causing the images to defocus when a constant speed of sound is assumed. Incorporating speed of sound and attenuation correction in the GPU-based SAFT reconstruction increases the image quality significantly [4,5], but leads also to a significant reduction of computational performance. A time of flight interpolation based GPU implementation (TOFI-SAFT) [6] was developed which accelerates our previous GPU implementation of speed of sound corrected SAFT by a factor of 7 with only minor reduction of image quality. The approximation allows reconstructing speed of sound and attenuation corrected SAFT images as fast as non-corrected SAFT. In this paper the applied methods for accelerating SAFT and some results of phantoms and clinical cases are shown.

2 Methods

2.1 3D synthetic aperture technique

The applied reconstruction algorithm for reflectivity images is the 3D synthetic aperture focusing technique (SAFT), which can be described by the following equation:

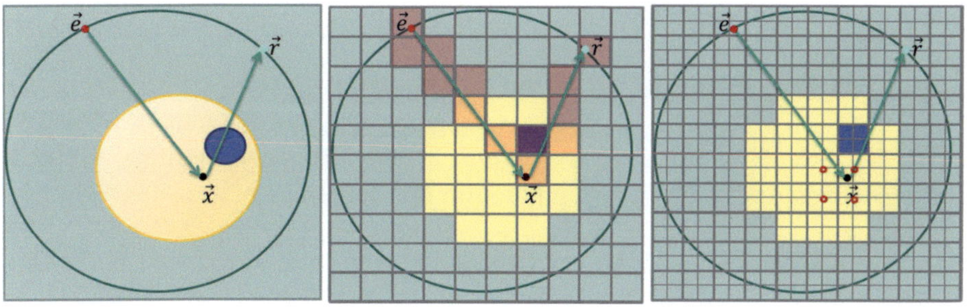

Figure 2: Simplified 2D diagrams of SAFT reconstruction: On the left the geometry with emitter $\vec{e}$, point $\vec{x}$ and receiver $\vec{x}$ and a circular breast (beige) with inclusion (blue). In the center the same geometry overlaid with low resolution speed of sound map and approximated paths for calculation of the average speed of sound. On the right overlaid with higher resolution grid for reflectivity imaging and red marks indicating the voxels of the speed of sound map used for interpolation of the average speed of sound $\hat{c}_{path(\vec{e},\vec{x},\vec{r})}$ for point $\vec{x}$.

$$I(\vec{x}) = \sum_{\forall(e,r)} \left(\frac{1}{att} T(A_{(e,r)} tof)\right) \text{ with } tof = \frac{\|\vec{e}-\vec{x}\|+\|\vec{x}-\vec{r}\|}{\hat{c}}, \quad (1)$$

where I denotes the reconstructed qualitative volume of local impedance-differences, $\vec{x}$ the reconstructed point, att is the attenuation of the ultrasound signal from emitter to point $\vec{x}$ to receiver, T contains the pre-processing steps, $A_{e,\mathrm{r}}$ is the A-scan acquired at emitting position $\vec{e}$ and receiving position $\vec{r}$. The time tof is the time of flight from emitter $\vec{e}$ to the point $\vec{x}$ and to receiver $\vec{r}$. The equation is valid for small attenuation, weak point scatterers, and spherical emittance. SAFT calculates at each image point the mean of all reflections which might originate from this position. Norton and Linzer [7] showed that for ideal conditions, i.e. continuous aperture, isotropic point scatterers and no attenuation, SAFT solves the inverse problem of calculating the local impedance differences. A simplified setup is shown in Figure 2 left.

For the simplest reconstruction, the harmonic mean of the speed of sound $\hat{c}$ may be assumed to be constant, e.g. the speed of sound of water at the temperature measured during image acquisition. Often the attenuation att is ignored, i.e. set to 1.

Acquiring unfocused ultrasound facilitates new possibilities for signal preprocessing, as the data can be accessed before the focus of emission is generated. For reconstruction of clinical cases we either use a matched filter only, or apply the preprocessing "Adapted Matched Filter" [8] described in the following, especially if images of lower resolution are reconstructed. First, a matched filter is applied to increase the signal-to-noise ratio, by correlating the signal with the known pulse shape. This is followed by an envelope transformation and detection of the local maxima. To cope with the phase aberrations the resulting signal is convoluted by a pulse with an adapted lower bandwidth.

In summary, the preprocessing is

$$T\big(A(t)\big) = locMax\big(\big|H\big(A(t) * p(t)\big)\big|\big) \otimes p_{opt,\tau_{new}}(t), \tag{2}$$

where $locMax$ denotes the local maximum, H the Hilbert transform, $*$ the cross-correlation operator, $p(t)$ the known pulse form, and $\otimes$the convolution operator.

The optimal pulse $p_{opt,\tau_{new}}(t)$ for reflectivity imaging was introduced by Norton and Linzer [7] with

$$p_{opt,\tau_{new}}(t) = \frac{2\sqrt{\pi}}{\tau_{new}{}^3}\left[1 - 2\left(\frac{\pi \cdot t}{\tau_{new}}\right)^2\right] \cdot e^{-\left(\frac{\pi \cdot t}{\tau_{new}}\right)^2}\ , \tag{3}$$

where τ_{new} is the new pulse duration, i.e. the main lobe of the optimum pulse. For example if the main lobe of the optimal pulse is set to 2 μs, this corresponds to a Full Width Half Maximum (FWHM) of the point spread function of approx. 1.5 mm, and is comparable to the resolution of an breast MR image.

2.2 Speed of sound and attenuation correction

Assuming constant speed of sound can lead in large objects with varying speed of sound to wrong scaling, spatial displacement and even defocusing of the image contents. For USCT approaches where the "paths" of the sounds, i.e. direction of the sound wave travelling through the object, vary greatly due to the wide spatial distribution of the transducers defocusing is prominent. For example Figure 6 left shows a cylindrical gelatin phantom (Ø 10 cm) with one embedded bonding wire (Ø 0.5 mm). The gelatin has a speed of sound of approx. 1550 m/s, the surrounding water 1490 m/s. Center left and right show slices of 3D SAFT reconstructions without and with sound speed correction. The improvement of the image quality is significant. For the KIT 3D USCT the real speed of sound may maximally deviate from the constant assumption by 0.28 m/s for high resolution reconstructions [9]. On the contrary not accounting for refraction effects does not significantly reduce the image quality when the speed of sound is corrected [10].

For 3D SAFT with speed of sound and attenuation correction the intensity $I(\vec{x})$ of a voxel at $\vec{x}$ is calculated by

$$I(\vec{x}) = \sum\nolimits_{\forall(e,r)} \left(\frac{1}{att_{path(\vec{e},\vec{x},\vec{r})}} T(A_{(e,r)} tof)\right) \text{ with } tof = \frac{\|\vec{e}-\vec{x}\|+\|\vec{x}-\vec{r}\|}{\hat{c}_{path(\vec{e},\vec{x},\vec{r})}}, \tag{4}$$

where $att_{path(\vec{e},\vec{x},\vec{r})}$ is the attenuation and $\hat{c}_{path(\vec{e},\vec{x},\vec{r})}$ is the mean sound speed on the direct path from $\vec{e}$ to $\vec{x}$ and $\vec{r}$, i.e. the average values are calculated from all voxels which lie on the straight lines connecting $\vec{e}$ and $\vec{x}$ and $\vec{r}$ and $\vec{x}$, respectively.

2.3 Acceleration using GPUs

Equation (1) shows that SAFT can be parallelized easily, i.e. each A-scan and / or each voxel can be calculated independently. The elementary operations of the reconstruction, i.e. addition, multiplication and even square root operations, can be implemented efficiently. However the large number of operations which are necessary for USCT applications causes SAFT to be computing intensive, as for each voxel of a breast sized volume in submillimeter resolution the delay tof of each A-scan has to be calculated. E.g. for a hemispherical breast of 10 cm radius, a voxel size of $(0.5\ \text{mm})^3$ and 5 million A-scans more than 10^{14} tof calculations are necessary.

Our GPU implementation of 3D SAFT without correction assumes $\hat{c}$ to be constant and $att = 1$. Acceleration is achieved by calculating the volumes with parallel GPUs. The maximum performance on eight GTX 590 is 107 GVA/s, where 1 GVA/s denotes 10^9 voxel and A-scans processed per second, and the calculation of the above example takes 37 min.

For high resolution SAFT images a speed of sound correction is necessary to focus the image content. Additionally, attenuation correction increases the contrast of the SAFT images. For corrected SAFT reconstruction $att_{path(\vec{e},\vec{x},\vec{r})}$ as the attenuation and $\hat{c}_{path(\vec{e},\vec{x},\vec{r})}$ as the mean sound speed on the path from $\vec{e}$ to $\vec{x}$ and $\vec{r}$ are calculated using reconstructed attenuation and speed of sound images from the same acquired data. For performant calculation of the corrected SAFT volumes on GPUs the paths are approximated by Bresenham's algorithm [11] and calculated on voxel grids of low resolution. In Figure 2 the center and right diagrams show an example. Path calculations using up to factor 20 lower resolution than the SAFT resolution still result in acceptable focusing [4]. With correction for speed of sound and attenuation variations, the performance on eight GTX 590 GPUs decreases to 34 GVA/s when using 128^3 voxels for the speed of sound and attenuation volumes [9] and the calculation takes 2 h.

2.4 Time of flight interpolated synthetic aperture focusing technique

For clinical studies or even clinical practice a 2 hour calculation poses a long delay between data acquisition and image availability. Hence a fast alternative is necessary, allowing the important speed of sound correction. Reducing the number of calculated tof would result in a lower resolution of the volumes, which is not desirable. The alternative is to reduce the amount of operations per tof calculation. TOFI-SAFT reduces the number of operations by calculating the exact tof only for a small subset of voxels, i. e. the tof calculation in equation (1) is only carried out for the voxels corresponding to the reduced speed of sound resolution. The tof of all other high resolution voxels is calculated by linear interpolation using the neighboring base points of exact tof values. Figure 3 shows an example for a simple 2D case.

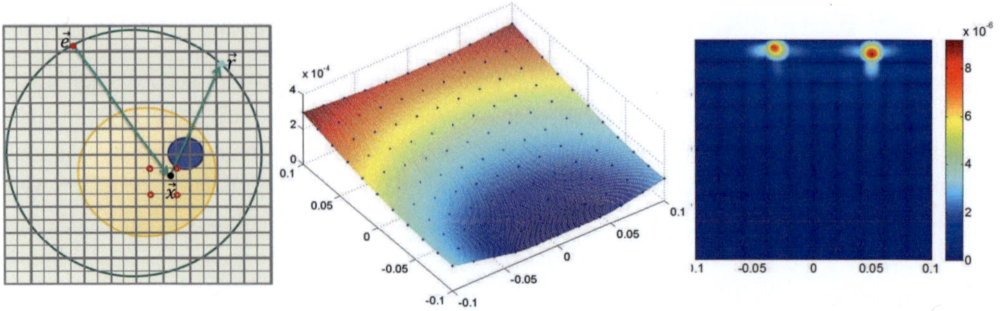

Figure 3: Principle of TOFI-SAFT simplified in 2D. Left: Emitter $\vec{e}$ and receiver $\vec{r}$ on a ring aperture with radius of 10 cm using the same setup as in Fig. 2. The tof of pixel $\vec{x}$ is interpolated for this emitter receiver combination. Overlay of grid of pixels with a low resolution speed of sound image (bold grey lines) and a high resolution SAFT image (thin grey lines). Red dots mark the spatial positions of neighboring base points with tof calculation from equation (4) applied for linear interpolation of tof for pixel $\vec{x}$. Center: $tof_{\overline{e,r}}(\vec{x})$ for the given example, the resolution of speed of sound is $(2\ \text{cm})^2$ and of SAFT is $(1\ \text{mm})^2$. Dark blue dots indicate the position of the base points. Right: Error map of calculated and linearly interpolated tof with mean of 0.6 µs, median of 0.4 µs and standard deviation of 0.7 µs. The areas of large errors up to 9 µs are located near the transducers and outside of the breast. Speed of sound is assumed to be constant at 1500 m/s.

A more general analysis in 3D of the errors made by this approximation showed that large errors are mainly located outside the breast as the error drops quickly with increasing distance to the transducers and does not significantly decrease the image quality [6].

For implementation of TOFI-SAFT within our GPU framework, the base points for exact tof calculations are chosen to coincide with the voxels of the speed of sound volume, which is applied for correction in lower resolution, i.e. factor 5 to 10. The tof of the high resolution voxels for the reflectivity volumes, which do not coincide with the base points, are linearly interpolated using the tof of neighboring base points. For GPU implementation the linear interpolation can be carried out very effectively in texture memory units.

TOFI-SAFT achieves a maximum performance of 104 GVA/s on the GPU server with eight GTX 590, which is a speed up of factor 3 compared to the corrected SAFT. It approaches the maximum performance of 107 GVA/s of the uncorrected SAFT reconstruction. Tested on one newer generation GPU, GTX Titan, TOFI-SAFT can be even faster than uncorrected SAFT: a GPU server of eight GTX Titans would result in a maximum performance of 210 GVA/s for uncorrected SAFT, 62 GVA/s for corrected SAFT and 442 GVA/s for TOFI-SAFT which is a speed up of more than factor 7. This increase in performance is due to 3.5 times more texture units in GTX Titan compared to GTX 590. Thus for the above example with a semispherical breast of 10 cm radius, a voxel size of $(0.05\ \text{mm})^3$, 5 million A-scans and 80^3 base points TOFI-SAFT could be calculated in 16 min on eight GTX Titan GPUs.

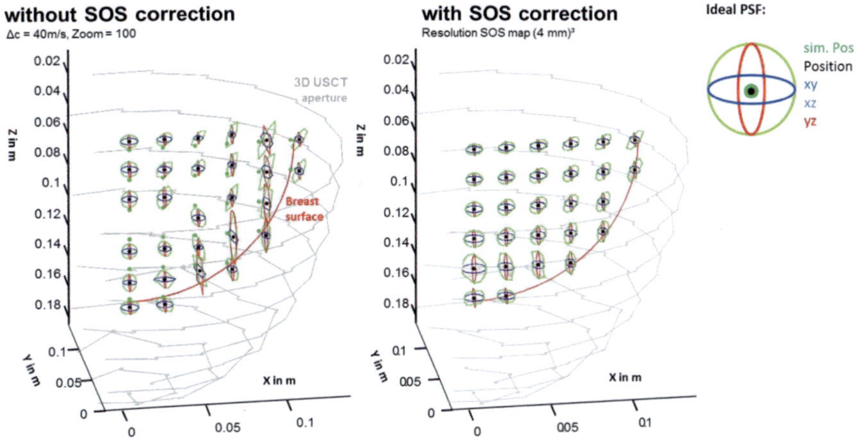

Figure 4: Resulting point spread functions of 28 simulated point scatterers within a hemispherical breast of 20 cm diameter and speed of sound of 1540 m/s in 1500 m/s water. The PSFs are scaled wit a factor of 100 for better visibility.

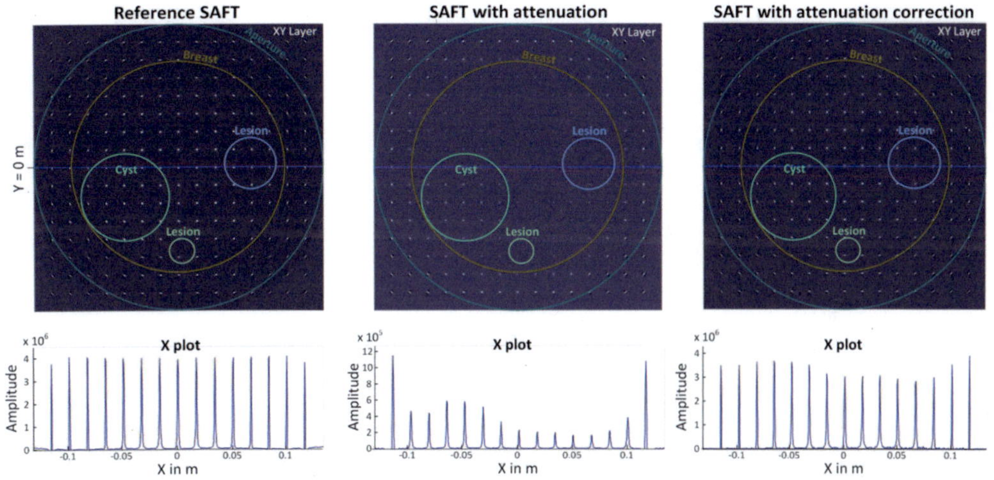

Figure 5: Comparison of reconstructions of 255 simulated point scatterers for (left) not attenuation, (center) attenuation simulated but not taken into account for the reconstruction, and (right) simulated and reconstructed attenuation. The top rows shows slice images of the reconstruction and the bottom row contour plots of the scatterers at y = 0m (blue line). The breast had 20 cm diameter and 0.5 dB/cm attenuation, the cyst 0.0009 dB/cm and 8 cm diameter, and the lesions 0.1 dB/cm and 2 and 4 cm diameter. No noise was added to the simulations.

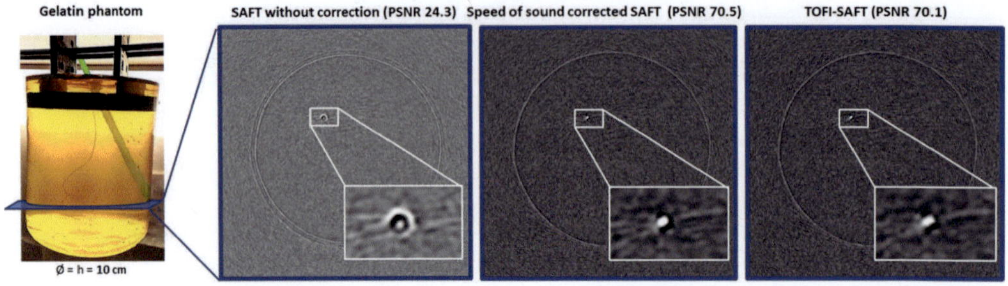

Figure 6: Comparison of SAFT reconstructions of the gelatin phantom with nylon thread. Left: Photo of Phantom. Center left: SAFT reconstruction without correction. Center right: Slice image with speed of sound corrected SAFT (PSNR 70.5). Right: Slice of TOFI-SAFT (PSNR 70.1).

3 Results

For evaluation of the speed of sound correction a simulation of a worst case scenario was used. Figure 4 shows a diagram of the resulting point spread functions (PSF) of 28 simulated point scatterers within a breast with 20 cm diameter and speed of sound of 1540 m/s in 1500 m/s water. The PSFs are scaled by a factor of 100 for better visibility. Without speed of sound correction the mean displacement of the points is 6 mm, the mean width of the PSF is 0.5 mm and the relative contrast, i.e. percentage of Peak-Signal-to-Noise-Ratio (PSNR, $PSNR = \frac{\max(I)}{\sigma(I)}$) to PSNR of the ground truth, i.e. reconstruction of simulation without speed of sound difference, is 16%. The speed of sound correction approach using a SOS map with $(4\text{ mm})^3$ resolution results in a mean displacement of the reconstructed points of 0.06 mm, a mean PSF of 0.28 mm, and a relative contrast of 85%. Figure 6 center left and center right show experimental results.

Similarly, for evaluation of the attenuation correction 255 point scatterers within a 20 cm breast were simulated. Resulting slice images and contour plots are shown in Figure 5. The breast tissue was simulated at 0.5 dB/cm attenuation, the cyst at 0.0009 dB/cm and had 8 cm diameter.The lesions had a diameter of 2 and 4 cm with an attenuation of 0.1 dB/cm. No noise was added to the simulations. The percentage of the relative standard deviation (STD) of the reflectivity of the scatterers was measured as quality metric and normalized to the maximum amplitude of the reconstructed point scatterers in the reference, i.e. no attenuation simulated. The measure resulted in 34 % of relative STD for the non-corrected SAFT and 9% for the corrected SAFT. For evaluation of TOFI-SAFT A-scans for 54 evenly distributed point scatters within one quarter of the maximum sized breast (hemisphere with 10 cm radius) were simulated for the 3D USCT aperture with speed of sound of the background of 1500 m/s and 1460 m/s for the breast tissue.

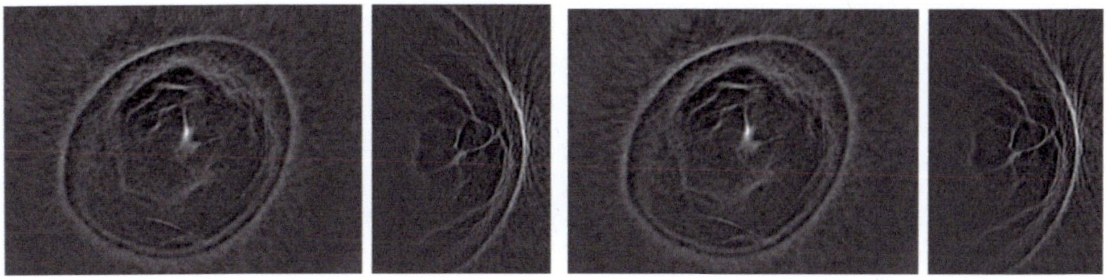

Figure 7: 3D USCT slice images of reflectivity volumes reconstructed with corrected SAFT (left) and with TOFI-SAFT (right) for patient data. The imaged breast has a maximum diameter of approx. 18 cm. The reduction of image contrast in terms of peak signal to noise ratio (PSNR from left to right: 32.1, 43.9, 32.1, 43.8) is very small.

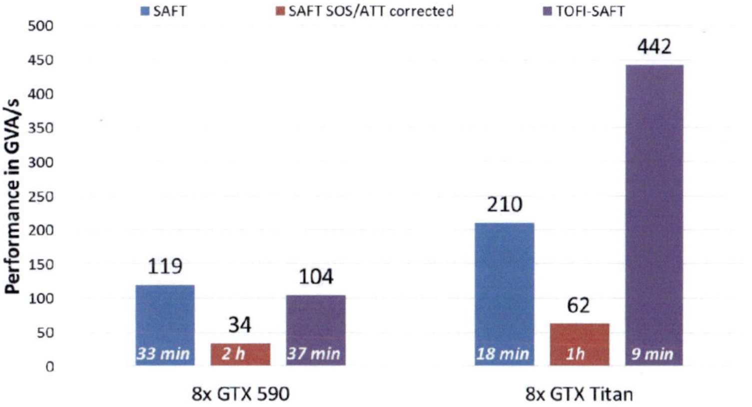

Figure 8: Performance of the three 3D SAFT approaches for two different generations of GPUs in GVA/s. The durations in minutes and hours respectively were calculated for an example of 444^2 x 266 voxels for reflectivity volumes with 128^3 base points, and 10^7 A-scans. The GTX Titan has a large number of texture units for interpolation, in this case the performance of TOFI-SAFT including speed of sound correction can even surpass the performance of SAFT without speed of sound correction.

The A-scans were then used to reconstruct speed of sound corrected SAFT volumes without and with TOFI approximation. The voxel size of the SAFT volumes was $(0.05\ \text{mm})^3$ and 128^3 base points were applied. The mean full width half maximum was 0.34 mm for TOFI-SAFT compared to 0.33 mm with full speed of sound corrected SAFT and the relative contrast was 0.98. Thus the errors introduced by the approximation are not significant for the resulting image quality.

For experimental evaluation a phantom consisting of a gelatin block of cylindrical shape (height and diameter 10 cm) containing a nylon thread of diameter of 0.2 mm, see Figure 6, was imaged. The phantom was reconstructed with a voxel size of $(0.4\ \text{mm})^3$ and 128^3 base points. The image contrast in terms of PSNR of the approximation was only reduced by 0.6%

compared to the full calculation of all tof. Comparing speed of sound corrected SAFT and TOFI-SAFT for clinical data resulted also in only small degradation of the image quality, see Figure 7.

Figure 8 summarizes the performance values for the different SAFT approaches. For calculation of the duration of SAFT the example setup was to reconstruct a SAFT volume of 444^2 x 266 voxels, with 128^3 base points, i.e. resolution of the attenuation and SOS maps, and 10^7 A-scans (N~900).

4 Discussion and conclusion

In this paper an overview of three approaches for fast calculation of 3D SAFT for 3D USCT at KIT was presented and the motivation to apply speed of sound and attenuation correction was given. For clinical applicability, i.e. calculation of breast volumes in a couple of minutes, a new approximation based approach for speed of sound corrected 3D SAFT enables a significant acceleration of reconstructions for reflectivity volumes with only minor reduction of image quality. The type of applied GPU limits the performance by increased memory requirements and texture units for interpolation, thus high end GPUs are required, especially when using TOFI-SAFT.

Using quad-core CPUs and a cluster of eight GPUs allowed us for the first time to calculate volumes in less than 10 min, enabling the application of the method in clinical studies. While readout of the full raw data is important during the development state, for clinical practice a stand-alone system outputting reconstructed images only would be sufficient. For application in clinical practice, however, we also considered reuse of the device's built-in FPGA-based data acquisition system (DAQ) through reconfiguration. Due to the dated FPGAs the speed up was only marginal. Yet 3D SAFT using new generation FPGAs was shown to be nearly as performant as using GPUs [12]. For future development of the 3D USCT technology scalability and a good performance-per-power ratio become very important. Therefore we will consider FPGAs for future applications. Today, with the available FPGA technology real-time imaging is not possible at reasonable efforts and costs. However, we expect that even real-time image reconstruction will be possible by the year 2020, roughly following Moore's law.

References

[1] Ruiter, N.V., Zapf, M., et al.: "First Results of a Clinical Study with 3D Ultrasound Computer Tomography." Proc. IEEE Internat. Ultrasonics Symp., (2013).

[2] Kretzek, E., Zapf, M., Birk, M., Gemmeke, H., Ruiter, N.V., "GPU based acceleration of 3D USCT image reconstruction with efficient integration into MATLAB," Proc. SPIE 8675, Medical Imaging 2013: Ultrasonic Imaging, Tomography, and Therapy, page 86750O (2013).

[3] Ruiter, N.V., Schnell, R., Zapf, M., Gemmeke, H., "Phase aberration correction for 3D Ultrasound Computer Tomography images," 2007 IEEE Ultrasonics Symposium, pps. 1808–11 (2007).

[4] Kretzek, E., Ruiter, N.V., "GPU based 3D SAFT reconstruction including phase aberration," Proc. SPIE 9040, Medical Imaging 2014: Ultrasonic Imaging and Tomography, pages 90400W (2014).

[5] Kretzek, E., Hopp, T., Ruiter, N.V., "GPU-based 3D SAFT reconstruction including attenuation correction," Proc. SPIE 9419, Medical Imaging 2015: Ultrasonic Imaging and Tomography, pages 94190E (2015).

[6] Ruiter, N.V., Kretzek, E, Zapf, M., Hopp, T., Gemmeke, H., "Time of flight interpolated synthetic aperture focusing technique," Proc. SPIE 10139, Medical Imaging 2017: Ultrasonic Imaging and Tomography, 101390Q (2017).

[7] Norton, S., Linzer, M., "Ultrasonic reflectivity imaging in three dimensions: Reconstruction with a spherical array," Ultrasonic Imaging, vol. 1 (3), pp. 21031, 1979.

[8] Ruiter, N.V., Schwarzenberg, G.F., Zapf, M., Gemmeke, H., "Improvement of 3D ultrasound computer tomography images by signal pre-processing," Proc. IEEE UFFC Symp., pp. 852-855, 2008.

[9] Kretzek, E., "Optimierung von Bildgebungsverfahren für die 3D-Ultraschall-Computertomographie," Ph.D Thesis, KIT, 2015.

[10] Hopp, T., Zapf, M., Gemmeke, H., Ruiter, N.V., "Experimental evaluation of straight ray and bent ray phase aberration correction for USCT SAFT imaging,", Proc. SPIE Medical Imaging 2018, in press.

[11] Bresenham, J.E., "Algorithm for computer control of a digital plotter," IBM Systems Journal, 4(1), pps. 25-30, (1965).

[12] Birk, M., Kretzek, E., Figuli, P., Weber, M., Becker, J., Ruiter, N.V., "High-Speed Medical Imaging in 3D Ultrasound Computer Tomography," in IEEE Transactions on Parallel and Distributed Systems, 27(2), pp. 455-67, 2016.

Minimum-variance beamforming for ultrasound computer tomography imaging

Shanshan Wang, Junjie Song, Liang Zhou, Peng Yang, Mingyue Ding, Ming Yuchi*

Department of Biomedical Engineering, School of Life Science and Technology, Key Laboratory of Molecular Biophysics of the Ministry of Education, Huazhong University of Science and Technology, Wuhan, Hubei, China
E-mail: m.yuchi@hust.edu.cn

Abstract

In recent years, a number of studies on ultrasound computed tomography (USCT) have been carried out for its application prospect in early detection of breast cancer. The traditional delay-and-sum (DAS) beamforming has been widely used in USCT imaging. However, DAS method has wide main lobe and high side lobe level. In this paper, minimum-variance (MV) beamforming method is applied to improve the image quality for USCT. MV beamformer adopts an adaptive strategy by maintaining a unity gain in the desired direction and reducing the interference from other directions. Through using the MV beamforming method, the USCT image is expected to have less noises and artifacts, and higher resolution and contrast. It was tested with the radio-frequency (RF) data of the breast phantom captured by the USCT system developed in the Medical Ultrasound Laboratory. The ring-type transducer has 1024 elements with a center frequency of 2.5MHz. Experimental results show that the reconstructed images of the breast phantom by the MV beamformer enhanced the image quality compared to DAS. The cysts in breast phantom are more clearly presented.

Keywords: ultrasound computer tomography, minimum-variance beamforming, ring array

1 Introduction

Ultrasound has been widely used in medical imaging because of its non-ionizing radiation and low cost. Ultrasound computed tomography (USCT) is a promising imaging tool for early breast cancer detection. Delay-and-sum beamforming (DAS) has been widely used in USCT imaging. The received signals from active channels are dynamically delayed and summed up in the beamformer. In contrast to the predetermined weight in DAS, the minimum-variance (MV) adaptive beamformer computes the optimal weights for each receive focal point based on MV algorithm [1-2]. Hence, MV can improve the lateral and contrast resolution since it can effectively reduce both the main lobe and clutter levels [3]. Several researchers have previously investigated the MV approach in medical ultrasound [4]. Mann and Walker introduced the basic structure of MV and used a constrained adaptive beamforming on experimental data of a single point target and a cyst phantom demonstrating improved contrast and resolution [5]. Sasso and Cohen-Bacrie used subaperture averaging to handle the coherent echoes, showing improved contrast in the reconstructed image [6]. Wang et al. presented a synthetic aperture focusing technique combining with robust MV beamformer[7]. In [8], babak et al. applied MV beamforming with adaptive coherence weighting to medical ultrasound imaging. In this paper, MV beamforming method is applied for USCT imaging. It aims to reduce the levels of side lobes and narrow the main lobes to improve the image quality.

The remainder of this paper is arranged as follows. Section 2 briefly describes the background and principle of the MV. The experimental setups are shown in section 3. The experimental results are shown and analyzed in Section 4. Finally, Section 5 is devoted to the conclusion.

2 Methods

In conventional data-and-sum (DAS) beamforming, time delay is applied to the received signals. Then, sum the delayed signals to construct the image. It is non-adaptive and blind beamformer whose weights are predetermined. In the MV beamformer, the weights are computed to optimally minimize the output power by maintaining a unity gain in the desired direction and reducing the interference from other directions.

2.1 The MV beamformer

Consider a USCT transducer array with M' elements. Here, the reflected echoes near the emitter are adopted to reconstruct USCT images. M element received signals are selected with each emission. After the time delay compensation, the sample output of each channel can be expressed in a vector,

$$\mathrm{X}[n] = [x_1(n)\; x_2(n) \ldots x_M(n)]^H , \qquad (1)$$

where $[\;]^T$ denotes the matrix transpose, $x_M[n]$ the received radio-frequency (RF) data of channel M after receive delays have been applied. The output of MV beamformer is

$$z[n] = \sum_{m=0}^{M-1} w_m[n]x_m[n] = \mathrm{w}[n]^H\, \mathrm{X}[n] , \qquad (2)$$

where $w_m[n]$ is a weighting value for the $x_m[n]$, $\mathrm{w}[n]=[w_1(n)\ w_2(n)\ldots w_M(n)]^H$. The variance of $z[n]$ can be written as

$$E[|z(n)|^2]=\mathrm{w}[n]^H\mathrm{R}[n]\mathrm{w}[n], \tag{3}$$

where $\mathrm{R}[n]=E[\mathrm{X}[n]\mathrm{X}[n]^H]$ is the spatial covariance matrix, $E[\cdot]$ the expectation operator. The optimal weight vector $\mathrm{w}[n]$ can be formulated as follows,

$$\min_{w[n]} \mathrm{w}[n]^H\mathrm{R}[n]\mathrm{w}[n] \quad \text{subject to } \mathrm{w}[n]^H\mathrm{a}=1, \tag{4}$$

where a is the equivalent of the steering vector. Assume the received data have been delayed appropriately, a is a vector of ones. The solution to (4) is given by

$$\mathrm{w}[n]=\frac{\mathrm{R}[n]^{-1}\mathrm{a}}{\mathrm{a}^{\mathrm{H}}\mathrm{R}[n]^{-1}\mathrm{a}}. \tag{5}$$

2.2 Estimation of the spatial covariance matrix

The spatial covariance matrix $\mathrm{R}[n]$ can not be obtained in practice. As the transmitted pulses are short and nonstationary in medical ultrasound image, $\mathrm{R}[n]$ changed with time rapidly and should be estimated. The spatial smoothing and temporal averaging have been used for covariance matrix estimation [8]. The array is first divided into overlapping subarrays with length of L and temporally averaged over $2K+1$ samples, then the corresponding covariance matrices are calculated to estimate the full covariance matrix. The estimated covariance matrix is given as follows,

$$\hat{\mathrm{R}}[n]=\frac{1}{2K+1}\frac{1}{M-L+1}\sum_{k=-K}^{K}\sum_{l=0}^{M-L}\overline{\mathrm{X}}_l[n-k]\overline{\mathrm{X}}_l[n-k]^H, \tag{6}$$

where $\overline{\mathrm{X}}_l[\mathrm{n}]=[\overline{\mathrm{x}}_l(n),\overline{\mathrm{x}}_{l+1}(n),\ldots,\overline{\mathrm{x}}_{l+L-1}(n)]^H$, L the subarray length. In this paper, Temporal averaging is not used, K=0. We selected forward and backward spatial averaging to obtain $\hat{\mathrm{R}}[n]$. The formula is given by

$$\hat{\mathrm{R}}_{FB}[n]=\frac{1}{2(M-L+1)}\left(\sum_{l=0}^{M-L}\overline{\mathrm{X}}_l[n]\overline{\mathrm{X}}_l[n]^H+\sum_{l=M-L}^{0}\overline{\mathrm{X}}_l^*[n]\overline{\mathrm{X}}_l^*[n]^H\right), \tag{7}$$

where $\overline{\mathrm{X}}_l^*[\mathrm{n}]=[\overline{\mathrm{x}}_{M-l-1}(n),\overline{\mathrm{x}}_{M-l-2}(n),\ldots,\overline{\mathrm{x}}_{M-l-L}(n)]^H$. Replace $\mathrm{R}[n]$ by $\hat{\mathrm{R}}_{FB}[n]$, the estimated amplitude is obtained by averaging over all subarrays

$$z(n) = \frac{1}{M-L+1} \sum_{l=0}^{M-L} \mathrm{w}(n)^H \overline{X}(n) . \tag{8}$$

There are two ways to increase robustness of the MV estimation: decreasing the subarray length L or diagonal loading of the estimated covariance matrix. If L=1, the MV becomes DAS. When L increased to form the covariance matrix, the resolution increased but the robustness get worse. The choice of L should ensure that the covariance matrix estimate is invertible. The limit of L is $L < M/2$ [9]. Diagonal loading means that using R[n]+εI to replace $\mathrm{R}[n]$. ε is chosen to be proportional to the power of the output,

$$\varepsilon = \Delta \cdot tr\{\mathrm{R}[n]\} , \tag{9}$$

where $tr\{\cdot\}$ is the trace operator. Δ is less than $1/L$. Here, Δ is set to be $1/(100L)$ ..

3 Result

A 1024-element ring array with the center frequency 2.5MHz was used to scan the breast phantom 052A (CIRSINC, USA) (Fig.1(a)). The diameter of ring array was 200 mm, and the sampling frequency was 12.5 MHz. Phantom 052A immersed in water were put in the center of the transducer. Fig.1(b) shows the data acquisition system (NI 5752, USA).

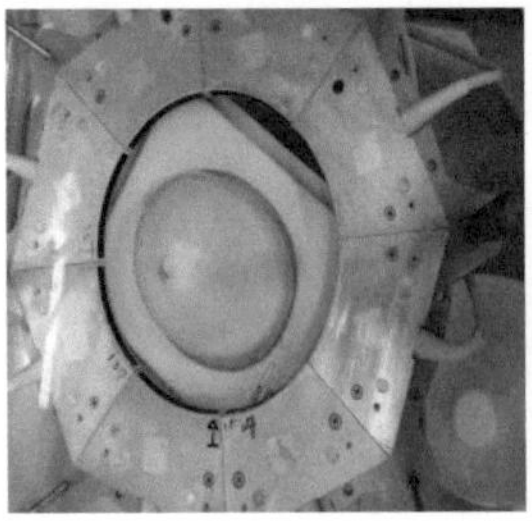

(a)

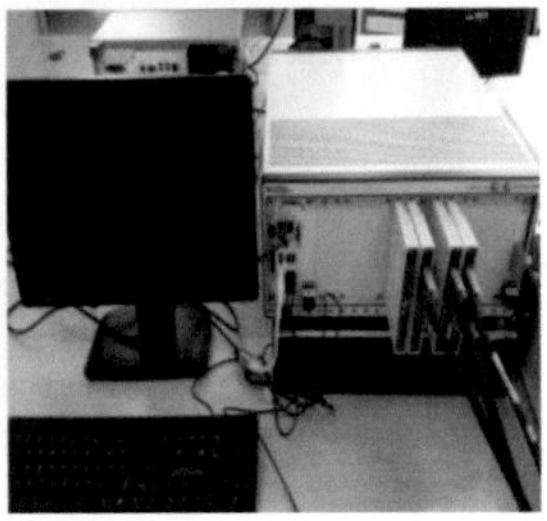

(b)

Fig. 1. (a) Ring array and phantom 052A; (b) NI data acquisition system.

One element emits the ultrasound impulse signal, while all the elements act as the receiver to capture the raw data. The reconstruction algorithm for reflectivity image is the synthetic aperture focusing technique (SAFT). For each focal point, the weighting factors were calculated in each emissions using the MV beamformer.

Fig.2 shows the B-mode images of breast phantom using traditional DAS and MV method. It can be found that MV (Fig.2b) can reduce the artifact around array boundary while the phantom are more clearly presented comparing with DAS (Fig.2a).

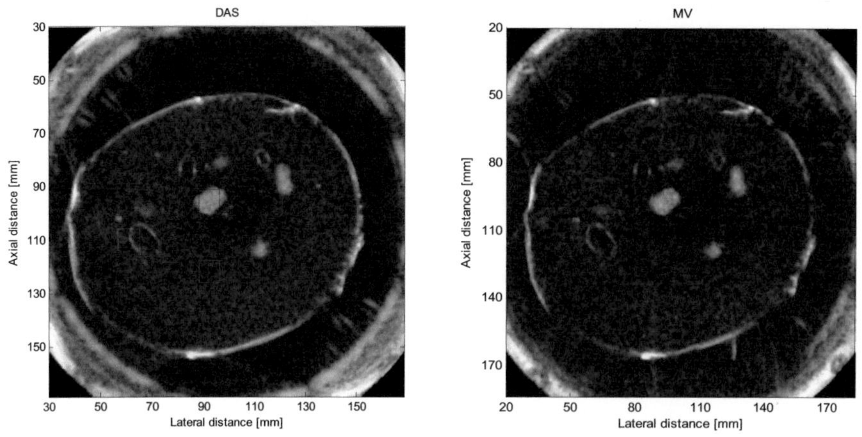

(a) (b)

Fig.2. The reconstructed images of breast phantom by (a) DAS; (b) MV.

	ROI1		**ROI2**	
Method	CR(dB)	CNR	CR(dB)	CNR
DAS	25.89	0.61	20.71	0.49
MV	30.632	0.75	17.35	0.43

Table 1. CR and CNR of the breast phantom images

	Black-box region		
Method	Mean(dB)	Std (dB)	SNR
DAS	31.88	6.97	1.09
MV	29.76	8.01	0.85

Table 2. Mean, standard deviation and SNR of the breast phantom images

Three common indices, the contrast ratio (CR), contrast to noise ratio (CNR) and speckle signal to noise ratio (SNR) were calculated using the image point values for these methods. These indicators are used to quantify the reconstructed image quality. *CR* is defined as $CR = |\mu_{ROI} - \mu_B|$ and CNR is the ratio of *CR* to the standard deviation of the background. It is defined as CNR= $CR/\sigma_B = |\mu_{ROI} - \mu_B|/\sigma_B$, where σ_B is the standard deviation of the background[10-11]. μ_B is the mean value of the background and μ_{ROI} is the mean value of the region-of-interest (ROI). SNR is defined as SNR= μ/σ [12]. It is the ratio between the mean value μ and the standard deviation σ. As shown in Fig.2 (a) (indicated by the white rectangle), the speckle pattern region without influenced by the weighting factors is chosen as the background. Therefore, three common indices for the ROI1 (indicated by the black dashed rectangle) and ROI2 (indicated by the white dashed rectangle) are calculated based on the previous formulas. The speckle pattern region (indicated by the black rectangle) is selected to computer signal to noise ratio. DAS gets the lower CR than MV method in ROI1 but higher in ROI2 and the strongest speckle intensity variations as shown in Table 1 and Table 2. The MV method removes the artifacts in the images more significantly and obtains improved speckle pattern near the boundary. The image quality enhances while suppressing clutter consequently.

4 Conclusion

The MV beamformer have been applied to improve spatial resolution and suppress clutters in USCT. The proposed method was evaluated by experimental results. The results showed that the reconstructed images of the breast phantom by the MV beamformer enhanced the image quality compared to DAS. The main disadvantage of MV beamforming method is the excessive computational complexity. In the future, the proposed methods will be testified with in-vivo data.).

References

[1] J. F. Synnevag, A. Austeng and S. Holm, Minimum variance adaptive beamforming applied to medical ultrasound imaging, IEEE Ultrasonics Symp. Pro., 1199-1201(2005).

[2] J. F. Synnevag, A. Austeng and S. Holm, Adaptive beamforming applied to medical ultrasound imaging, IEEE trans. Ultrason. Ferroelectr. Freq. Control, 54(8), 1606-1613(2007)

[3] M. Bae, S. B. Park, and S. J. Kwon, Fast minimum variance beamforming bsed on legendre polynomials, IEEE trans. Ultrason. Ferroelectr. Freq. Control, 63(9), 1422-1431(2016)

[4] S. Mehdizadeh, A. Austeng, T.F.Johansen, and S. Holm, Eigenspace based minimum variance beamforming applied to ultrasound imaging of acoustically hard tissues. IEEE trans. Med. Imag.,31(10), 1912-1921(2012)

[5] J.A.Mann and W.F.Walker, A constrained adaptive beamformer for medical ultrasound:initial results, IEEE Ultrasonics Symp. Pro., 1807-1810(2002)
[6] M.Sasso and C. Cohen-Bacrie, Medical ultrasound imaging using the fully adaptive beamformer, Int.Conf. Acoustics, Speech and Signal processing,489-492(2005)
[7] Z. Wang, J. Li, and R. Wu, Time delay and time reversal-based robust capon beamformers for ultrasound imaging, IEEE trans. Med. Imag.,24, 1308-1322(2005)
[8] J. F. Synnevag, C.I.C.Nilsen, and S.Holm,Speckle statistics in adaptive beamforming, IEEE Ultrasonics Symp. Pro., 1545-1548(2007)
[9] P. Stoica and R. Moses, Introduction to spectral analysis. Englewood cliffs, NJ: Prentice-Hall, 1997
[10] C.J. Lou, M.L. Xu, M.Y. Ding, and M. Yuchi, Spatial smoothing coherence factor for ultrasound computed tomography, SPIE Medical Imaging, 979008(2016).
[11] S. Krishnan, K. W. Rigby, and M. O'Donnell, Improved estimation of phase aberration profiles, IEEE trans. Ultrason. Ferroelectr. Freq. Control, 44, 701-713(1997)
[12] M. Lediju, G. E. trahey, B. C. Byram, and J. J. Dahl, Short-lag spatial coherence of backscattered echoes: imaging characteristics, IEEE trans. Ultrason. Ferroelectr. Freq. Control, 58, 1377-1388(2011)

Piezofibre composite transducers for next generation 3D USCT

M. Zapf[1], K. Hohlfeld[2], P. Pfistner[1], C. Imbracio Liberman[1], K.W.A. van Dongen[4], H. Gemmeke[1], N.V. Ruiter[1], A. Michaelis[2,3], S. Gebhardt[3]

[1] *1Karlsruhe Institute of Technology, Institute for Data Processing and Electronics, Karlsruhe, Germany*
E-mail: michael.zapf@kit.edu

[2] *Institute of Materials Science, TU Dresden, Dresden, Germany*

[3] *IKTS, Fraunhofer Institute for Ceramic Technologies and Systems, Dresden, Germany*

[4] *Department of Imaging Physics, Faculty of Applied Sciences, Delft University of Technology, Delft, the Netherlands*

Abstract

At the Karlsruhe Institue of Technology (KIT), a 3D-Ultrasound Computer Tomography (3D-USCT) medical imaging system for early breast cancer detection is currently developed. With the next generation of 3D-USCT 2.5, the current region of interest (ROI) of 10 x 10 x 10 cm^3 shall be increased to 20 x 20 x 20 cm^3 to allow reliable imaging results also for bigger female breasts. Therefore, the opening angle (OA) of the future transducers should be increased to approx. 60 ° at 3 dB while other characteristics such as bandwidth (BW) and resonance frequency should be preserved or even improved. Based on Fraunhofer IKTS Piezofibre composites utilized for transducer production, an optimization is performed on piezoelectric sensor geometry and size, type and structure of matching and backing layer and interconnection technology of the several parts of the transducer

Keywords: US transducer, composite materials, SAFT imaging, piezo fibre composite

1 Introduction

Breast cancer is the most common cancer in females in the world [1, 2].The spreading probability of the tumor and thus the chances of survival are correlated to its size [3]. Therefore, early detection plays a vital role in reducing the mortality of breast cancer.

KIT developed a 3D USCT imaging system for early breast cancer detection [4] [5] [6]. Imaging is achieved by Synthetic Aperture Focusing Technique (SAFT) using a multistatic setup of 2041 ultrasound transducers, grouped in 157 Transducer Array Systems (TAS) embedded in a semi-elliposoidal aperture (Figure 1). A center frequency of 2.5 MHz is applied. The bandwidth (BW) and opening angle (OA) at 3 dB amount to 1 MHz and 36°, respectively. The fundamental connection between an ultrasound transducer's emission and reception sensitivity in the azimuth and elevation angle space is the tranducer's aperture size.

Finite element (FE) simulations have shown that a reduction in size of the current generation transducer elements by roughly a factor 2 from 900 μm to 500 μm is required to realize an OA of 60 ° at 3 dB. Wave simulations also revealed that a circular instead of the current rectangular aperture will result in additional homogeneity of the sound field.

As circular sensors are difficult to produce in the dice-and-fill approach, octagon shaped transducers are built for USCT 2.5. The octagon shape can be achieved with the established dice-and-fill technique by adding 2 sawing cuts. Furthermore, inspired by compressive sensing, an irregular distribution of the sensor elements on the TAS is applied which covers almost the full surface area of US transducer. Further improvements are introduced regarding connectivity and bandwidth.

2 Motivation

2.1 3D USCT 2.0 current status

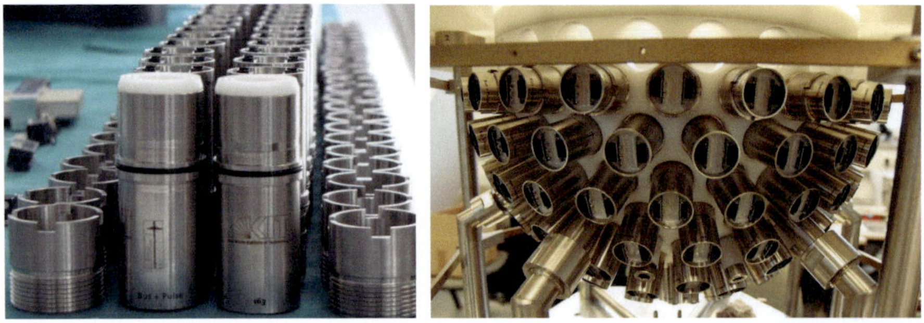

Figure 1: Left: USCT 2.0 TAS systems transducers before assembly in the final system. Right: Semi-ellipsoidal aperture of USCT 2.0

The current USCT 2.0 system covers a ROI of 10 x 10 x 10 cm^3. Results from the clinical trial with the University hospital Jena indicated that a bigger ROI is beneficial to cover a broader range of breasts and adapt also to the buoyance broadening effect of floating breasts [5]. Each of the 157 TAS consists of 13 rectangular transducer elements 0.9 x 0.9 mm in size

[7]. One TAS consists of four emitters, nine receivers which are regularly distributed in a square grid, covering just the inner part of the TAS (Figure 2).

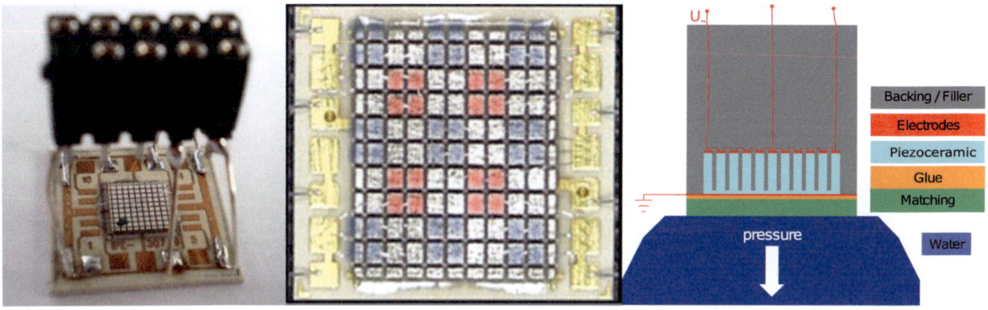

Figure 2: Left: Inner part of one TAS of USCT 2.0. Middle: Closer view on the piezoelectric elements. Four squares are connected to form one receiver (blue) or emitter (red). Right: Schematic side-view on one TAS of USCT 2.0.

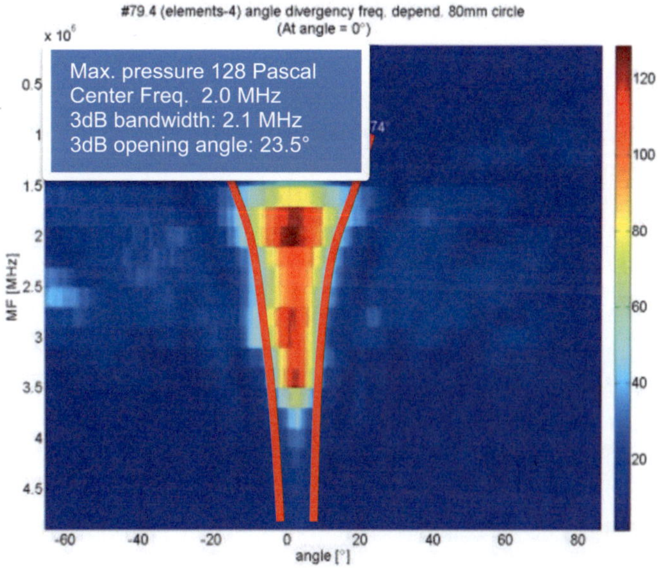

Figure 3: Frequency over angle for one element of one TAS of USCT 2.0. Given with red-lines approx. the frequency dependend 3dB opening angle.

2.2 Design considerations for next generation 3D USCT

For next generation 3D USCT (called 3D USCT 2.5) several should be improved contribute to a homogenous illumination and imaging contrast.

2.2.1 Opening angle (OA)

The benefit of an increased OA is schematically shown in Figure 4.

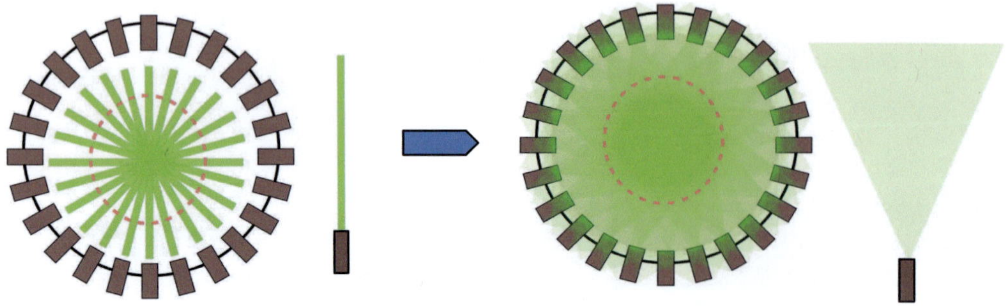

Figure 4: Illumination of an exemplary 3D-USCT system (top down view) for transducers with a small OA (left) compared to transducers with a larger OA (right).

2.2.2 Bandwidth

The BW of the transducers should be increased, as a larger BW better contrast in SAFT images, see Fig. 6. An increased coverage of the K-space, the spatial Fourier domain, can be achieved by broadening the bandwidth of the transducers. [8] Also, full wave inversion schemes and transmission tomography benefits from lower frequency components included in a broader bandwidth which covers also lower frequency down to 0.5 MHz.

2.2.3 Irregular distribution of sensor

An irregular distribution of the elements leads to greater coverage of the ROI and more homogeneous illumination. This is inspired by the "compressive sampling" concept now utilized in many apertures of various imaging systems as also ultra sound imaging systems.

2.2.4 Reduction in sparsity of sampling

An upgrade from 13 to 17 elements is performed. There are still nine receivers but the number of emitters has been doubled from four to eight emitters. Electronic constraints inhibit an upgrade to 9 emitters for symmetric emitter/receiver distribution. More emitters reduce the sparsity in imaging, leading to a more homogeneous coverage of the ROI. The final transducer distribution is shown in Figure 14.

2.3 Simulations

2.3.1 MATLAB

Ultrasound wavefield emission simulations for different surface geometries ("transducer apertures") have been performed as "piston model". As it is well known from antenna and transducer design, there is a reciprocal relationship between the element / aperture size, and the directivity / opening angle of the sound beam. A reduction in transducer sidelength / diameter from 900 µm to 550 µm should lead to an increase in OA to 50°-60° at 3 dB.

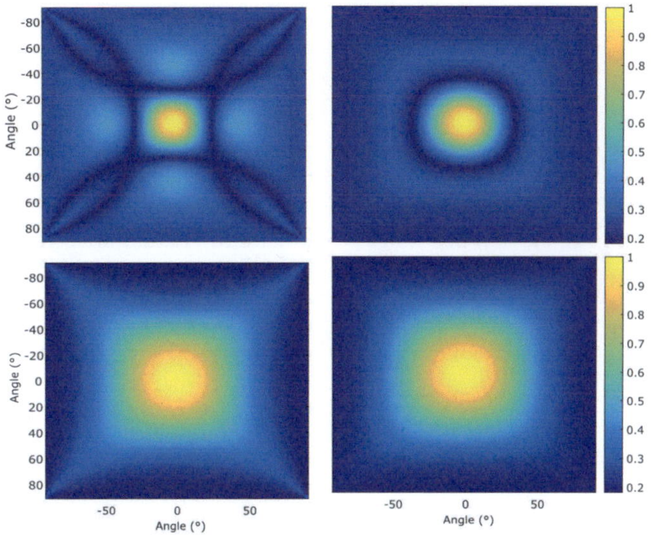

Figure 5: MATLAB aperture piston model simulations: US sound field for rectangular 0.9 mm (upper left), rectangular 0.4 mm (lower left), circular 0.94 mm (upper right) and circular 0.45 mm (lower right).

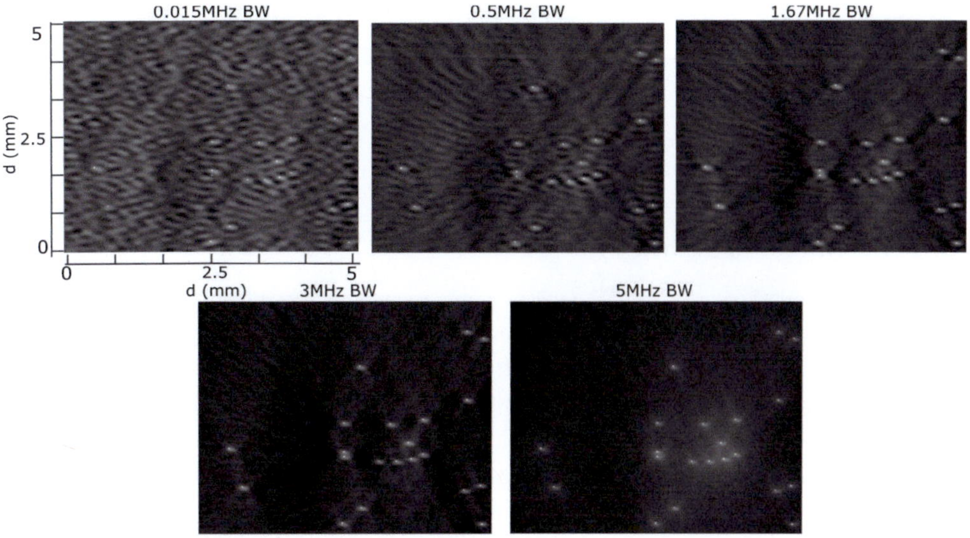

Figure 6: SAFT simulations for many point scatterers for varying BW. Contrast increases for broader bandwidth, while the resolution is more or less retained.

Circular elements express a more homogeneous sound over field compared to rectangular elements. (Figure 5).

SAFT simulations have been performed on point scatterers with varying BW (Figure 6). The results show that for SAFT image reconstruction, more BW leads to higher contrast in the images.

2.3.2 KLM

KLM simulations have been performed to find the ideal matching layer thickness for a broad BW. Simulations on TMM4 as a matching layer are shown in Figure 7. In the given configuration the resonance was the broadest for a 200 μm TMM4 layer due to two resonance peaks.

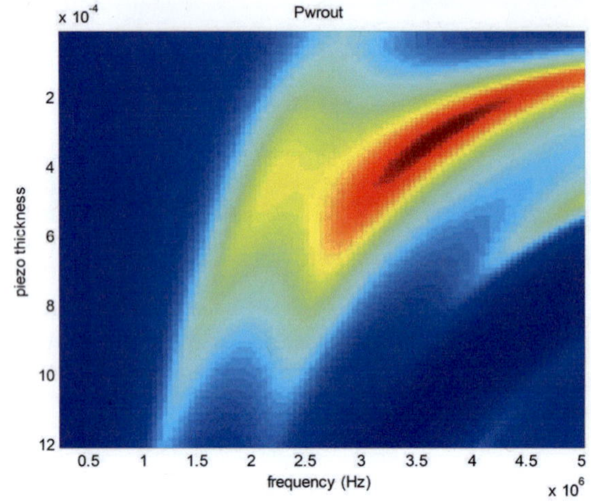

Figure 7: KLM model showing piezo thickness over frequency for a 200μm TMM4 matching layer with varying PZT thickness on the Y axis. X axis give the frequency range.

2.3.3 Finite element simulation

As 1D KLM simulations are insufficient to analyze lateral and shear wave effects of a design, a higher spatial dimensional simulation was utilized. Finite element (FE) simulations in 3D and 2D were performed. Also the impact of various materials on the Transducer performance were analyzed. PZflex was used as standard tool for piezoactive materials and non-piezoactive materials. The spatial properties of the transducer design was meshed with at least 3 times spatial sampling. Temporla sampling was derived automatically by the simulation tool, exported was the sound pressure field in each element in the water in the farfield in 2 to 6 cm distance.

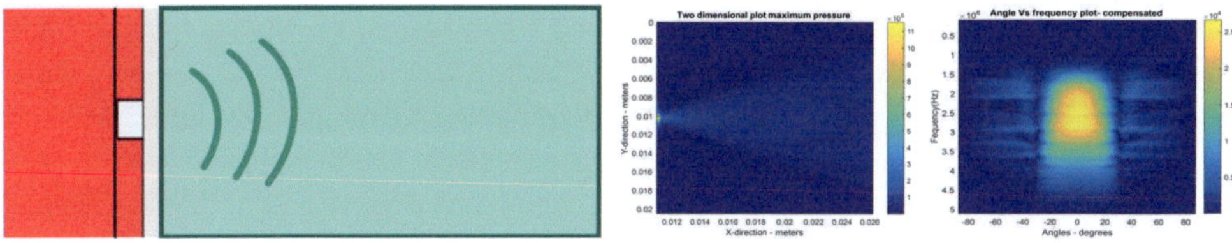

Figure 8: Left: Exemplary 2D PZFlex simulation model spanning 6cm in x and 2 cm in Y: Red: Backing + filling PU + Tungsten (12 MRayl): Red + bright blue: Piezofibrecompositedisc. (CeramTec Sonox 505 14.2 MRayl). Grey: Matching (TMM4 ca. 6.3 MRayl). Blue: Water (1.5 MRayl). Middle: Left: two-dimensional pressure plot X over Y, simulated by PZFlex for the setup described. Right: frequency over angle plot for the same setup.

3 Approach and method

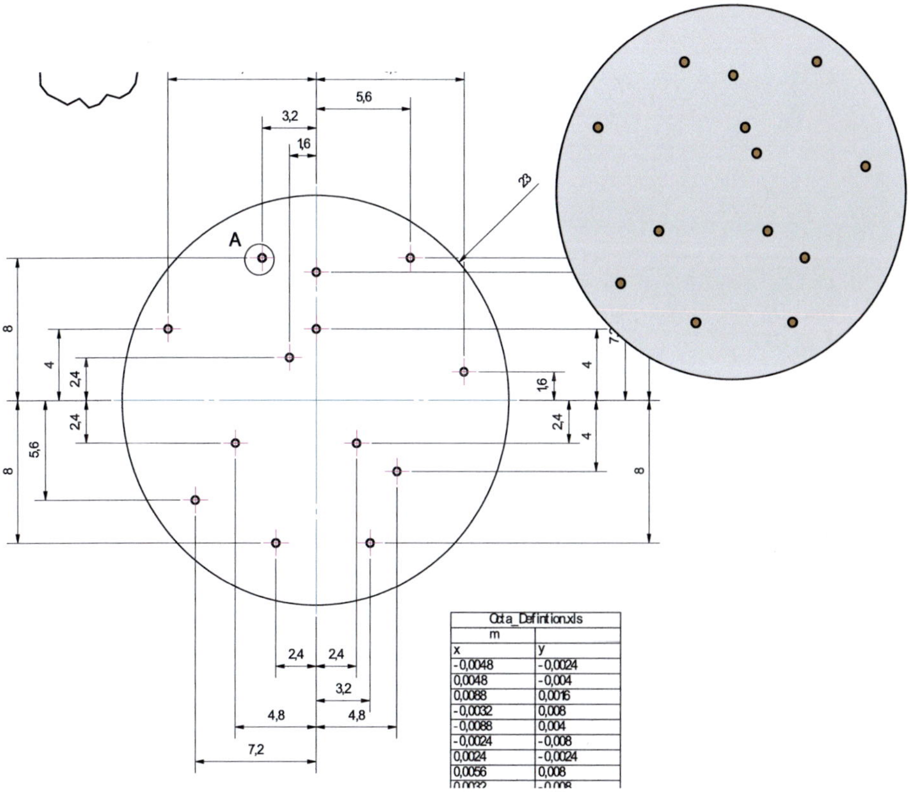

Figure 9: Definition of a pseudo random transducer distribution on the piezofibre disc. Original 13 element design (later extended to 17 elements).

The selected design is a pseudo-random distribution which should be homogenous distribution over thc surface of the whole transducer array, while being irregular and non-periodic to minimize side lobes; this is inspired by compressive sampling techniques; see figure 9.

3.1 Piezofibre disc production

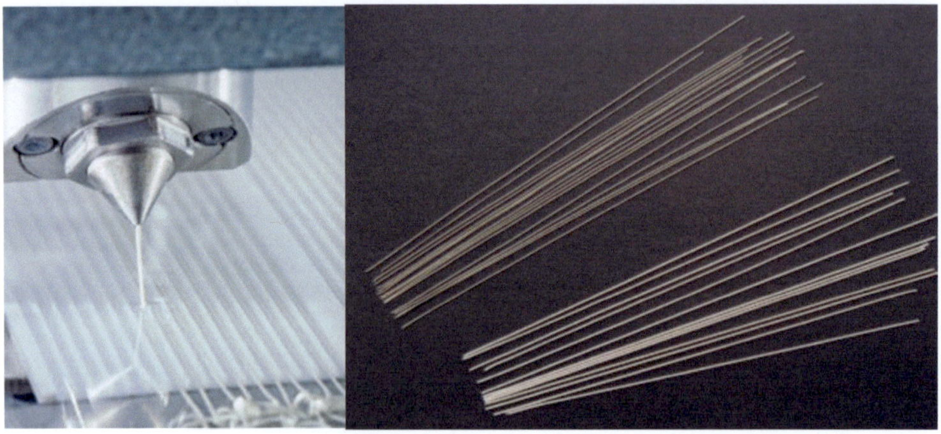

Figure 10: IKTS Piezofibre production process.

The FhG IKTS fiezofibre production process promises a cost reliable, reproducible and accurate build of arbitrary placed and sparse 2d transducer geometries. Additionally, a homogenous performance is to be expected due to production from a small number of fibres and piezo production batches.

The process starts from slicker with a liquid solvent which is pushed with a dispenser in a water bath and cures instantely in a green piezo fibre. These fibres are cured and hardened in a plumbum enriched atmosphere sinter oven [15,16].

The next steps is the placing of the pre-shrinked to ~470μm diameter fibres in metallic mask, see figure 4 top left. The mask with the piezo fibres is placed in a moulding container and filled with the epoxy substrate. The resulting block is milled to a round rod of approx. 14cm length and 2.3cm thickness. Two such rods are sufficient to satisfy the required 200 discs for an USCT. The rod is than sawed in discs of the desired thickness: for this analyzis 400, 550, 750, 1050, 1450, and 2050 μm thick discs were sawed with an in-hole saw.

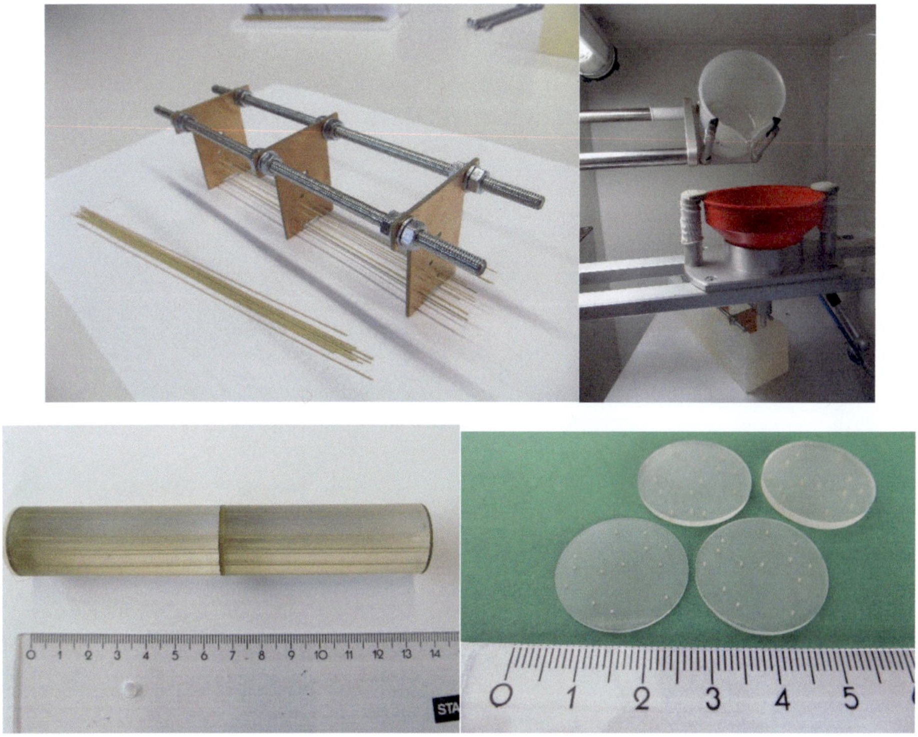

Figure 11: Fibre composite disc production: top left putting the sintered piezo fibres into the mask, top right: filling the mould with epoxy as substrate, bottom left: cured and mround milled rod, bottom right: sawed to four different thicknesses piezo discs

Then, the discs got a front common ground electrode by sputtering and individual connections per fibre. Then the discs weres poled with approx. 2kV/mm.

3.2 Transducer design and built up process

The prototypes are built piezofibre from the piezofibre discs glueing them to a TMM 26.75mm diameter front matchin plate of 470µm thickness Rogers TMM4 disc, a high-frequency aluminium oxid based PCB material. The glueding was done with conductive silver-glue also providing the common ground connection, see Figure 12 top right.

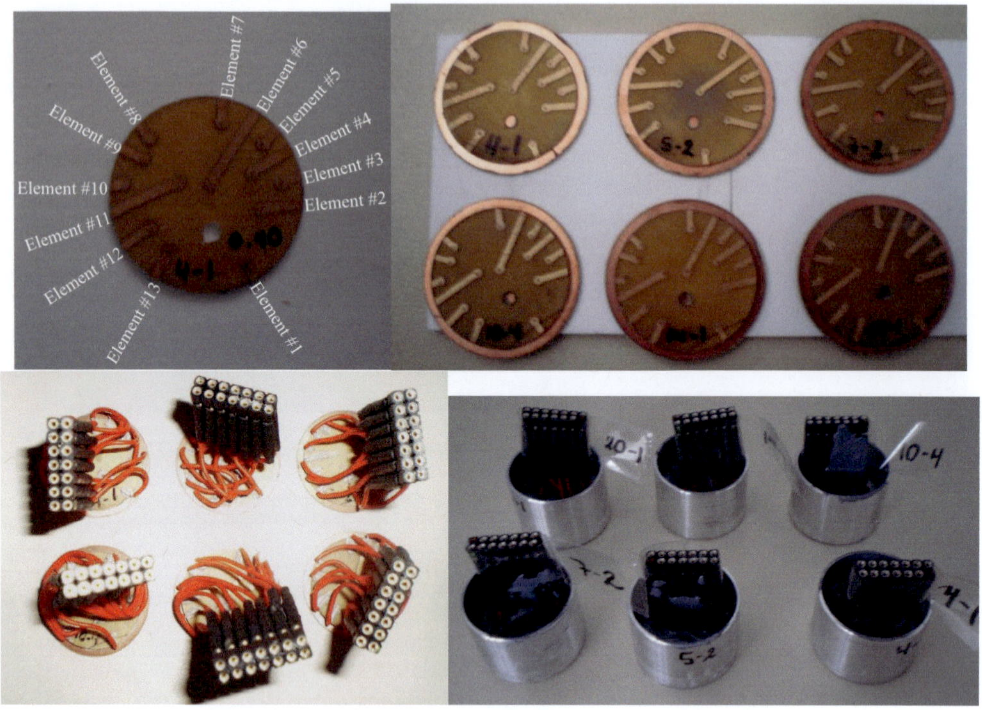

Figure 12: Schematic of the whole build-up process for the six transducer prototypes.

3.3 PCB design

A Flexprint design was choosen as PCB base for electrical connectivity for the transducers (not shown in the prototypes).

The design has many holes acting as pinholes for X-Y position accuracy (~0.05mm) and for later underfilling and getting rid of air. The backsite has substrate defined pads of 400µm diameter. The layout and final product are shown in Figure 13.

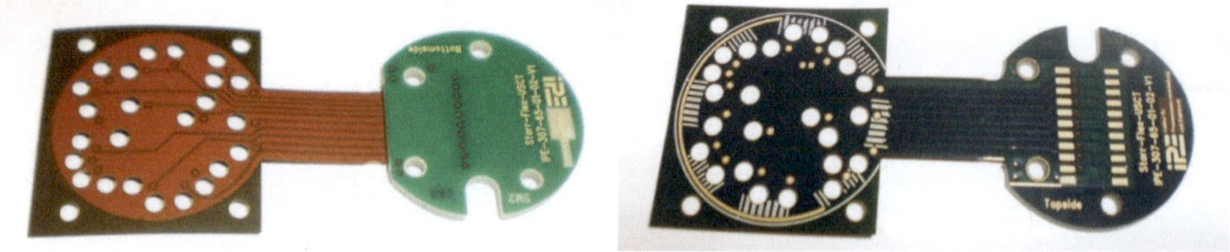

Figure 13: Flexprint PCB layout top side (left) and flex-print PCB backside (right).

3.4 Backing

3.4.1 Tungsten + PU backing

As backing some improved formula of the 3D USCT II baking was used: 1g VOSSFlex 2k Polyurethane filled with 2.5g Tungsten with 10µm particle size [10]. This resulted in a strongly attenuating composite of PU and tungsten powder which is also a well matching with an acoustic impedance values of approx. 11 MRayl. The mixing process was supported by 1% defoamer, the mixture was extensively, manually (~30min) degassed in vacuum chamber going to ca 50mbar.

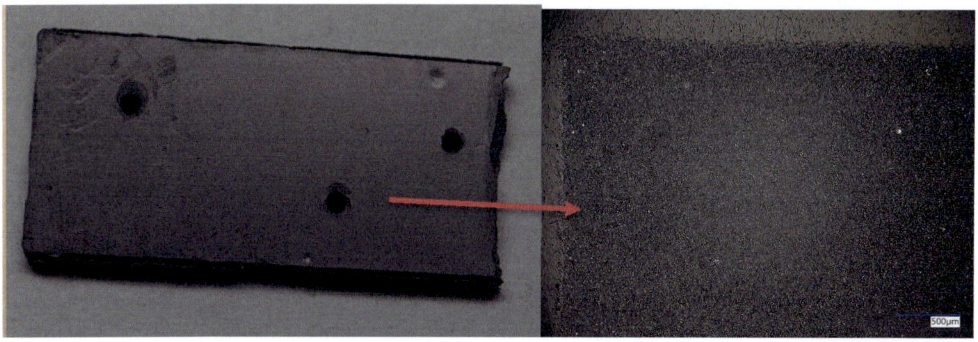

Figure 14: (left) PU-tungsten composite material, (right) its lower part under the microscope. Degassing is effective; no major air inclusions are visible (left).

3.5 Gluing and electrical connectivity

1K Heraeus PC3000 silver glue is used to electrical connect the individual elements. Curing is achieved with 100C° for half an hour on n temperature regulated heating plate.

A sieve printing mask test of 400µm, 500µm, 600µm dots diameter sizes was developed to analyze and optimize the individual element connect.

3.6 Matching and glueing

3.6.1 TMM4

The acoustic impedance of Rogers TMM4 an aluminum oxide composite with of 6.4 MRayl acoustic impedance is near optimal for a single-layer matching between PZT and water. TMM4 is a very stiff, mechanical mil-and drillable material and exhibits low water absorption. Besides being a strong electrical insulator, thermal conductivity of TMM4 is quite high. This is helpful for correct water temperature measurements, as the USCT temperature sensors are situated behind the TMM4 plate. Final waterproofing will be achieved with a thin layer of parylene.

4 Evaluations and results

4.1 Electrical Characterization

The sputtered piezofibre discs were analyzed with a fast electrical characterization in phase (see Fig. 15) and impedance between 500 kHz and 6 MHz. The HP 4194 phase analysator was calibrated before usage and every element of the 13 elements was measured of the selected six piezofibre discs shown in Fig.16.

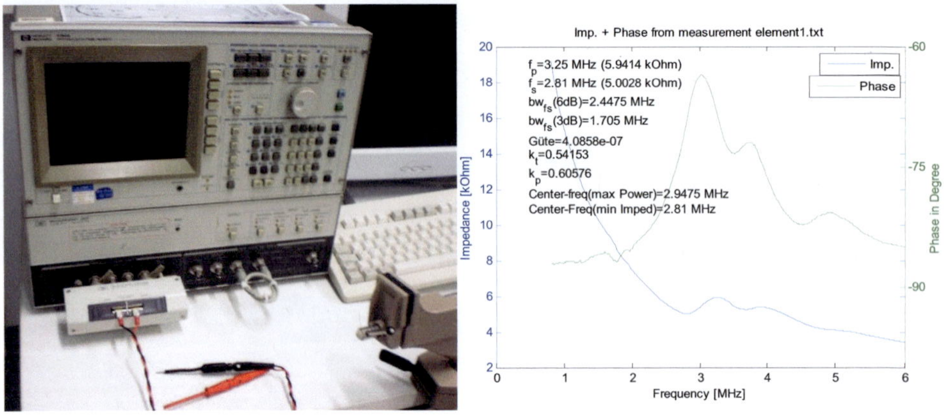

Figure 15: Impedance spectroscop used to characterize the build up prototypes (left). Example impedance and phase measurement graph of one element (right).

As result of the electrical characterization the thicknesses 400, 550, and 750μm were considered for further analysis; thicker disc thickness were not analyzed further due to poor performance and low sound pressure.

Thickness of disc (in µm)	**Center freq. (in MHz @max. Power, mean/std.)**	**BW (max. Power@ 3dB/6dB)**	**Phase (in degree@max. Power)**	**Kt (mean/std.)**	**Working (kt >0.1)**
400	3.01 (0.24)	1.69 / 2.34	-69.98°	0.56 (0.17)	**11/13**
550	2.54 (0.07)	1.57 / 1.99	-72.24	0.84 (0.06)	**12/13**
750	2.06 (0.11)	1.23 / 1.34	-74.53	0.90 (0.01)	**13/13**
1050	3.56 (1.29)	0.17 / 0.17	-85.08	0.91 (0.03)	**4/13**
1450	3.34 (0.07)	1.62 / 2.54	-85.22	0.11 (0.24)	**1/13**
2050	2.53 (0.04)	1.25 / 1.73	-85.30	0.00 (0.00)	**1/13**

Figure 16: Table of the results of the impedance phase measurement of the analyzed 6 piezofibre discs.

4.2 Acoustical measurements

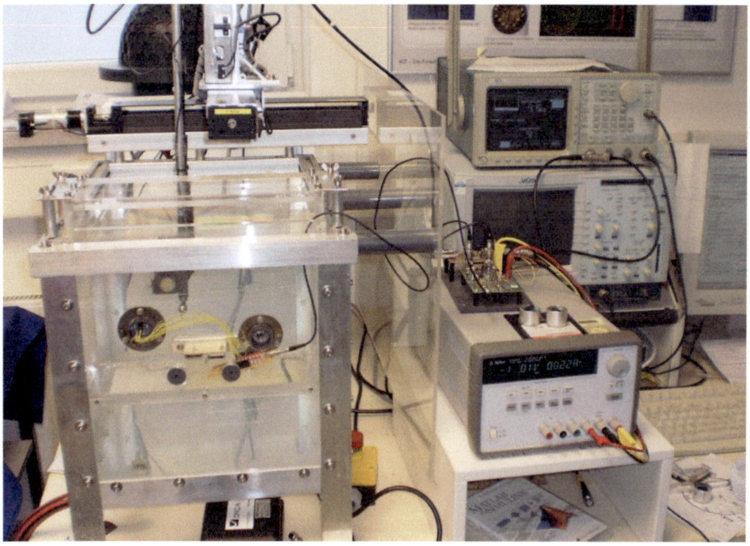

Figure 17: Left: measurement container (30 x 30 x 50 cm), top: 3-movement axis with stepper-motors and mounted hydrophone, bottom left: sockets for transducers, right: AWG, HV amplifier, DAQ, and control PC.

Ultrasound characteristics were evaluated quantitatively with a hydrophone in a 3-axis water tank for selected sample transducers [8, 9].

The measurement tank is a self-built system. The excitation voltage used was +-/100Vpp for a frequency sweep with chirps of 0.5MHz to 5.5MHz in 250kHz steps. A calibrated Onda HNC-400 hydrophone (up to 10MHz) with a 20dB pre-Amplifier was used. In the measuremenet procedure 16x averaging of the measurement was used to achieve a 4x SNR gain. The measured signal digitization length was 400µs with as sampling rate of 20MHz. Overall measurement time per prototype was several hours. The resulting performance for the thicknesses 400, 550, and 750µm can be seen in Fig. 18.

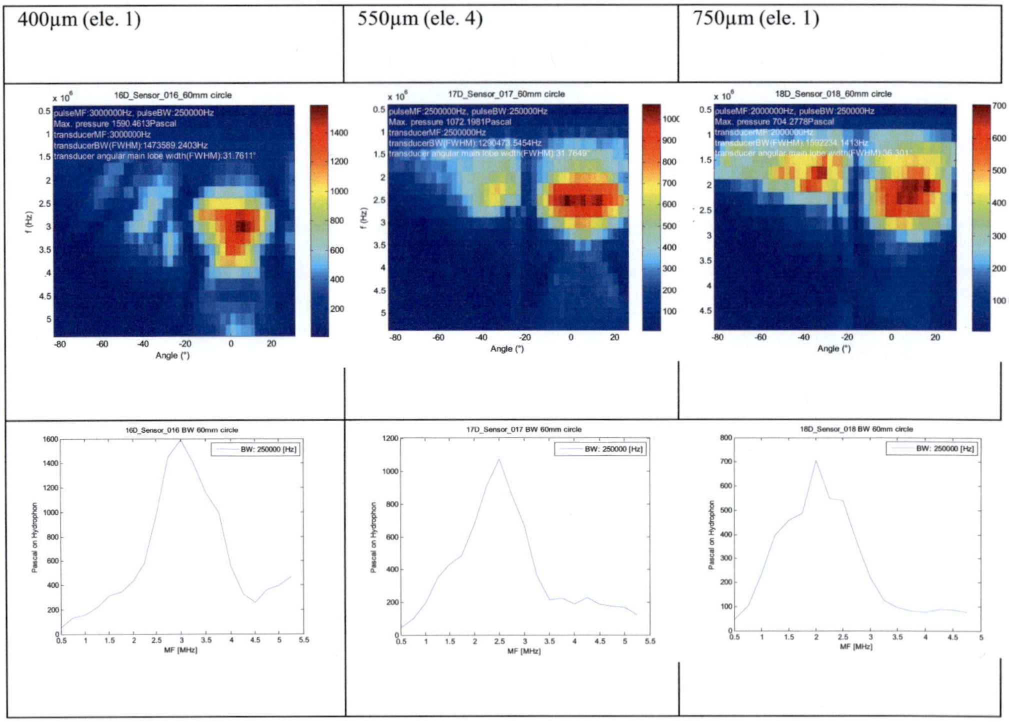

Figure 18: Acoustical characterization of transducer prototypes of varying dic thickness, top row: sound pressure over angle and frequency, bottom row frequency characteristic.

5 Discussion and conclusion

Funtionality and reliability of the piezofibre discs as analyzed with a phase impedance analysator and the reliability of >92% was encouraging. Then six prototypes of varying dis were build up to select the preferred center frequency and bandwidth; the 750µm thickness was selected. The developed PU-tungsten composite backing material led to a significant increase in BW through improved acoustic matching to the rear of the transducer in co-maprision to the original 3D USCT transducer design. This it can be seen in the acoustical measurements in fig. 18. Also, future by USCT utilized imaging techniques like paraxial wave inversion approaches benefit greatly from lower frequency <1MHz (down to approx. 0.5MHz) now available due to the extended bandwidth.

Analysis of the integration and connectivity process of the TMM4 ceramic matchin layer is ongoing. The curently semi-automatized process leads still to variations and in result to the failure of a signifcant portion of the transducer elements; especially in the glueing and filling step. This is currently under intensive investigation with further test prototypes. Final step to adapt and integrate the electronic front-end board (pre-amp and MUX) and the housing are the next steps in finalizing the production process.

References

[1] [Online]. Available: http://www.wcrf.org/int/cancer-facts-figures/data-specific-cancers/breast-cancer-statistics.

[2] [Online]. Available: http://www.who.int/cancer/detection/breastcancer/en/index1.html..

[3] James S Michaelson et al., „"Predicting the survival of patients with breast carcinoma causing tumor size,“ Cancer, 2002.

[4] Ruiter et al., „Realization of an optimized 3D USCT,“ SPIE 7968, Medical Imaging 2011: Ultrasonic Imaging, Tomography, and Therapy,, 2011.

[5] T. H. M. Z. C. K. N. R. H. Gemmeke, „3D ultrasound computer tomography. hardware setup, reconstruction methods and first clinical results.".Nuclear Instruments and Methods in Physics Research Section A: Accelerators, Spectrometers, Detectors and Associated Equipment.

[6] Gemmeke et al., „An improved 3D Ultrasound Computer Tomography system". IEEE International Ultrasonics Symposium., 2014.

[7] G. Göbel, „Entwicklung von Ultraschallsensorarrays mit miniaturisierten Komponenten,“ Diploma, KIT, 2002.

[8] M. Zapf, „Simulation eines Ultraschalltomographen im k-space,“ in Master thesis for Hochschule Karlsruhe (University of Applied Science), Karlsruhe, 2010.

[9] L. Petzold, „Aufbau eines Messplatzes zur Ermittlung der Schallfeldcharakteristik,“ Master thesis, KIT, 2006.

[10] G. Shah, „Auto-Calibration of Ultrasound Transducer Characterization Setup,“ Master thesis, KIT, 2015.

[11] P. Pfistner, „Composite-based ultrasound transducers for a 3D-Ultrasound computer tomograph,“ Master thesis, KIT, 2017.

[12] B. Kohout, „Finite Elemente Simulation von Ultraschallwandlersystemen für die Ultraschall Computertomographie,“ KIT, Diploma , 2010.

[13] G. S. M.Zapf, „Aperture optimization for 3D ultrasound computer,“ IEEE UFFC Symp., 2007.
[14] N. R. H. Gemmeke, „3D ultrasound computer tomography for medical,“ Nuclear Instruments and Methods in Physics Research Section A: Accelerators, Spectrometers, Detectors and Associated Equipment, 2007.
[15] K. Hohlfeld, S. Gebhardt, A. Schönecker, A. Michaelis: „PZT components derived from polysulphone spinning process“. In: Advances in Applied Ceramics 2015; 114(4), 231-237.
[16] M. Zapf, K. Hohlfeld, G. Shah, S. Gebhardt, H. Gemmeke, A. Michaelis, N. V. Ruiter: „Evaluation of piezo composite based omnidirectional single fibre transducers for 3D USCT“. In: Proc. IEEE Int. Ultrasonics Symp., October 21-24, 2015, Taipei (Taiwan).

Improved temperature measurement and modeling for 3D USCT II

Michael Zapf, Anirudh Patel, Alexander Menshikov, Nicole Ruiter

Karlsruhe Institute of Technology, Karlsruhe, Germany
E-mail: michael.zapf@kit.edu

Abstract

Medical visualization plays a key role in the early diagnosis and detection of symptoms related to breast cancer. However, currently doctors must struggle to extract accurate and relevant information from the 2D models on which the medical field still relies. The problem is that 2D models lack the spatial definition necessary to extract all of the information a doctor might want. In order to address this gap, we are developing a machine capable of performing ultrasound computer tomography and reconstructing 3D images of the breasts - the KIT 3D USCT II.

In order to accurately reconstruct the 3D image using ultrasound, we must first have an accurate temperature model. This is because the speed of sound varies significantly based on the temperature of the medium (in our case, water). We address this issue in three steps: so-called super-sampling, calibration, and modeling. Using these three steps, we were able to improve the accuracy of the hardware from ±1°C to just under 0.1°C.

Keywords: Temperature modelling, calibration, super resolution

1 Introduction

Breast cancer is the most common form of the affliction that there is, affecting more than 1.7 million women in 2012 alone. There is still a major problem with breast cancer screenings, as the images collected using the most common method, mammography, are two-dimensional. They therefore lack the spatial information that is often necessary for an accurate and confident judgement. At KIT, we seek to address this problem. Our novel imaging method uses ultra-sounds computer tomography to reconstruct a 3D image of the breast. The prototype of this technology is currently being used in a clinical study called 3D-USCT II.

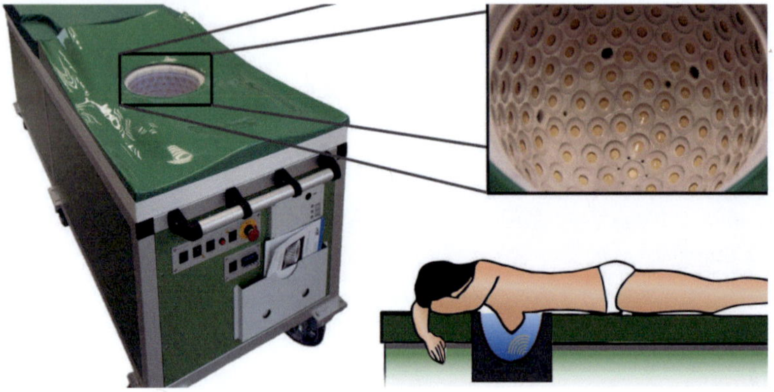

Figure 1: KIT 3D USCT II demonstrator (left), aperture (right top) and schematic

This technology functions based on the use of 3D synthetic aperture focusing, or SAFT, applied to unfocused spherical waves that are iteratively emitted and received by individual transducers. The measurement of these waves takes place in a semi-ellipsoidal water-filled container (17cm x 24 centimeters, height x width), which can be both lifted and rotated. Thousands of transducers have been strategically placed along the walls to form the imaging aperture. These transducers have a resonant frequency of 2.5 MHz at 50% relative bandwidth and a directivity of ±23° at 6dB. The system images and processes the data based on several imaging techniques, such as the previously-mentioned SAFT technique and transmission tomography-based approaches [1].

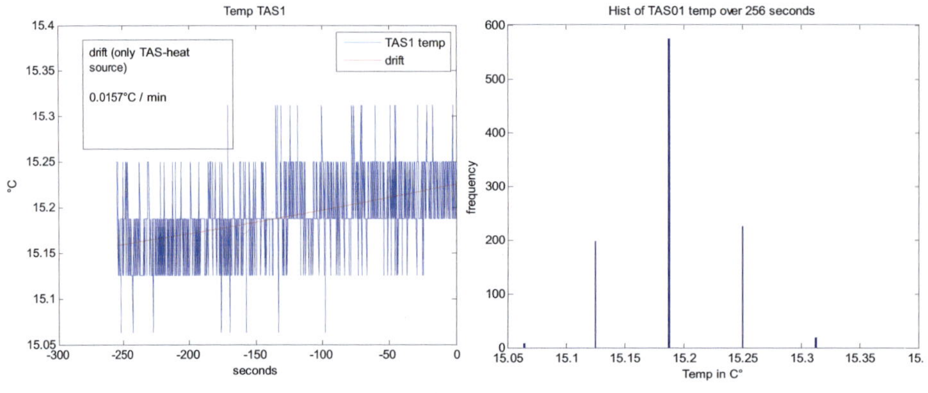

Figure 2: Left: temperature measurement over four minutes (blue curve). Visible noise and temperature drift. Red curve is the low order polynomial fit. Right: histogram of the measurement

2 Motivation

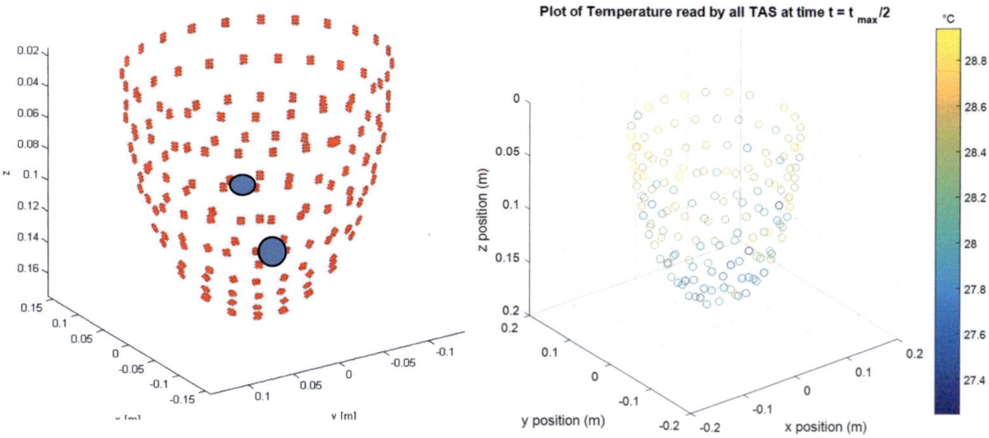

Figure 3: Left: Distribution of temperatures sensors, red dots indicate TAS temperature sensor position in space, blue dots are the 2 high quality JUMO sensors; right: temperature distribution over aperture surface and sensors.

The key point about the previous paragraph to understand for this paper is that the imaging techniques mentioned require accurate time-of-arrival and speed of sound values such that they can calculate back to identify the depths of possible lesions and cysts. The fidelity of these values is called into question by several factors. However, by far the biggest culprit in engendering errors is the variation of the speed of sound due to variations in medium temperature. The speed of ultrasound waves in water is significantly temperature-dependent [1].

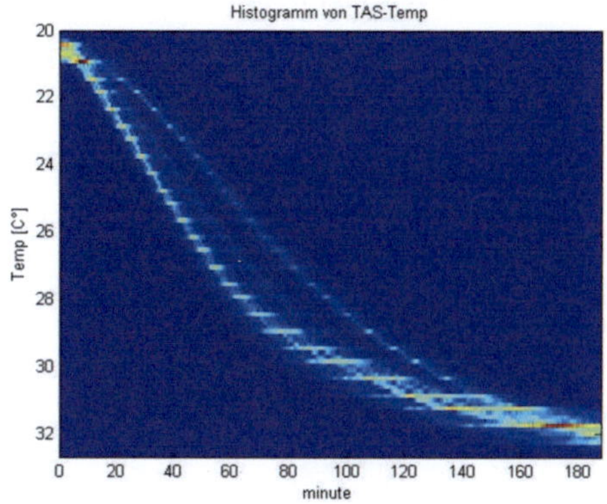

Figure 4: Temperature drift and spatial spread as 2D histogram over all TAS temperature sensors during 3D USCT heat up. X-axis is time, y-axis is temperature, color coding frequency of temperature. Around minute 80 the spread is the biggest, the system has "settled" after three hours.

There are several factors that may lead to poor temperature data. These include the outside air temperature, heating due to the systems DAQ electronics (roughly 1kW), heat dissipation at the water's surface, heating from the patient's body (roughly 100W), and mixing of the water due to the patient's motion.

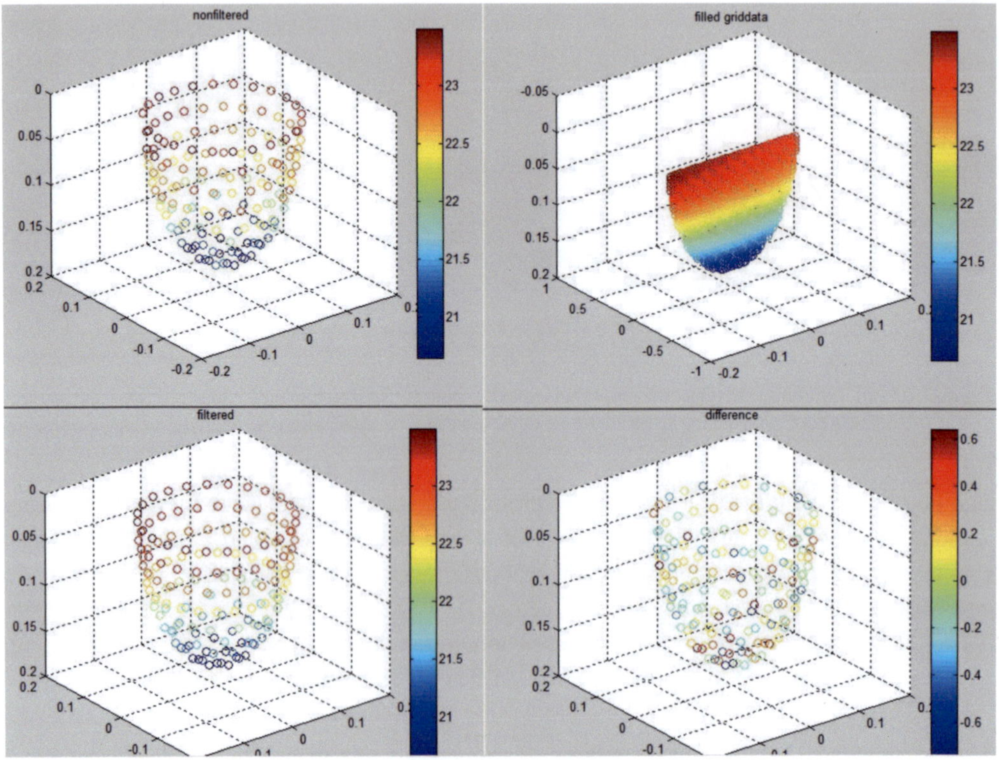

Figure 5: top left: raw temperature distribution, bottom right: filtered temperature, top right modelled and extrapolated for the water, bottom right: difference temperature filtered vs unfiltered

We pre-heat the water to match the patient's body temperature to mitigate the effects of the patient's body temperature as much as possible. However, even this is often impractical in the dynamic situations presented in hospital environments.

To summarize, the behavior of the temperature of the water is complicated and difficult to regulate into the required margins. As a result, we found it necessary to actively collect temperature data across space and time to develop a robust temperature model with which the images can be accurately reconstructed.

3 Hardware Setup

The USCT system utilizes 157 Transducer Array Sensors (TAS), each of which is outfitted with nine receivers, four emitters, and one MAX6627 temperature sensor. According to its datasheet, the MAX6627, hereafter referred to as TAS, has an accuracy of ±1°C and offers 12-bit resolution. It therefore has a temperature resolution of 0.0625°C-per-bit. The temperature measurement cadence is limited to about 320 milliseconds.

The system additionally contains two, high-accuracy temperature sensors, the JUMO dTRANS T03 B Typ 707031 Pt100 (DIN EN 60751), hereafter referred to as JUMOs. The datasheet reports the JUMOs‘ accuracy as 0.08°C and offers 10-bit resolution. This makes its temperature resolution similar to that of the TAS.

3.1 Constraints and Requirements

We have estimated that our required speed of sound accuracy should be within 1m/s. This translates to a temperature-accuracy of approximately 0.1°C, as opposed to the ±1°C offered by the TAS. Another constraint is that the collection of temperature information should not disturb or slow down the overall USCT measurement process, which, for a typical patient, is on the order of several minutes.

4 Methods

We take three steps in order that the necessary resolution and temperature accuracy are acquired. The path of the data is as follows. We begin with the raw temperature data from the 157 TAS. This raw data is passed through our super-resolution step, which is meant to increase accuracy and compensate for drift. The compensated data is then passed into the calibration step, in which we attempt to mitigate the effects of the hardware parameters of the TAS. The calibrated data then moves into our final step in which we determine a suitable spatial and temporal temperature model and remove outliers. These steps are described in more detail in the following sections.[2]

4.1 Super-Resolution

The analog-to-digital converter (ADC) has a standard deviation of 0.0405°C. This value correlates to having a standard-error-derived confidence interval and reliability of 68% at 0.081°C (1.29 bits) and to having a reliable of 95.5% at 0.162°C (2.59 bits).

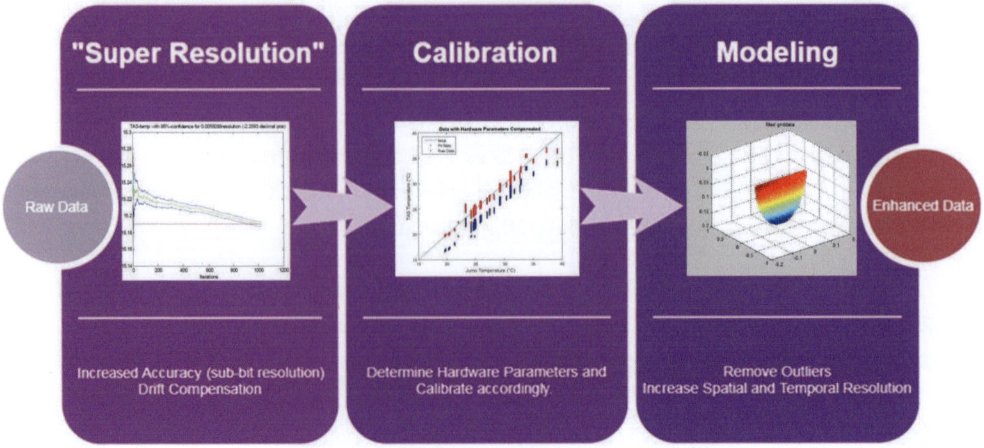

Figure 6: 3 step process for temperature data handling

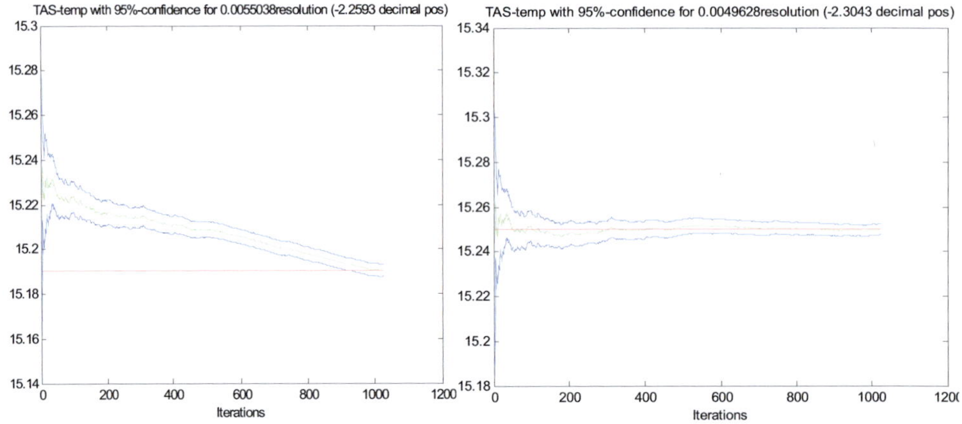

Figure 7: Blue lines 95% confidence interval, green line actual temperature measurement value, red line final end result. Left: Temperature measurement without drift compensation, red line leaves the confidence interval. Right: with drift compensation, the red line is always inside the confidence interval.

We know from signal processing and sampling theory that oversampling by simply averaging over time can achieve a higher reliability and accuracy, given that the noise is distributed normally. However, due to us having a limited measurement read-out speed, and as we expect to see a significant effect of drift over time, we cannot apply simple averaging. Rather, we must begin by compensating for the observed drift.

In order to do so, we began by changing the modus operandi of the temperature measurement from a synchronous on-demand action to an autonomous measurement. This process is handled by the TAS internal TI430 microcontroller, which fills in an internal memory buffer at a 0.5 second cadence.

We then used this data to model the drift with a first-order polynomial fit over the measurement time. This substitute of the simple averaging technique suggested by signal processing and results in an improved accuracy as well as super-resolution (resolution below 1 bit).

4.2 Calibration

After the applying the previous step to all TAS measurements, we pass the compensated data into our calibration step. The TAS temperature data suffers from a significant offset due to hardware parameters. This is in large part due to bad coupling with the water medium, as each TAS is insulated by a 0.4 millimeter ceramic plate. We have also noticed that the TAS see small heating effects from the DAQ electronics surrounding them. When compared with the generally good temperature measurements of the JUMO sensors, which are topped with a stainless steel tip that extends directly into the water, the TAS measurements need to be significantly adjusted.

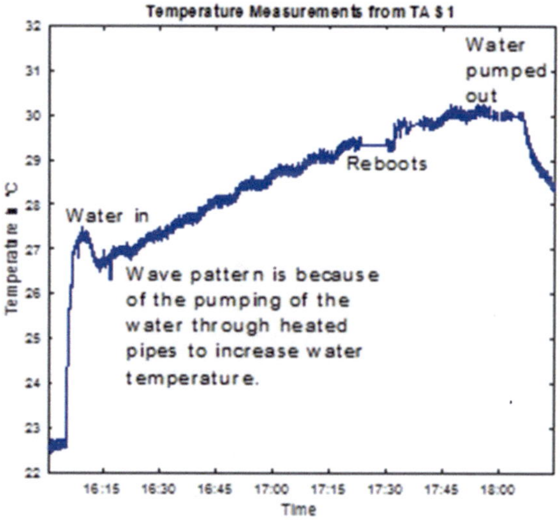

Figure 8: Temperature measurement monitoring the heat up of the system. Approx. over three hours.

4.3 Spatial and Temporal Temperature Modeling

Our final step begins with us removing the outliers from our newly calibrated data. We do this by removing the TAS measurements that are more than ten standard deviations away from the median of its 10 closest neighbors‘ temperatures. Having removed outliers, we can now begin to determine an overarching temperature model. We apply a second-order polynomial fit over the spatial domain, which assumes that the temperature change happens very slowly over space. This has been experimentally shown to be a safe assumption.

5 Results

Our process increases the accuracy and prevision of the TAS temperature measurements by more than an order of magnitude, 36.3x and 12.6x, respectively. This is well beyond the original 1 bit resolution. Though the datasheet specifies ±1°C for the TAS, for a 512 second measurement period with 1024 samples, we achieves 0.00496°C with a 95% confidence interval.

6 Conclusion and Future Work

Though we have, for the most part, achieved the goal, which we had set out to achieve, when we plot the temperatures seen by our TAS, we see layering effects. These layering effects are quite significant, up to around 1°C. We are currently investigating the possible causes of such a phenomenon. We have recently begun to collect more data about possible confounding variables such as air temperature above the ellipsoid, air temperature around the ellipsoid, heating due to the DAQs and piping that run around the ellipsoid, and initial water temperature. We are currently using manual sensors with the same accuracy as the JUMOS (0.08°C) to measure these effects and correlate them to patterns we see in our TAS data.

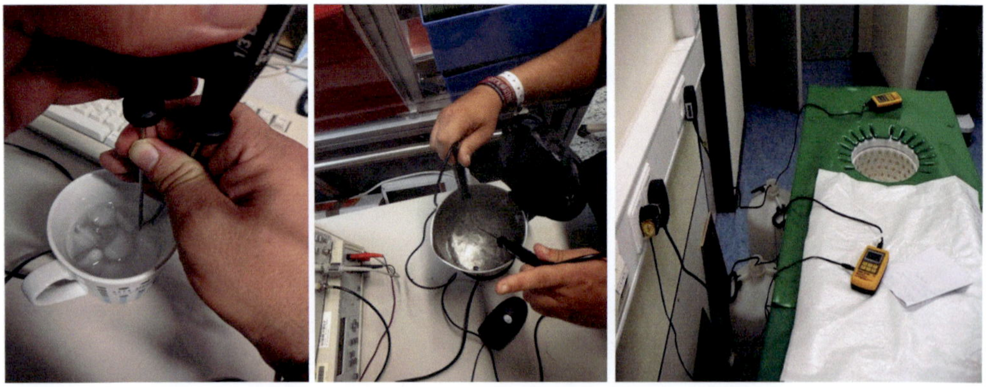

Figure 9: left and middle: calibration of Greisinger temperature measurement probes, right: setup for measuring the heat-up of the 3D USCT 2.0 and air temperature for improved calibration

References

[1] Ruiter et al., „Realization of an optimized 3D USCT," *SPIE 7968, Medical Imaging 2011: Ultrasonic Imaging, Tomography, and Therapy,,* 2011.

[2] Zapf, Michael & Menshikov, Alexander & Ruiter, Nicole. (2016). Temperature model for 3D ultrasound computer tomography. 1-4. 10.1109/ULTSYM.2016.7728723.

Visualisation of Ultrasound Computer Tomography Breast Dataset

Nicholas Tan Jerome[1], Zhassulan Ateyev[1,2], Vladislav Lebedev[1,2], Torsten Hopp[1], Michael Zapf[1], Suren Chilingaryan[1], and Andreas Kopmann[1]

[1] *Karlsruhe Institute of Technology, Eggenstein-Leopoldshafen, Germany*
E-mail: nicholas.jerome@kit.edu
[2] *Tomsk Polytechnic University, Tomsk, Russia*

Abstract

Medical visualisation plays a vital role in diagnosing and detecting early symptoms. In particular, visualising the anatomy of breast model allows doctors or practitioners to identify first signs of the breast cancer. However, despite the advancement in visualisation techniques, most standard visualisation approaches in the medical field still rely on analysing 2D images which lack spatial information. In this paper, we present an interactive web-based 3D visualisation tool for ultrasound computer tomography (USCT) breast dataset. We base our implementation on the Web-based Graphics Language (WebGL) technology that utilises the GPU parallel architecture. The tool serves as a common platform among research collaborators to analyse and share findings on their dataset. We render the data using state-of-the-art algorithms of interactive computer graphics and produce results with quality comparable to the desktop application. Aside from that, our tool enables researchers to perform arbitrary view slicing, modality thresholding and multiple rendering modes. In the evaluation, our tool maintains an interactive frame rate above 30 fps on a standard desktop.

Keywords: Web-based Visualization, Scientific Visualization, Multiresolution Slicemap, Normal fusion

1 Introduction

A most common cancer among woman is the breast cancer [1]. In the United States, the breast cancer continues to rank second after lung cancer [2], and significant efforts have been undertaken to improve early breast cancer detection. Primarily due to the improvement in screening methods and treatments, the mortality from breast cancer has declined steadily since 1995 [3].

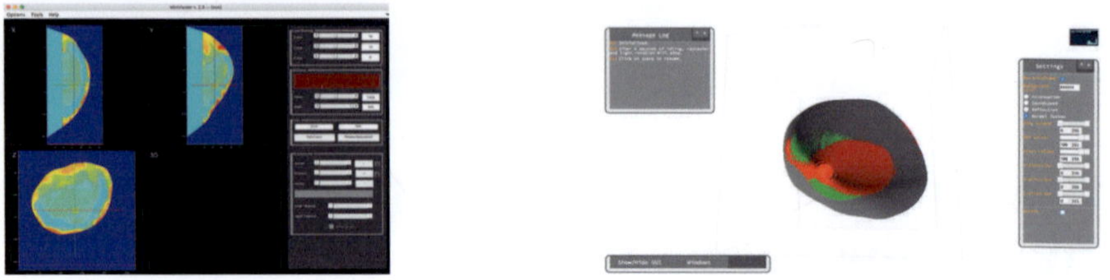

(a) (b)

Figure 1: The left image shows the Matlab MiniViewer user interface [5] showing the speed of sound modality ranging from 1300 $\mathrm{m\,s^{-1}}$ to 1600 $\mathrm{m\,s^{-1}}$. The right image shows the screenshot of the 3D web-based visualisation tool [15].

A somewhat new and attractive screening method is the ultrasound computer tomography method (USCT) which does not use any ionisation radiation, and yet produces high-quality 3D dataset using the 3D synthetic aperture focusing technique [4].

Despite the benefits of the USCT method, most of the research focused on comparing the screening results to the more familiar mammography screening methods [6, 7]. Although visualisation is a crucial step in diagnosing the dataset, less attention was given to improving visualisation techniques which could potentially improve data interpretation. The current state of visualisation tools still bases on analysing a stack of 2D slice images and rely on specific software dependencies, i.e., Matlab MiniViewer [5]. Such approach requires doctors to mentally imagine the breast anatomy based on a series of 2D images which could lead to mental fatigue.

Our goal is to create a web-based 3D visualisation of the breast dataset which allows remote and collaborative visualisation. On the one hand, we compromise for lesser quality on client devices with low GPU requirements. On the other hand, we adopted the state-of-the-art algorithms in computer graphics to interactively render the breast dataset using direct volume rendering and surface rendering on client devices with high GPU requirements. To aid the analysis process, we integrated data fusion methods where we merge multimodal information into a single volume. In particular, we integrated the *normal fusion* approach [12] which projects the region of interest along the *normal* direction on top of the surface, and the *image level intermixing* approach [16] which blends the multimodal information by varying its opacity level. Furthermore, our tool allows users to perform arbitrary view slicing, modality grey values thresholding and multiple rendering modes.

In this paper, we present a web-based visualisation tool (Figure 1b) that incorporates interactive rendering of the USCT data. The tool can serve a broad range of client devices, ranging from mobile phone to powerful workstation.

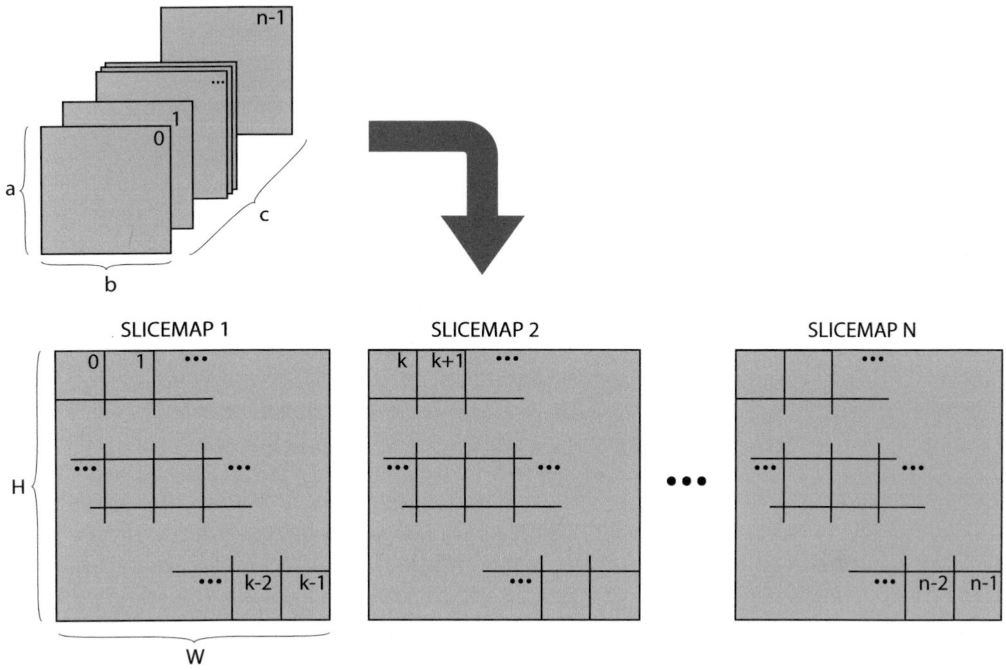

Figure 2: The composition of slicemaps: A 3D volume (image slices) is arranged into multiple slicemaps.

2 Methods

Our approach to design a web-based visualisation tool follows an overarching principle: visual quality and interactive scalability should be limited by the capability of the target client and network. With varying computational resources at the client side, no single visualisation method provides the best performance and the best rendering quality at the same time. Moreover, the limited network bandwidth is also a primary consideration. Although rendering original data may yield the best visual quality, but transferring large size of data may result in a less responsive tool. In this section, we first describe our approaches to find a balance between visual quality and interactive response. The latter parts cover the visualisation approaches and user interactions that are integrated into our tool.

2.1 Input Data

Often, a tomographic dataset presents itself as a stack of image slices, with each slice containing a cross-sectional image that represents an intersection of the volume. Using the standard volume rendering technique, we often load the data into the GPU 3D texture to take advantage of the hardware interpolation which is fast and efficient. However, not all browser supports

3D texture which motivates us to emulate the feature in the Graphics Processing Unit (GPU) shaders [14, 15]. A straightforward approach would be loading input data into the 2D texture memory, but the browser technology further limits the number of images (*texture unit*) and size of each image (*texture size*). These limitations vary across different client devices. For instance, a *Nexus 5* Android phone (GPU: Adreno 330) can accept up to 16 images with each image must not exceed the image resolution of 4096^2 texels.

Hence, we transform the image slices into *slicemap* [15] which comprises a series of 2D cross-section images stacked in a mosaic gridded format. Figure 2 shows the composition of slicemaps from a series of image slices. Here, we generate multiple slicemaps to maximise the capacity of the allowable texture memory in the GPU. Figure 3 shows a slicemap created from the USCT dataset. The USCT dataset consists of three modalities: *sound speed*, *attenuation*, and *reflection*. To this end, we map each modality into its respective colour channel. We express the colour representation of the pixel within the slicemap by a three-tuple $(R,G,B) \in [0,1]$, where $SoundSpeed \mapsto R$, $attenuation \mapsto G$, and $reflection \mapsto B$.

To address the diverse client requirements, we introduce the use of multiresolution slicemap—a hierachy of mutiresolution slicemaps differing in image resolution. The main idea is to transfer a suitable size of data that the best performance at the client. We characterise the client by its *texture unit* and *texture size* properties. To deal with the bandwidth limitation, we included the load-on-demand approach where low-resolution data is firstly served followed by a high-resolution data loading in the background [15].

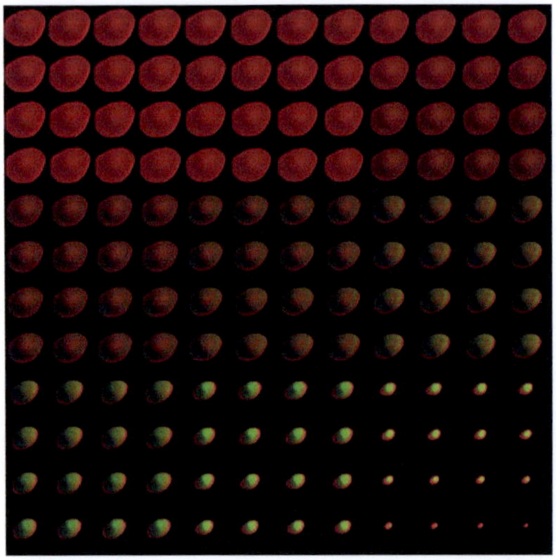

Figure 3: A 12×12 slicemap of a breast dataset. A mosaic-format image comprises a stack of 2D slice images. The iteration of the stack images is from left-right and top-bottom. Each slice consists of three modalities—*sound speed*, *attenuation* and *reflection*—that are mapped onto the colour channels respectively.

2.2 Visualisation Methods

2.2.1 Direct Volume Rendering

The objective of visualising the USCT dataset is to allow doctors or researchers to identify possible tumour regions efficiently. Hence, showing the spatial information of the dataset is crucial. For this reason, we incorporate direct volume and surface renderings as the main visualisation methods. The direct volume rendering is commonly used to display the scientific dataset [8]. In particular, we adopted the particle model variation described by Max [9] where the intensity at each sampled position is constant along the viewing ray direction. Thus, resulting in an image similar to an X-ray negative—brightest where the data is most dense but saturates at the maximum intensity as can be seen in Figure 4a.

Furthermore, we further improve the visual quality by adopting the real-world light simulations — reflection and refraction. In particular, we include the empirical Phong illumination model which describes the light interaction on each surface point [10]. Inspired by the lighting setup in photography studio [11], we mimic the lighting setup to provide an adequate lighting source to the data model. Since our model lies within a bounding box, we place our lights at the corners of the box (Figure 4a). The lighting design consists three light components: (1) key light, (2) fill light, and (3) back light (Figure 4b). Typically in a photography studio, the lightings and the model are static while the photographer moves around the model to find the best shooting angle. In contrast to our setup, the viewer is static while the lightings and model rotate along the model axes.

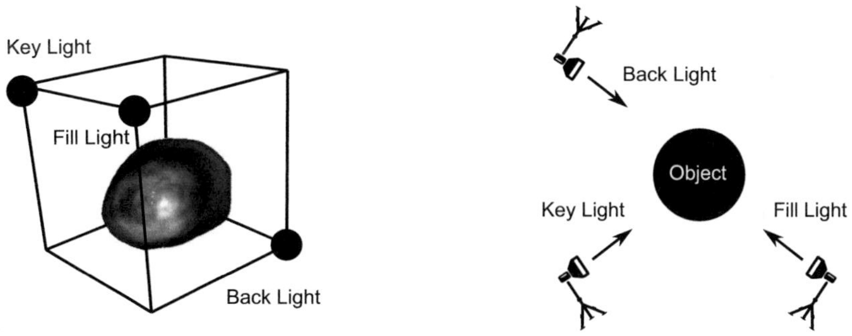

(a) (b)

Figure 4: The lighting positions within the bounding box. The key light, fill light and back light are attached to the three corners of our model to provide adequate lightings on the data.

2.2.2 Data Fusion Approach

Whenever we visualise the multimodal USCT dataset, we get three full range of volumes—each volume representing each modality. Despite having 3D models, manually analysing multiple datasets is cumbersome. Instead, we merge the three modalities into a single representation for better data interpretation (data fusion). Mainly, we allow fusion scheme which determines the projection of each modality, i.e., Ranger's fusion scheme [6]. In this section, we will discuss on two data fusion approaches where we utilise both surface and volume rendering techniques interchangeably: the *normal fusion* approach [12] and the *image level intermixing* approach [16] (Figure 5). Throughout the data fusion approaches, we label thresholded region of *sound speed* as orange colour and *attenuation* as green colour.

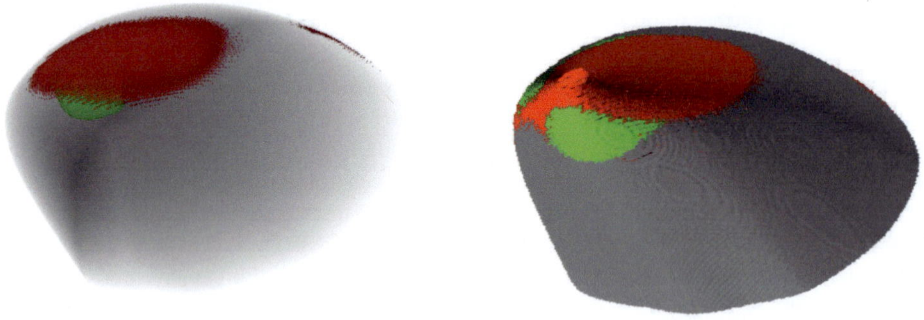

(a) (b)

Figure 5: The data fusion approaches: (a) *image level intermixing* and (b) *normal fusion*.

The image level intermixing: In the rendering process (Algorithm 1), we combine the information stored in the slicemap to produce the final image. Mainly, we use the direct volume rendering and extend the classification step where we choose values at each point selectively. The *sound speed* modality is prioritised first, followed by the *attenuation* modality and lastly the *reflection* modality. Firstly, we set the opacity of the background base on the *reflection* modality where the structure of the data can be determined. Then, we look at whether the *sound speed* or the *attenuation* falls within the predefined threshold regions (regions of interest). In the case where any of the two modalities are within the region, we set the colour and opacity of the voxel to the corresponding modality opacity and its predefined colour according to the modality priority.

The normal fusion approach: Algorithm 2 describes the process of projecting the interior information of the volume onto the surface. Here, we utilise volume rendering to collect information within the volume and surface rendering to produce a realistic image. Similar to the *image level intermixing*, we prioritise the *sound speed* modality over *attenuation* modality, and we use *reflection* modality to present the structure information. However, if there is an overlapping region, we show the *sound speed* modality only. To produce the final *normal fusion* result, we firstly cast a ray into the bounding box until we hit the surface of the object. Then, we calculate the normal vector at the intersection point. Rather than continuing in the ray direction, we continue to traverse further in the normal direction instead (secondary ray). Along the secondary ray, we return the orange label if we detect any *sound speed* within the predefined threshold. Otherwise, we return green label if we find *attenuation* within the predefined threshold with no *sound speed* presence. With the colour label ready, we perform the surface rendering using the returned label as our ambient colour.

```
Ray setup (entry position and ray direction);
while ray in volume do
    Interpolate data value at current position;
    if current value (sound speed) within sound speed threshold then
        colour ← orange;
        opacity ← current sound speed opacity;
    else
        if current value (attenuation) within attenuation threshold then
            colour ← green;
            opacity ← current attenuation opacity;
        else
            colour ← grey;
            opacity ← current reflection opacity;
        end
    end
    Perform compositing (colour and opacity);
    Propagate position along ray;
end
```

Algorithm 1: Image level intermixing: pseudo code

2.3 Data Interactions

To study and explore the data, we enable arbitrary model view slicing, grey values thresholding, and multiple rendering modes. Since interesting information often lies within the volume, we allow users to slice and inspect the interior of the volume. The slicing angle can be any arbitrary position which the user can freely define. Given the many visualisation approaches adopted within the tool, we allow the user to change the visualisation mode interactively. Aside, the user can select the grey value threshold and show only the region of interest. Depending on the visualisation mode, the threshold parameter may filter out data from the view or define a particular region to be displayed. We also allow the user to interact with the 3D model by including rotation and zoom features.

```
Ray setup (entry position and ray direction);
Define W as length of the cube;
while ray in volume do
    if intersect then
        calculate normal direction;
        read current position and value;
        output ← grey;
        Secondary ray setup(current position and normal direction);
        while secondary ray less than W/2 do
            if current value within sound speed threshold then
                output ← orange;
                break;
            end
            if current value within attenuation threshold then
                output ← green;
            end
        end
        ambient ← output;
        Perform compositing (ambient + diffuse + specular);
        break;
    else
        propagate position along ray
    end
end
```

Algorithm 2: Normal fusion: pseudo code

3 Evaluations

The basis for all frame rate comparison is the client's local server which is primarily affected by its available GPU resource. Hence, to measure the efficiency and performance of our tool, we evaluate the mentioned visualisation methods—direct volume rendering (DVR), the *image level intermixing* approach (ILI), the *normal fusion* approach (NF)—on several clients with different GPU resources. The methods are tested on (i) a mobile phone (GPU: Adreno 510), (ii) a standard desktop (GPU: integrated graphics card HD4000), (iii) a laptop (GPU: GT750M), and (iv) a powerful workstation (GPU: Tesla C2). We use the USCT data with the size of $256 \times 256 \times 144$ which is transformed into a single slicemap (Figure 3). The three modalities are encoded into the colour channels of the slicemap.

Base on the results shown in Figure 6, the direct volume rendering has the best performance due to its simplicity. There is no classification step nor any fusion scheme involved. In the case of the ILI and NF, both fusion methods involve priority-based modality selection to determine the visual output. The ILI is based solely on volume rendering algorithm and extends the classification step; whereas the NF consists of both volume and surface renderings. Moreover, the NF approach involves a primary ray in the view direction and a secondary ray in the normal direction. In comparision with the ILI approach, the addtional secondary ray in the NF approach results in higher traversal steps. However, the performance of the ILI and NF is comparable which suggests the priority-based selection in the NF serves as an *early secondary ray termination*—the secondary ray terminates upon the detection of *sound speed* modality.

With exception to the mobile device, our tool resulted in an overall frame rate higher than 30 fps which suggest the suitability of our tool in clinic or laboratory environments. Worth noting is the performance shown by the desktop with only an integrated graphics card (integrated GPU HD4000) with no dedicated GPU. Hence, we can conclude that our tool is capable of running on any modern desktop with acceptable performance. On the other hand, the usage of the web-based 3D tool in mobile phones in the current state is not feasible. We can optimise the existing algorithm by reducing the sampling step number along with the primary ray. Also, we can adopt less resource demanding algorithm such as additive blending. To minimise the processing load at the client, we can shift the data-intensive operation to the server side such as precalculating normal vectors. Also, reducing the data size can improve the client side performance immensely but at the cost of the visual quality [15].

4 Conclusions and Future Work

We have presented a web-based 3D visualisation tool that can be served by a broad range of client devices. Our tool supports the direct volume rendering, the *image level intermixing* approach, and the *normal fusion* approach which are useful in identifying the interesting region of the USCT data. Not only web-based platform encourages collaborative research, but the visual results were promising and comparable to desktop applications.

Future work of our tool encompasses several opportunities. Firstly, given the simple geometry of the USCT dataset, fusing the multimodal data is much more interesting. In this paper, we have shown a small fraction of the many multimodality visualisations imaginable. For example, we can consider the work by Bramon [17] to fuse multimodal data using the mutual information approach which requires probability map of the interested anatomy features. Since our input data are inherently images, we can improve the network latency by introducing compression schemes such as LZO algorithm.

Throughout this paper, we assume a simple client-server architecture with no high-performance computer (HPC). With hardware commodity being affordable, it is an exciting prospect to improve the image quality and network latency by deploying an image streaming approach, which the approach shifts computation intensive processes to the server and send the resulting image—small memory footprint—to the client. Furthermore, a new trend arises where many applications are emphasising on the visual analytic system. Having only multimodality visualisation is maybe useful, but integrating more domain knowledge into the visualisation system can enlighten the doctors or practitioners in their daily work.

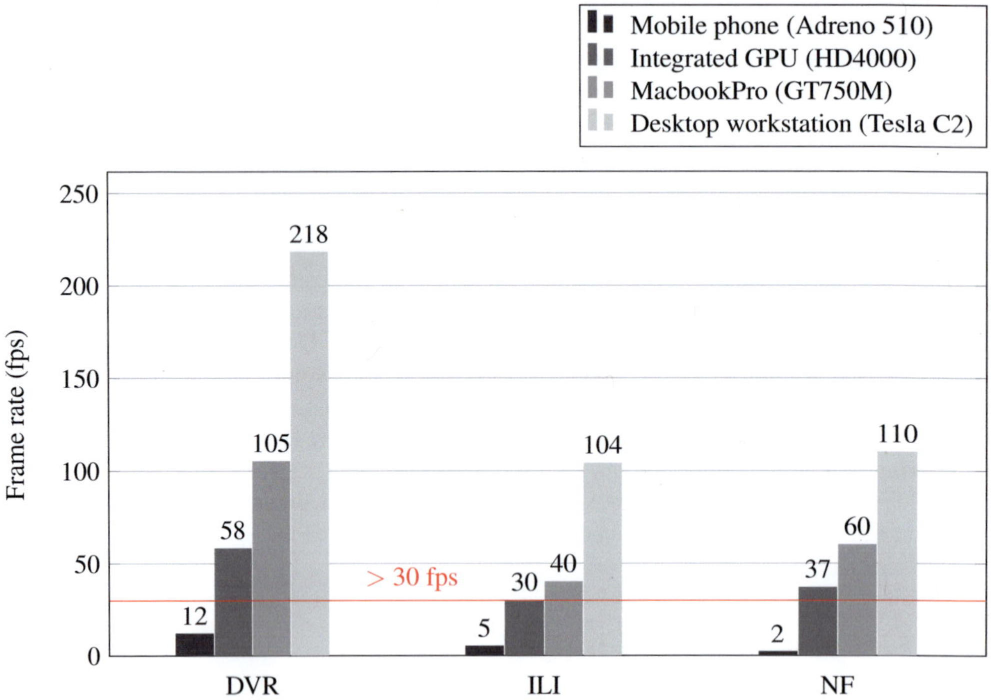

Figure 6: The frame rate of three visualisation methods—the direct volume rendering (DVR), the image level intermixing (ILI) and the normal fusion approach (NF)—tested on the mobile phone, the desktop with integrated GPU, the MacbookPro and the powerful workstation. The higher the frame rate, the better.

References

[1] L. A. Torre, F. Bray, R. L. Siegel, J. Ferlay, J. Lortet-Tieulent, A. Jemal.: Global cancer statistics, 2012. CA: a cancer journal for clinicians 65(2) (2015) 87-108.

[2] K. C. Oeffinger, E. T. Fontham, R. Etzioni, A. Herzig, J. S. Michaelson, Y.-C. T. Shih, L. C. Walter, T. R. Church, C. R. Flowers, S. J. Lamonte, A. M. Wolf.: Breast cancer screening for women at average risk: 2015 guideline update from the american cancer society. Jama 314 (2015) 1599-1614.

[3] R. L. Siegel, K. D. Miller, A. Jemal.: Cancer statistics, 2016. CA: A Cancer Journal for Clinicians 66 (2016) 7-30.

[4] H. Gemmeke, T. Hopp, M. Zapf, C. Kaiser, N. V. Ruiter.: 3D ultrasound computer tomography: Hardware setup, reconstruction methods and first clinical results. Nuclear Instruments and Methods in Physics Research Section A: Accelerators, Spectrometers, Detectors and Associated Equipment, (2017).

[5] T. Hopp, G. Schwarzenberg, M. Zapf, N. V. Ruiter.: A MATLAB GUI for the analysis and exploration of signal and image data of an ultrasound computer tomograph. IEEE Advances in Computer-Human Interaction (2008) 53-58.

[6] B. Ranger, P. J. Littrup, N. Duric, P. Chandiwala-Mody, C. Li, S. Schmidt, J. Lupinacci.: Breast ultrasound tomography versus MRI for clinical display of anatomy and tumor rendering: preliminary results. American Journal of Roentgenology 198 (2012) 233-239.

[7] N. V. Ruiter, M. Zapf, R. Dapp, T. Hopp, W. Kaiser, H. Gemmeke.: First results of a clinical study with 3D ultrasound computer tomography. IEEE International Ultrasonics Symposium (2013) 651-654.

[8] M. Levoy.: Display of surfaces from volume data. IEEE Computer graphics and Applications 8 (1988) 29-37.

[9] N. Max.: Optical models for direct volume rendering. IEEE Transactions on Visualization and Computer Graphics 1 (1995) 99-108.

[10] B. T. PHONG, Illumination for computer generated pictures, Commun. ACM, 18 (1975), pp. 311-317.

[11] Y. Zhang, K.-L. Ma.: Lighting design for globally illuminated volume rendering. IEEE transactions on visualization and computer graphics 19 (2013) 2946-2955.

[12] R. Stokking, K. J. Zuiderveld, M. A. Viergever.: Integrated volume visualization of functional image data and anatomical surfaces using normal fusion. Human Brain Mapping 12 (2001) 203-218.

[13] S. D. Roth.: Ray casting for modeling solids. Computer graphics and image processing 18 (1982) 109-144.

[14] J. Congote, A. Segura, L. Kabongo, A. Moreno, J. Posada, O. Ruiz.: Interactive visualization of volumetric data with webgl in real-time. ACM. Proceedings of the 16th International Conference on 3D Web Technology (2011) 137-146.

[15] N. Tan Jerome, S. Chilingaryan, A. Shkarin, A. Kopmann, M. Zapf, A. Lizin, T. Bergmann.: WAVE: A 3D online previewing framework for big data archives. INSTICC SciTePress. Proceedings of the 12th International Joint Conference on Computer Vision, Imaging and Computer Graphics Theory and Applications 3 (2017) 152-163.

[16] W. Cai, G. Sakas.: Data Intermixing and Multivolume Rendering. Blackwell Publishers Ltd. In Computer Graphics Forum 18(3) (1999) 359-368.

[17] R. Bramon, I. Boada, A. Bardera, J. Rodriguez, M. Feixas, J. Puig, M. Sbert.: Multimodal data fusion based on mutual information. IEEE Transactions on Visualization and Computer Graphics 18(9) (2012) 1574-1587.

Comparison of registration strategies for USCT-MRI image fusion: preliminary results

T. Hopp, P. Cotic Smole, and N.V. Ruiter

Karlsruhe Institute of Technology, Institute for Data Processing and Electronics, Karlsruhe, Germany
E-mail: torsten.hopp@kit.edu

Abstract

Comparing Ultrasound Computer Tomography (USCT) to the well-known Magnetic Resonance Imaging (MRI) is an essential step in evaluating the clinical value of USCT. Yet the different conditions of the breast either embedded in water (USCT) or in air (MRI) prevent direct comparison. In this work we compare two strategies for image registration based on biomechanical modeling to automatically establish spatial correspondence: a) by applying buoyancy to the MRI, or b) by removing buoyancy from the USCT. The registration was applied to 9 datasets from 8 patients. Both registration strategies revealed similar registration accuracies (MRI to USCT: mean = 5.6 mm, median = 5.6 mm, USCT to MRI: mean = 6.6 mm, median = 5.7 mm). Image registration of USCT and MRI allows to delineate corresponding tissue structures in both modalities in the same or nearby slices. Our preliminary results indicate that both simulation strategies seem to perform similarly. Yet the newly developed deformation of the USCT volume is less computationally demanding: As the breast is subjected to buoyancy it can thereby serve as the unloaded state while for the contrary strategy we have to solve an inverse problem.

Keywords: Image registration, Biomechanical breast model, Ultrasound Computer Tomography, Magnetic Resonance Imaging

1 Introduction

Among other Ultrasound Computer Tomography (USCT) systems, e.g. [1, 2], KIT's full 3D USCT system is currently being tested in clinical trials [3]. In this development state of a novel imaging modality it is essential to correlate the images to well-known imaging modalities in order to learn the imaging characteristics and evaluate the diagnostic value of USCT. In our clinical studies we use Magnetic Resonance Imaging (MRI) as a three-dimensional modality of choice for comparison to 3D USCT images. Yet the different environmental conditions of the breast either embedded in water (USCT) or in air (MRI) and the contact of the breast with the MRI breast coils lead to different non-linear deformations of the breast in 3D, which result in a challenging correlation of tissue structures.

In our previous work [4] we presented an automated image registration method to overcome these considerable differences during the image acquisition. The challenging non-linear deformations of the soft tissue are tackled by applying patient-specific biomechanical breast models. The models are until now generated based on the MRI volumes and the registration process simulates the effect of buoyancy to create deformed MRI volumes which are directly comparable to the USCT volume. The buoyancy simulation is approximated by estimating the unloaded state of the breast, i.e. to remove the gravity that is acting on the breast during MRI acquisition. Hence we have to solve an inverse problem of estimating the unknown unloaded state from a loaded state, which can be derived by an iterative procedure [5] and is therefore time consuming. In this work we consider the opposite strategy: deforming the breast imaged in USCT to match the breast shape in the MRI. Due to assuming the breast imaged in USCT as the approximate unloaded state this might be beneficial for biomechanical modeling as only the forward problem of applying gravity has to be solved. This papers describes the developed methods and presents the preliminary results comparing both registration strategies.

2 Methods

The key difference between USCT and MRI is the breast positioning in water respectively air. In particular the gravity which is present during MRI acquisition causes an elongation of the breast in anteroposterior direction and a contraction in mediolateral respectively craniocaudal direction. In contrast, the breast shape during USCT image acquisition approximately equals the gravity-free state as buoyancy and gravity are in equilibrium. In our previous approach - here denoted as strategy A - the general idea is to simulate the buoyancy effect by estimating the gravity-free state of the breast from the MRI (Figure 1). In the new approach - here denoted as strategy B - the breast imaged in USCT is assumed to be in a gravity-free state and we simulate the gravity effect (Figure 2). For both strategies we apply patient-specific biomechanical models and Finite Element simulations to estimate the large deformation. Following the biomechanical model based deformation, a cubic B-spline based free form deformation is applied to refine the surface overlap of the breasts in MRI and USCT respectively. Both registration steps rely on the breast surfaces detected in MRI and USCT images and do not consider additional landmarks to drive the registration.

A biomechanical model is constructed from the segmented MRI (strategy A) or USCT (strategy B) volume. The MRI based model requires a preprocessing of the MRI volume which includes a segmentation of the breast from the background using an automated state of the art segmentation method based on fuzzy C-means clustering [6]. As the MRI volume contains a whole cross-section of the patients body which is not relevant for the breast image registration, the volume is cropped at the sternum in anteroposterior direction, which is detected automatically from the image. Furthermore the volume is resampled to an isotropic voxel size by a linear interpolation to overcome the gap between slices. The USCT based model is constructed by segmenting the breast from the background using a semi-automated edge detection and surface fitting approach [7].

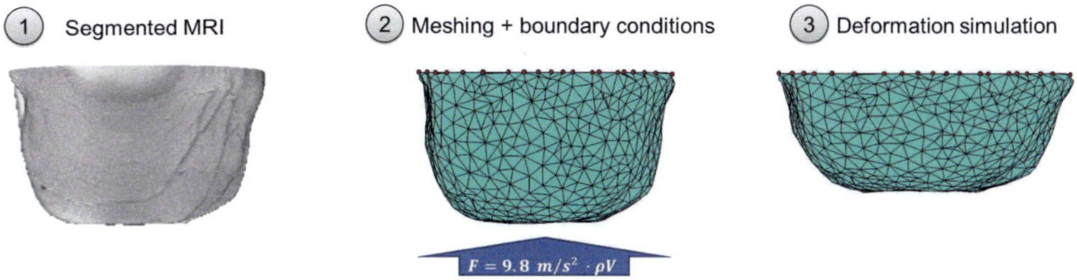

Figure 1: Illustration of image registration strategy A: a buoyancy simulation is applied to the breast acquired in MRI to obtain the loading configuration of the breast during imaging in USCT. Note that the illustration refers to the simplified buoyancy simulation using a simple body load. For the full resolution simulation an iterative approach is applied: a gravity load is applied iteratively and the estimate of the node positions in the unloaded state are updated to solve the inverse problem.

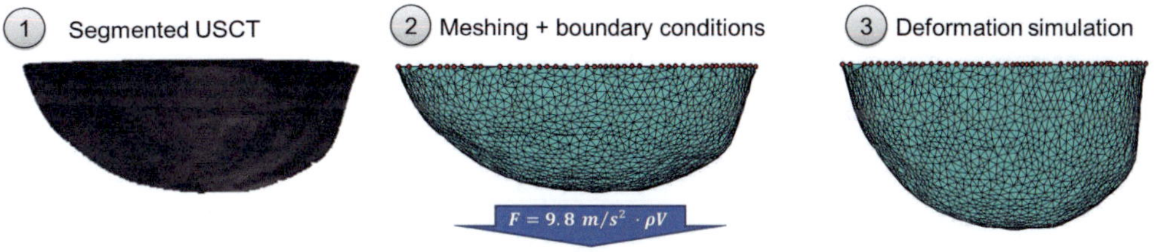

Figure 2: Illustration of image registration strategy B: a gravity simulation is applied to the breast acquired in USCT to obtain the gravity loaded configuration of the breast during prone MRI acquisition

The geometry of the biomechanical models is generated by a meshing algorithm [8] using 4-node tetrahedrons. A hyperelastic neo-hookean material model is applied. The breast tissue is assumed to be nearly incompressible by applying a Poissons ratio of 0.49. The material stiffness parameters, i.e. the Young's modulus E for fatty tissue (E_{FAT}), are initially applied constant for all patients. They are converted to the neo-hookean material constants using the relationship between the Young's modulus and the shear and bulk modulus as described in e.g. *Bower* [9].

Buoyancy is simulated by applying a body load with an acceleration of $g = 9.81\,m/s^2$, in posterior direction on the entire breast while posterior-most nodes of the mesh are held in position to model the fixation of the breast at the chest wall (strategy A). The resulting force F is given by $F = mg$ with m the mass of the water replaced by the breast volume V, i.e. $m = \rho V$ with the density of water $\rho = 1000\,kg/m^3$. Gravity is simulated vice versa: a body load is applied in anterior direction on the entire model assuming an average density of the breast of $\rho = 1000\,kg/m^3$, while posterior-most nodes are fixed (strategy B). To compute the biomechanical simulation, the commercial Finite Element Method (FEM) package ABAQUS [10] is used.

To enable a patient-specific registration, the material stiffness parameters as well as dataset rotation and cropping are automatically optimized using simulated annealing with bound constraints. The optimization criterion is the surface agreement between the deformed breast after buoyancy respectively gravity simulation and the corresponding breast in the USCT respectively MRI volume. The surface agreement is calculated as the average distance of closest points on both breast surfaces, which becomes minimal for perfectly overlapping breast images. An empirically chosen maximum of 50 iterations is used as a stopping criterion.

The image resolution of datasets included in this study was $(0.75\,mm)^3$ for the USCT volume and $0.91\,mm \times 0.91\,mm \times 3.0\,mm$ for the MRI volume. To accelerate the overall registration process, the parameter optimization is performed on images downsampled by factor two. After the optimization of the material parameters, the cropping and the rotation, the optimized parameters are used for a simulation in full resolution. In the case of strategy A, an iterative simulation similar to *Carter et al.*[5] to approximate the true unloaded state of the breast is applied for the full resolution simulation.

Due to simplifications of the biomechanical model compared to the unknown real biomechanics of the breast such as neglecting connective tissue structures like Cooper ligaments [11], the deformed images usually do not fully overlap. Furthermore the predeformation caused by a possible contact between the breast and the MRI breast coil may cause additional differences in the breast shape. Therefore an additional simulation step is performed to bring the MRI and USCT volumes in full overlap. The deformed MRI (strategy A) respectively deformed USCT (strategy B) after biomechanical simulation is rigidly aligned with the contrary modality based on both centers of mass in mediolateral direction and the chest wall in anteroposterior direction. Afterwards a 3D free form deformation with cubic B-splines is applied [12]. Again the surface agreement of deformed MRI and USCT is used as a penalty function for the optimization process that drives the free form deformation. Supporting grid point distances of the B-splines were manually chosen as a tradeoff between the local and global deformation of the breast.

To measure the accuracy of the registration, landmarks like lesions, predominant connective tissue structures or breast implants which could be clearly delineated in MRI as well as in USCT, were manually annotated in the unregistered MRI and the USCT volume by circumscribing the border of the structure with a freehand tool in 3D. The Target Registration Error (TRE) is defined as the average of Euclidean distances of closest points between the annotations in the unregistered and the compared modality.

3 Results

The registration was applied to nine datasets from eight patients of our first clinical study with the KIT 3D USCT [3]. The datasets were chosen such that at least one correlating tissue structure could be clearly delineated in one USCT volume and the MRI volume before the registration was carried out. In total 11 correlating tissue structures were annotated. In case of more than one marking in a breast the TRE was averaged for the particular volume image to estimate an error per registered dataset.

The TRE was analyzed for all processing steps:

(1) before the registration was carried out, i.e. applying a matching of the amount of tissue present in both images as well as a three-dimensional rigid alignment.

(2) after the buoyancy respectively gravity simulation was carried out.

(3) using the final registered state after applying the buoyancy respectively gravity simulation and the surface-refinement by the free form deformation.

The mean TRE before the registration was carried out (analysis 1) was $9.7\,mm$ (median: $7.2\,mm$, standard deviation SD: $7.3\,mm$) for strategy A and $9.9\,mm$ (median: $7.4\,mm$, standard deviation SD: $7.6\,mm$) for strategy B. The slight difference is due to the search for the closest point on the contrary modality.

When applying the buoyancy simulation in strategy A, the mean TRE reduces to $6.9\,mm$ (median: $6.5\,mm$, SD: $2.7\,mm$). In contrary the strategy B reduces the TRE to an average of $7.9\,mm$ (median: $5.9\,mm$, SD: $4.2\,mm$) when applying the gravity simulation.

After performing the additional surface-refinement by the free-form deformation, the average TRE for strategy A was $5.6\,mm$ (median: $5.6\,mm$, SD: $2.4\,mm$) and the average TRE for strategy B was $6.6\,mm$ (median: $5.6\,mm$, SD $4.0\,mm$).

Both registration strategies revealed similar registration accuracies. Compared to the simple alignment of datasets (analysis 1) the TRE is reduced by nearly factor 2 (analysis 3). Figures 3 and 4 show the registration results for the same patient for strategy A and strategy B respectively.

The parameter optimization resulted in similar average material stiffnesses for both registration strategies: the average E_{FAT} was $1792\,Pa$ (median: $2172\,Pa$, SD: $794\,Pa$) for strategy A and $1853\,Pa$ (median: $1200\,Pa$, SD: $1318\,Pa$) for strategy B.

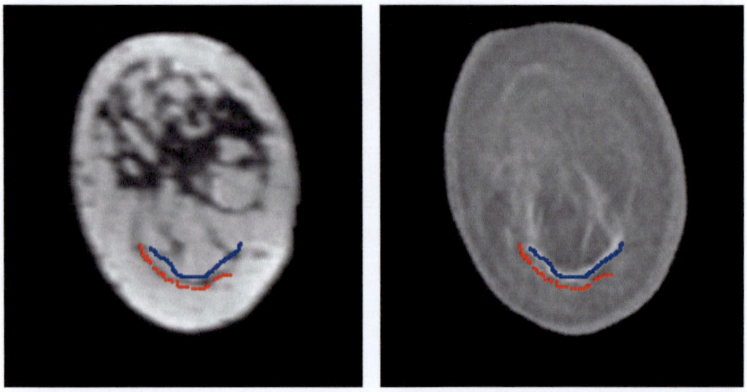

Figure 3: Result of the registration with strategy A. MRI (left) and USCT (right), each with markings of a connective tissue structure, which served as a basis for evaluation of the TRE. Blue denotes the surface points of the marking in USCT, red denotes the surface points of the marking in MRI. Note that both images show the same coronal slice from the 3D volumes.

4 Discussion and conclusion

Our proposed registration method is aimed at improving visual and quantitative comparison of tissue structures in USCT and MRI as it spatially correlates the images of both modalities automatically. We previously successfully developed, applied and evaluated a method for registration of MRI and USCT volumes which allows to delineate corresponding tissue structures more easily [4]. In this paper we preliminarily evaluated two registration strategies: either simulating the buoyancy effect to deform the MRI or removing the buoyancy effect to deform the USCT.

Both strategies lead to similar results with respect to the TRE. The previous method (strategy A) results in a slightly lower average TRE when using only the biomechanical model simulation without the additional surface-refinement by the free-form deformation (analysis 2), however the median values are comparable, i.e. there is only one outlier which causes the increase in the average TRE. With both strategies the median TREs vary by max. $0.6mm$ in all analyzed processing steps. A limitation of the current study is the low number of datasets, which limits the analysis of statistical significance of the results. Furthermore the experiments were carried out with simplified homogeneous biomechanical models, which do not distinguish between different types of tissue within the breast. In a future analysis we are planning to test more sophisticated models, e.g. similar to *Cotic Smole et al.* [13] for strategy A or similar to *Hopp et al.* [14] for strategy B.

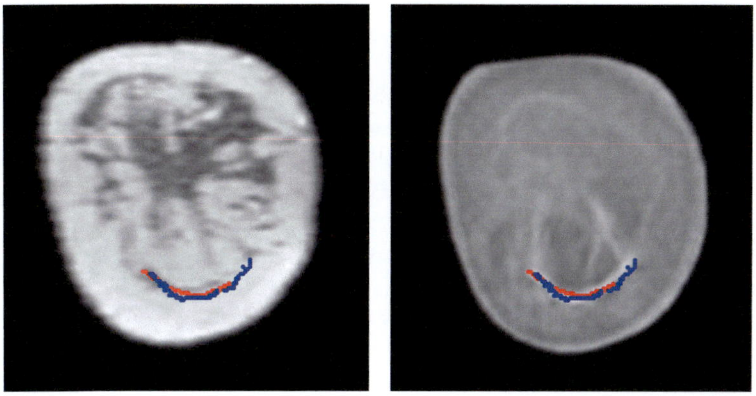

Figure 4: Result of the registration with strategy B. MRI (left) and USCT (right), each with markings of a connective tissue structure, which served as a basis for evaluation of the TRE. Blue denotes the surface points of the marking in USCT, red denotes the surface points of the marking in MRI. Note that both images show the same coronal slice from the 3D volumes.

While both strategies perform approximately equal with respect to their accuracy we assume less computational demand for strategy B as the forward problem of applying gravity to an unloaded configuration of the breast needs to be carried out only once, while for the inverse problem an iterative procedure with multiple applications of the forward problem is usually the method of choice. In the previous and present work we overcome the majority of the additional computational burden of the inverse problem by applying the iterative procedure only once with the optimal parameters. Yet, the optimization might result in even better parameters if also the iterative procedure is applied in each optimization step. For strategy B a similar trade-off was not necessary. Further analysis in future will test these hypotheses. Furthermore the strategy B could easily be extended by further boundary conditions, e.g. by modeling the MRI breast coils to cope for additional deformations when the breast is in contact with them.

In conclusion, we have developed the initial methods to compare two registration strategies in order to estimate the spatial correspondence between MRI and USCT and presented the preliminary results. The spatial correspondence allows to delineate corresponding tissue structures in both modalities in the same or nearby slices (Figures 3 and 4). It therefore can serve as a major tool for further analysis of USCT images, e.g. for human reader studies, quantitative analysis of sound speed and attenuation parameters similar to *Hopp et al.*[14] and for the development of computer aided detection (CADe) tools using classification of tissue types based on extracted image parameters.

References

[1] N. Duric, P. Littrup, P. Chandiwala-Mody, C. Li, S. Schmidt, L. Myc, O. Rama, L. Bey-Knight, J. Lupinacci, B. Ranger, A. Szczepanski, E. West: In-vivo imaging results with ultrasound tomography: Report on an ongoing study at the Karmanos Cancer Institute. Proc. SPIE Medical Imaging 7629 (2010), 76290M

[2] J. Wiskin, D. Borup, S. Johnson, M. Berggren, D. Robinson, J. Smith, J. Chen, Y. Parisky, J. Klock: Inverse Scattering and Refraction Corrected Reflection for Breast Cancer Imaging Proc. SPIE Medical Imaging 7629 (2010) 76290K

[3] N. Ruiter, M. Zapf, R. Dapp, T. Hopp, W. Kaiser, H. Gemmeke: First Results of Clinical Study with 3D Ultrasound Computer Tomography. Proc. IEEE Ultrasonics Symposium (2013), 651654

[4] T. Hopp, R. Dapp, M. Zapf, E. Kretzek, H. Gemmeke, N.V. Ruiter: Registration of 3D Ultrasound Computer Tomography and MRI for evaluation of tissue correspondences, Proc. SPIE Medical Imaging 9419 (2015), 941925

[5] T. Carter, C. Tanner, N. Beechey-Newman, D. Barratt, D. Hawkes: MR Navigated Breast Surgery: Method and Initial Clinical Experience. Medical Image Computing and Computer-Assisted Intervention MICCAI 2008, 5242 (2008) 356363.

[6] J.C. Bezdek: Pattern Recognition with Fuzzy Objective Function Algorithms. Norwell, MA, USA: Kluwer Academic Publishers (1981).

[7] T. Hopp, M. Zapf, N.V. Ruiter: Segmentation of 3D Ultrasound Computer Tomography Reflection Images using Edge Detection and Surface Fitting, Proc. SPIE Medical Imaging 9040 (2014), 904066

[8] Q. Fang, D.A. Boas: Tetrahedral mesh generation from volumetric binary and grayscale images. IEEE International Symposium on Biomedical Imaging: From Nano to Macro (2009) 11421145.

[9] A. F. Bower, Applied Mechanics of Solids. Taylor and Francis (2011)

[10] Dassault Systemes Simulia Corp.: ABAQUS Analysis User's Manual (2014)

[11] A.P. Cooper: On the anatomy of the breast. Longman, London (1840)

[12] A. Myronenko, A. Song: Intensity-based image registration by minimizing residual complexity, IEEE Transactions on Medical Imaging 29(11) (2010), 18821891

[13] P. Cotic Smole, C. Kaiser, J. Krammer, N.V. Ruiter, T. Hopp: A comparison of biomechanical models for MRI to digital breast tomosynthesis 3D registration. Proceedings MICCAI Workshop on Computational Biomechanics for Medicine XII (in press).

[14] T. Hopp, N. Duric, N.V. Ruiter: Image fusion of Ultrasound Computer Tomography volumes with X-ray mammograms using a biomechanical model based 2D/3D registration. Computerized Medical Imaging and Graphics 40 (2015), 170-181

Measurement of the speed of sound, attenuation and mass density of fresh breast tissue

L. Keijzer[1]*, M. Lagendijk[2]*, N. Stigter[1], C.H.M. van Deurzen[3], C. Verhoef[2], W. van Lankeren[4], L.B.Koppert[2], K.W.A. van Dongen[1]

Both authors contributed equally to the manuscript.

[1] *Department of Imaging Physics, Laboratory of Acoustical Wavefield Imaging, Delft University of Technology, Delft, the Netherlands*

[2] *Department of Surgical Oncology, Erasmus MC, Rotterdam, the Netherlands*

[3] *Department of pathology, Erasmus MC, Rotterdam, the Netherlands*

[4] *Department of Radiology, Erasmus MC, Rotterdam, the Netherlands*

Abstract

An improved distinction between benign or malignant lesions in breast ultrasonography is needed to enhance diagnostic accuracy. This can be achieved when acoustic characterization of different tissues within the breast is improved. To measure the speed of sound, attenuation and mass density of breast tissue, two experimental methods are developed and evaluated. The first uses pulse-echo measurements to simultaneously measure the speed of sound and frequency dependent attenuation; the second uses a pycnometer to measure the mass density. To overcome problems associated with positioning the samples during the pulse-echo measurements, a novel sample holder using a vacuum pump is developed. For fresh samples of fat, skin, glandular tissue and nipple, the following average values are found for the speed of sound 1456±23 m/s, 1559±27 m/s, 1564±18 m/s and 1574±7 m/s; for the frequency dependent attenuation 5.7±1.1 Np/m $MHz^{-1.3\pm0.2}$, 4.8±1.1 Np/m $MHz^{-1.7\pm0.2}$, 10.5±0.8 Np/m $MHz^{-1.5\pm0.06}$ and 4.6±2.3 Np/m $MHz^{-2.0\pm0.05}$; and for the mass density 869±25 kg/m^3, 970±4 kg/m^3, 874±58 kg/m^3, 987±9 kg/m^3, respectively. Significant differences are observed when comparing these results with those in literature. It is proposed that these are caused by variances in applied measurement method. Factors such as sample preparation, sample holder and choice of background medium contribute to the observed variances. In addition, it is shown that the sample size influences the observed mass density.

Keywords: Acoustic medium parameters, fresh breast tissue

1 Introduction

1.1 Breast ultrasonography and acoustic medium parameters

Breast ultrasonography is a commonly applied diagnostic modality, used to evaluate patients who experience breast symptoms. Ultrasonography has the advantages that it is pain free, non-ionising and real-time. It is also sensitive in dense breast(s). As a result, the interest for breast ultrasonography is ongoing (1, 2). An improved distinction between benign and malignant lesions is necessary to enhance the diagnostic accuracy of breast ultrasonography. The possible need for additionaly performed invasive cytological or histopathological evaluation may then be diminished.

An improved distinction is obtained when a better quantitative characterization of the different tissues within the breast is achieved. This requires accurate knowledge about the values of the acoustic medium parameters. This knowledge also aids in the design of new ultrasound imaging modalities and the development of new imaging methods that are typically tested on simulated data. Consequently, reliable knowledge of acoustic medium parameters such as speed of sound, attenuation and mass density for different tissue types will help to optimize and to make more efficient use of ultrasonic imaging techniques (3). Unfortunately, as will be shown next, current data on values of acoustic medium parameters for breast tissue is inconsistent due to large variations in applied measurement protocols.

1.2 Literature-based measurement protocols and acoustic medium parameters

1.2.1 Speed of sound and attenuation

Many protocols are described in literature for the measurement of speed of sound and attenuation. Some protocols described in vivo measurements, using the complete breast (2, 4-6). A shortcoming than is that only average values for the complete breast can be computed since the wave travels through the breast and passes through multiple tissue types of unknown thickness. This drawback also holds for some results obtained from ex vivo measurements using a whole breast (7, 8).

Two methods are used for ex vivo measurements on breast tissues; pulse-echo and through-transmission. Both methods have been used in different studies (see Supplementary, Table S1). An advantage of pulse-echo over the through-transmission is that the wave propagates through the samples twice, making small variations in tissue properties more distinguishable. This makes it feasible to use relatively thin samples, which have the advantage that it is valid to assume that the waves only propagate through one type of tissue. While some authors measured only average values (9-11), others made an entire scan of the sample (12, 13). An advantage of the latter is that spatial variations within a sample can be investigated.

Differences are also found in the fixation of ex vivo tissue. This fixation is essential as samples otherwise float. Samples are for example; I) pinched between the branches of a clamp (9), II) enclosed in a certain shape (10-15), III) mounted with wires (16) or IV) pinned on a layer of paraffin (7). Considering fresh breast tissue and the inherent difficulty to cut thin slices with planar surfaces, important limitations are found for compressing the tissue. The difficulty of cutting planar surfaces results in thickness variations and surface irregularities. A sample holder, which covers the complete surface, will compress the sample differently along its surface and thus affects the outcome. Leydier et al (17) stated that uncertainties in sample thickness have led to inaccurate values for the speed of sound in biological tissues. For example, Foster et al. (12) used an average sample thickness when scanning sample slices, while Leydier et al (17) proposed the use of two coupling fluids as a solution. The latter approach seems less suitable, as during scanning small shifts in the alignment of the sample in the fluids can occur, making the measurements meaningless.

1.2.2 Sample preparation

Sample conditions listed in literature often deviate strongly from in vivo conditions. First, for several experiments tissues were initially frozen or fixed which eases the slicing process (12, 13, 15). Second, measurements were often performed at a temperature other than 37°C (4, 7, 8). Bamber (3) showed that temperature influences the attenuation values in breast tissues; an increase in temperature led to an increase in attenuation for parenchyma and fat, and a decrease for carcinoma. Additionally, the speed of sound in carcinoma and parenchyma increased with temperature, while the sound speed in fatty tissue decreased. Bamber and Hill (18) described the effects of temperature variances on the attenuation coefficients and showed that these effects were different in fresh versus fixed tissues. Therefore, to adequately mimic in vivo conditions, it can be stated that it is important to perform the measurements at 37°C. Third, a wide time span between tissue excision and ex vivo measurements was observed in several studies (3, 4, 7, 8, 15, 19). Foster et al. (12) did not find any effect with respect to the length of the time interval between mastectomy and the measurements on the sound speed and attenuation. However, for this study frozen instead of fresh samples were used. Based on these findings, Edmonds et al. (11) and Weiwad et al. (9) were most successful in adequately mimicking in vivo conditions.

Additional differences are found for the liquids used to submerge the samples in. For example, a (buffered) formalin solution (11) and (pure, distilled and / or degassed) water (9, 10, 12, 13, 16) was used by many authors. Although Kelly Fry et al. (7) stated that it is valid to use samples that are fixed in formalin, contrasting results were obtained by Bamber and Hill (18). They reported an increase of 10% in attenuation at 1 MHz and of 50% at 7 MHz for bovine tissues, and a small decrease in the speed of sound due to formalin fixation. Other studies have shown that formalin fixation affects the speed of sound in other tissues types and changes the acoustic properties of tissues due to a reduction of the lipid content (20).

1.2.3 Measuring mass density

Relatively few articles are found, without overlap in protocols, that refer to mass density measurements of breast tissues (19, 21, 22). Lipkin and Hardy (22) used the radiation method, which uses the interaction of gamma radiation with matter to measure mass densities via direct transmission or backscattering. Robinson et al (19) applied Archimedes' method, which is based on buoyancy forces. Another method based on buoyancy principles is the use of a density gradient column, in which floating samples reach a equilibrium position depending on their mass density. A last alternative is the use of a pycnometer; a glass container with a precisely defined volume. This method determines the density more accurately than the column-density gradient method for specimens with a volume of 0.12 ml or more (23).

Available data on values for speed of sound, attenuation and mass density of breast tissues is inconsistent. The inconsistence is caused by variances between samples and applied protocols (3). The latter is a direct consequence of the fact that, an up-to-date and well-defined standardized measurement protocol is missing. In particular, research studies have made different choices with respect to measurement methods, reference medium, sample storage and sample size. An overview of current data on acoustic medium parameters of fresh breast tissue is presented together with results using the proposed measurement methods.

2 Methods

2.1 Patients and samples

The study protocol was approved by the local ethics committee. Following informed consent, three patients scheduled for mastectomy, were included in the study. Freshly excised tissues were analysed directly after evaluation by the pathologist. Based on macroscopic evaluation of the specimens, slices were obtained for the evaluation of different breast tissues. Tissue types that were analysed are: skin, nipple, intra-glandular fat, glandular tissue and breast carcinoma. To lower the heterogeneity of samples, a sample thickness of approximately 5 mm was desired (if applicable). In vivo conditions were mimicked by measuring at 37°C.

2.2 Experimental measurement protocols

Based on the pros and cons of the different protocols, two methods are proposed. The first to measure the speed of sound and frequency dependent attenuation simultaneously and the second to measure the mass density.

2.2.1 Set up for measuring speed of sound and attenuation

An ultrasound macroscope, similar to the one designed by Foster et al. (12), was developed to measure speed of sound and frequency dependent attenuation. In this macroscope, small samples are scanned in two directions by a single transducer (V309-SU-F1.5, Olympus, Antwerp, Belgium) that operates simultaneously as a source and a receiver. The spherically focused transducer has a centre frequency of 5 MHz and a focal length of 38 mm. A sketch of the set-up is shown in Figure 1.The transducer is connected to a square wave pulser and receiver (Panametrics-NDT 5077PR, Olympus NDT), which is read out using an oscilloscope (Agilent DSO 7054A, Keysight Technologies). The position of the transducer is controlled using a XY-Raster Scanner (SMH42600 motors and Compax3 controllers, Parker Automation). Compared to the set-up used by Foster et al (12), two important adjustments are made to better mimic in vivo conditions. First, the membrane used to prevent the specimen from floating (through pressing the specimen on the reflector plate) is replaced by a pumping system. The pumping system includes a pump (Eheim 1048-219 pump, EHEIM GmbH & Co KG, Deizisau, Germany) connected to a copper box with small holes in the top. Due to a small under pressure in the box, water flows downwards through these holes, positioning the samples in a stable flat way on the top of the box, which acts as a reflector plate. An advantage of this novelty is that the sample thickness can be obtained at each grid point separately without compressing the tissue. A second difference is that a physiological-phosphate-buffered saline (PBS) solution of 37°C was used to prevent absorbing effects.

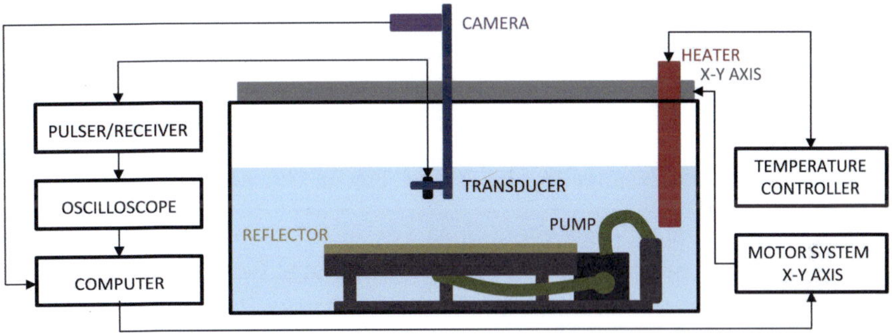

Figure 1: Schematic overview of the experimental set-up used to measure the speed of sound and frequency dependent attenuation in samples of breast tissue.

All data analysis has been executed by using MATLAB (version R2016a). To determine the speed of sound at each raster point (x,y), the travel time $t_2(x,y)$ of the wave propagating through the sample at a raster point is compared with the travel time $t_0(x,y)$ of a reference measurement made in absence of a sample at that same raster point, see Figure 2. This corrects for any irregularities or misalignments of the reflector plate. The thickness of the sample is computed at each point by comparing the travel time $t_1(x,y)$ of the wave reflecting on top of the sample, with the travel time $t_0(x,y)$ of the reference measurement. The frequency dependent attenuation is computed by comparing the Fourier spectrum A(x,y,f) of the wave propagating through the sample, with the spectrum $A_0(x,y,f)$ of a reference measurement. There are three effects that could be taken into account. Firstly, for acquisitions with the sample in place, each transmitted signal will interact with the interface between the background medium and the sample twice. These interactions are not present in the reference measurements. Secondly, the reflection coefficients $R_0(x,y)$ and $R_2(x,y)$ at the interfaces of the metal reflector plate in absence and in presence of the sample are not identical. Thirdly, the reflection and transmission coefficients of lossy media such as breast tissue are frequency dependent. The models tested in this work are categorized as follows: 1) all the effects caused by passing interfaces between media are neglected; 2) all amplitude and frequency dependent effects are included. A disadvantage of model 2) is that it requires accurate knowledge about the medium parameters of the background medium, sample and reflector. Moreover, small errors in these parameters may potentially lead to higher uncertainties.

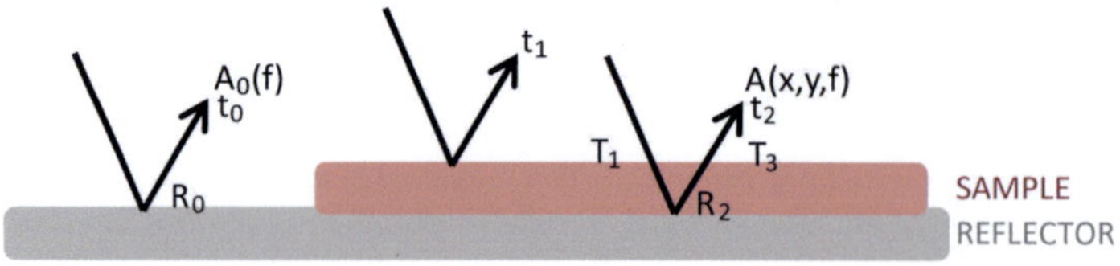

Figure 2: Overview of the travel times (t0, t1, t2) needed to compute the sample thickness and the speed of sound, of the different reflection (R0, R2) and transmission (T1, T3) coefficients and of the Fourier spectra (A, A0) used to compute the frequency dependent attenuation in samples of breast tissue.

2.2.2 Set-up for measuring mass density

The pycnometer (2.170 ml, Witeg Labortechnik GmbH, Germany) is found to be the most suitable tool to measure the mass density, since this method is suitable for small samples and expected to be more accurate than methods based on buoyancy principles. To evaluate the effect of storing the sample, the mass density was obtained for fresh samples, samples submerged in PBS for 24 hours, samples stored in the refrigerator for 24 hours and for samples that have been submerged in formalin for 24 hours. Of the samples submerged in PBS, mass density was assessed prior to the submersion of the samples. To investigate the short-term effect of submerging fat samples, the density of four different fat samples is measured after submerging the sample for 0, 30, 40 or 50 minutes in PBS.

3 Results

3.1 Patients and samples

Two patients in the study underwent a bilateral mastectomy for an invasive breast carcinoma Due to a high familial risk of breast cancer both breast were removed. The first two patients, aged 47 and 51 years, both had an invasive ductal carcinoma of <0.5 cm and were therefore excluded for analysis of the tumour tissue. The third patient was 81 years of age and had a unilateral mastectomy for an invasive ductal carcinoma of the breast of 2.1 cm.

3.2 Acoustic medium parameters

3.2.1 Speed of sound

Individual measurements of the speed of sound and their average values are shown in Figure 3. These values are compared with literature values in Figure 4. Samples of the left and right breasts of three women are included (Supplementary file, Table S2).

3.2.2 Frequency dependent attenuation

An overview of the results for the frequency dependent attenuation for fat, skin, glandular tissue and nipple, respectively, after using Model 1 and 2 is shown in Figure 5 and Table 1. To enable a comparison between the two models, only those samples on which both models are applied, were used to calculate the average values.

Higher (average) values are found for Model 2 compared to Model 1 for all types of breast tissue. Model 2 shows most attenuation for glandular tissue, followed by skin, nipple and fat. The same order is found with Model 1, except from the curve corresponding to nipple, who shows the highest attenuation at frequencies above 5 MHz.

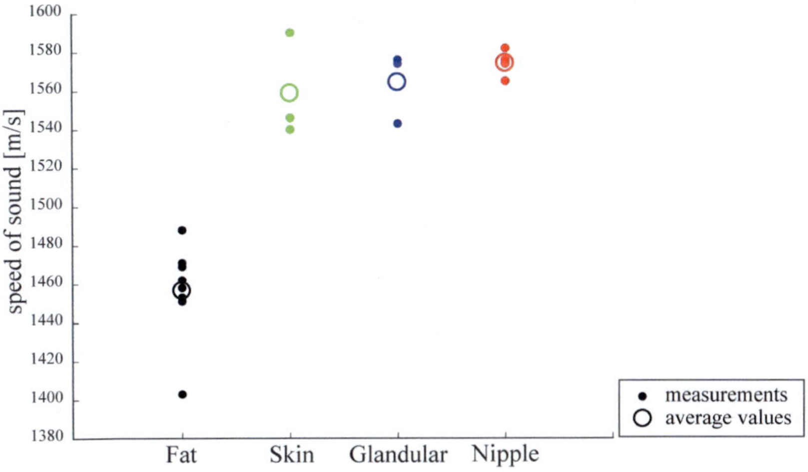

Figure 3: Overview of the results of the speed of sound and their average values. Fresh samples of fat, skin, glandular tissue and nipple from left and right breast from three women are included.

3.2.3 Density of mass

An overview of the mass density as a function of sample mass for different tissues is displayed in Figure 6. The samples originated from three women. Average values of 869±25 kg/m³, 970±4 kg/m³, 874±58 kg/m³, 987±9 kg/m³ are found for the mass density of fresh samples of fat, skin, glandular tissue and nipple respectively. Higher density values are found when using larger samples. The dotted lines in Figure 6 connect identical tissue samples that are measured twice; before and after being submerged in PBS. For these samples an increase in density is observed. On the contrary, the figure shows similar values for fresh samples as for samples cooled for 24 hours in the refrigerator or submerged for 24 hours in formalin.

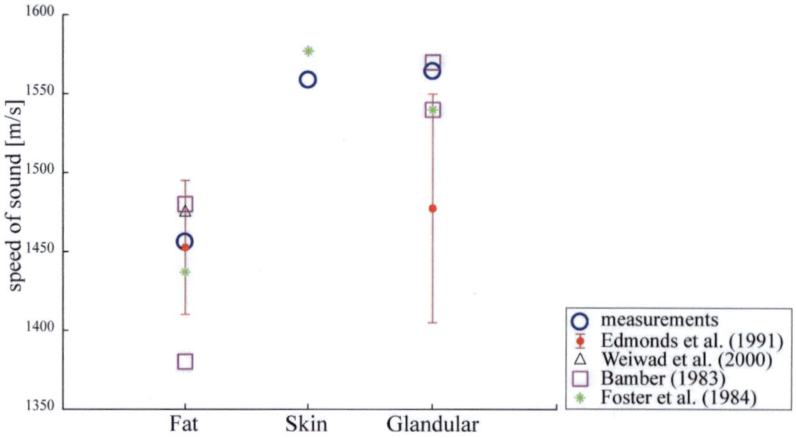

Figure 4: Comparison of the average values measured for the speed of sound in fat, skin and glandular tissue with literature values.

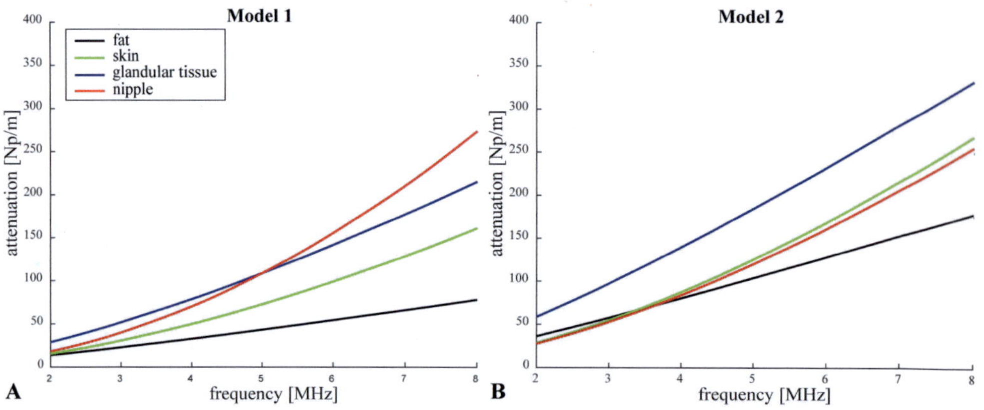

Figure 5: Average values found for the frequency dependent attenuation in fresh samples of fat, skin, glandular tissue and nipple after using Model 1 (Figure 5a) and Model 2 (Figure 5b).

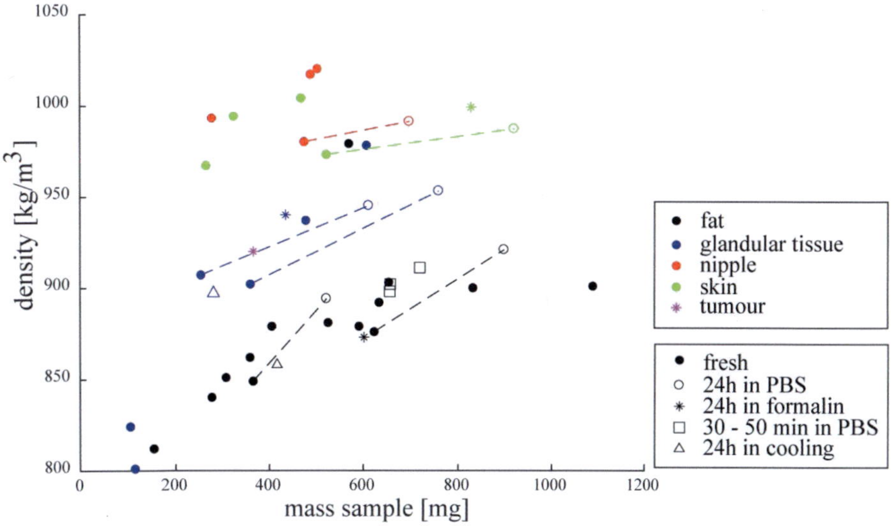

Figure 6: Mass density as a function of sample mass for fat, glandular tissue, nipple, skin and tumour.The overview also shows the effect of submerging the samples in PBS or formalin and of cooling the samples in a refrigerator. The dotted line connects identical samples which are measured twice; fresh and after 24 hours.

4 Discussion

Results are obtained for the speed of sound, frequency dependent attenuation and mass density for different types of fresh breast tissues. For the frequency dependent attenuation, large variations are found in the obtained results. Also variations are found in the measurements of the speed of sound and mass density. The latter is found to be strongly affected by the mass of the sample. The results show that the measurement protocols influence the obtained values for the acoustic medium parameters.

Measurements of the attenuation coefficients show large differences in the results by applying different computational models. For example, for fat the obtained average values are 5.7±1.1 Np/m $MHz^{-1.3\pm0.2}$ and 16.3±3.8 Np/m $MHz^{-1.2\pm0.04}$ for Model 1 and 2 respectively. This is consistent with the large variations found between the results presented in literature; D'Astous and Foster (13) found for the attenuation in fat 1.82±0.3 Np/m $MHz^{-1.7}$ while Edmonds et al. (11) measured 23.0±5.5 Np/m MHz^{-1}. Theoretically Model 2 is more accurate than Model 1, as it takes into account some frequency dependency effects. However, our results suggest that the error caused by using incorrect values for the reflection and transmission coefficients (partly explained by surface irregularities of fresh samples) is larger than the errors induced when neglecting these frequency dependent effects as is done with Model 1. Consequently, Model 1 is recommended for future studies.

These applied approximations may also have affected the reconstructed speed of sound, as any phase shift occurring at the interfaces is currently not taken into account when computing the speed of sound of the tissue. Fortunately, the effect of these phase shifts may be negligible. This is supported by the observation that differences with literature values are smaller for the speed of sound than for the attenuation coefficients. However large variations in acoustic values are possibly explained by variations in the applied measurement methods, the applied approximations or variances between individuals.

There are difficulties when using fresh breast tissue. Due to the weak structure of fresh breast tissue, it is difficult to obtain single-tissue samples with planar smooth surfaces. It is important that the sample slices are cut thin to avoid the intermingling of different types of tissue. Conversely, the slices should have a minimum thickness in the order of five to ten wavelengths corresponding to the centre frequency of the probing signal. This is needed to get sufficient response and to enable the discrimination between the wave reflecting from the water-tissue interface and the wave reflecting at the tissue-plate interface. One may freeze or fix the samples to ease the cutting process. However, it is expected that this will affect the sample quality and lead to erroneous results, and should therefore be avoided. In general, the difficulty of cutting tissue with planar surfaces leads to unavoidable thickness variations and surface irregularities. These should be taken into account in the error considerations.

Difficulties are also present in the positioning of the tissue since samples tend to float. The use of a sample holder is not an ideal option as the inherent surface irregularities will lead to a spatially varying compression of the sample. Additionally, further interfaces become present in the sample and reference measurements. These interfaces are neglected by both Mc Daniel (15) and D'Astous and Foster (13). As an alternative method, a pumping system was used to hold the samples in place. The speed of sound and attenuation values should be computed at each location of the sample to account for thickness variations. It is noted that the pumping system should be strong enough to prevent the tissues from floating, but weak enough to avoid strong currents near the sample that could disturb the measurements.

4.1 Mass density

The average values found for the mass density are low compared to literature values. In addition, these values are not distinct enough to be discriminative for the different tissue types. For all breast tissue samples a higher density is obtained when measuring larger samples, while in theory the sample size should not have any effect. For fat and glandular tissue this effect is found to be larger than for nipple and skin.

A PBS solution was chosen to minimize absorbing effects. However, measurements done, but not shown, with fat samples that were submerged in PBS for 0, 30, 40 and 50 minutes, indicate that the weight and the measured density increase with submersion time. The increase in density can be explained by difference in osmolarity between fat and PBS. The measured effects are smaller for skin and nipple than for glandular tissue and fat.

Comparable values to the fresh tissue values were observed for the samples stored in the refrigerator for 24 hours and those submerged in formalin for 24 hours. It is therefore hypothesized that temperature effects are negligible and that it takes longer than 24 hours before tissue imbibes formalin. However, since the samples used to test the effects of cooling and the use of formalin, were not measured beforehand, we cannot draw these conclusion with absolute certainty.

The results suggest that formalin can be a suitable alternative. However as stated above, previous studies performed by Bamber and Hill (11, 18) found an effect of formalin fixation on the measured medium parameters. Also with the use of distilled, degassed or pure water differences in osmolarity occur and therefore still absorbing effects are expected. Since samples are submerged for a longer period of time when measuring the speed of sound and attenuation, than when measuring mass density, absorbing effects disturbing these measurements are expected to be larger. It is thus necessary to search for an alternative solution.

5 Conclusions

For fresh samples of fat, skin, glandular tissue and nipple, the applied protocols reveal the following average values for the speed of sound 1456±23 m/s, 1559±27 m/s, 1564±18 m/s and 1574±7 m/s; for the frequency dependent attenuation 5.7±1.1 Np/m $MHz^{-1.3\pm0.2}$, 4.8±1.1 Np/m $MHz^{-1.7\pm0.2}$, 10.5±0.8 Np/m $MHz^{-1.5\pm0.06}$ and 4.6±2.3 Np/m $MHz^{-2.0\pm0.05}$; and for the mass density 869±25 kg/m^3, 970±4 kg/m^3, 874±58 kg/m^3, 987±9 kg/m^3. The literature review and the obtained results show that measurement protocols strongly affect the results for the acoustic parameters. It is concluded that further work is required to verify these values. To accurately measure the acoustic medium parameters, it is recommended; 1) to mimic in vivo conditions by using only fresh samples and perform the measurements at 37°C, 2) to avoid using a sample holder that deform the samples, 3) to minimize the submersion time for samples in order to reduce absorption effects, 4) to measure sample properties at each sample location separately and 5) to achieve consistent sample thickness and regularity in the slicing process. The results suggest that PBS is not suitable as a reference medium and that formalin may represent a good alternative.

References

[1] Ozmen N, Dapp R, Zapf M, Gemmeke H, Ruiter NV, van Dongen KWA. Comparing different ultrasound imaging methods for breast cancer detection. Ultrasonics, Ferroelectrics, and Frequency Control, IEEE Transactions on. 2015;62(4):637-46.

[2] Glover GH. Computerized time-of flight ultrasonic tomography for breast examination. Ultrasound Med Biol. 1977;3(2-3):117-27.

[3] Bamber JC. Ultrasonic Propagation Properties of the Breast. Ultrasonic examination of the Breast. 1983:37-44.

[4] Kossoff G, Fry EK, Jellins J. Average velocity of ultrasound in the human female breast. J Acoust Soc Am. 1973;53(6):1730-6.

[5] Katz-Hanani I, Rothstein T, Gaitini D, Gallimidi Z, Azhari H. Age-related ultrasonic properties of breast tissue in vivo. Ultrasound Med Biol. 2014;40(9):2265-71.

[6] Chang CH, Huang SW, Yang HC, Chou YH, Li PC. Reconstruction of ultrasonic sound velocity and attenuation coefficient using linear arrays: clinical assessment. Ultrasound Med Biol. 2007;33(11):1681-7.

[7] Kelly Fry E, Sanghvi NT, Frey FJ. Frequency dependent attenuation of malignant breast tumors studied by the fast fourier transform technique. Ultrasonic Tissue Characterization II. 1979:85-91.

[8] Greenleaf JF, Johnson SA, Bahn RC, editors. Quantitative Cross-Sectional Imaging of Ultrasound Parameters. Ultrasonics Symposium, 1977; 1977 1977.

[9] Weiwad W, Heinig A, Goetz L, Hartmann H, Lampe D, Buchmann J, et al. Direct measurement of sound velocity in various specimens of breast tissue. Invest Radiol. 2000;35(12):721-6.

[10] Landini L, Sarnelli R, Squartini F. Frequency-dependent attenuation in breast tissue characterization. Ultrasound Med Biol. 1985;11(4):599-603.

[11] Edmonds PD, Mortensen CL, Hill JR, Holland SK, Jensen JF, Schattner P, et al. Ultrasound tissue characterization of breast biopsy specimens. Ultrason Imaging. 1991;13(2):162-85.

[12] Foster FS, Strban M, Austin G. The Ultrasound Macroscope: Initial Studies of Breast Tissue. Ultrason Imaging. 1984;6(3):243-61.

[13] D'Astous FT, Foster FS. Frequency dependence of ultrasound attenuation and backscatter in breast tissue. Ultrasound Med Biol. 1986;12(10):795-808.

[14] Foster FS, Hunt JW. Transmission of ultrasound beams through human tissue--focusing and attenuation studies. Ultrasound Med Biol. 1979;5(3):257-68.

[15] McDaniel. Ultrasonic attenuation measurements on excised breast carcinoma at frequencies from 6 to 10 MHz. Ultrasonic Symposium Proceedings, IEEE. 1977;cat.377CH1264-1SU:234-6.

[16] Calderon C, Vilkomerson D, Mezrich R, Etzold KF, Kingsley B, Haskin M. Differences in the attenuation of ultrasound by normal, benign, and malignant breast tissue. J Clin Ultrasound. 1976;4(4):249-54.

[17] Leydier A, Mathieu J, Despaux G. The two coupling fluids method for ultrasonic velocity measurement. Application to biological tissues. Measurement Science and Technology. 2009;20(9):095801.

[18] Bamber JC, Hill CR. Ultrasonic attenuation and propagation speed in mammalian tissues as a function of temperature. Ultrasound Med Biol. 1979;5(2):149-57.

[19] Robinson MP, Richardson MJ, Green JL, Preece AW. New materials for dielectric simulation of tissues. Phys Med Biol. 1991;36(12):1565-71.

[20] Brewin MP, Srodon PD, Greenwald SE, Birch MJ. Carotid atherosclerotic plaque characterisation by measurement of ultrasound sound speed in vitro at high frequency, 20 MHz. Ultrasonics. 2014;54(2):428-41.

[21] Johns PC, Yaffe MJ. X-ray characterisation of normal and neoplastic breast tissues. Phys Med Biol. 1987;32(6):675-95.

[22] Lipkin M, Hardy JD. Measurement of some thermal properties of human tissues. J Appl Physiol. 1954;7(2):212-7.

[23] DiResta GR, Lee J, Lau N, Ali F, Galicich JH, Arbit E. Measurement of brain tissue density using pycnometry. Acta Neurochir Suppl (Wien). 1990;51:34-6.

Supplementary

Article	Protocol	Samples	Tissue Type	Speed of Sound [m/s]
Edmonds, Mortensen (12)	P.T., acoustoelectric transducer used to prevent phase cancellations, 3 – 8 MHz, 37 °C, tank with formalin, speed of sound measurements after attenuation measurements	Fresh biopsy specimens, manipulated in 37 °C buffered formalin to expel air, positioned in sample holder, thickness defined by chosen spacer of sample holder	Benign tissue	1430 - 1605[(a)]
			Fat	1410 - 1495[(a)]
			Fatty parenchyma	1405 - 1550[(a)]
			Fibrodenoma	1565 - 1600[(a)]
			Malignant tissue	1470 - 1605[(a)]
			Normal tissue	1405 - 1550[(a)]
Weiwad, Heinig (10)	P.T., room temperature, pure/distilled water	Freshly excised tissues, 30 minutes after excision, sample cut in blocks of 0.5 x 1 x 1.5 cm, samples between branches of a clamp	Carcinoma	1527.4 ± 11.1
			Benign changes or glandular/fibrous tissue	1526.8 ± 9.7
			Benign changes, hyperplastic or proliferative	1527.5 ± 12.6
			Benign changes, predominantly fibrous no proliferative	1526.4 ± 7.5
			Fatty tissue	1475.0 ± 6.1
			Fibroadenoma	1531.6 ± 3.6
			Compound tissue	1504.3 ± 9.7
			Phylloides tumour	1526.2
			Inflammation	1521.5
Bamber (4)	P.E., 10 MHz, 20 or 37 °C	Excised, >60 years, entire breast cooled to 4 °C for 2 hours, sliced with thickness of 7 mm, stored in saline at 4 °C for 14 – 18 hours to remove air bubbles	Carcinoma	1535 (20 °C)[(b)], 1625 (37 °C)[(b)]
			Fat	1480 (20 °C)[(b)], 1380 (37 °C)[(b)]
			Parenchyma	1540 (20 °C)[(b)], 1570 (37 °C)[(b)]
Foster, Strban (13)	P.E., scan of sample 13 MHz, 37 °C, tank with distilled and degassed water	Excised, frozen, sliced with rotary meat slicer, samples placed between Quartz mirror and Mylar membrane	Carcinoma	1572 ± 8
			Fat	1437 ± 13
			Parenchyma	1540 ± 20
			Skin	1577 ±18

Article	Protocol	Samples	Tissue Type	Attenuation [dB/cm]
Landini, Sarnelli (11)	P.T., S.A., 2 – 8 MHz, 21 °C, water	Fresh samples, moulded into a cylindrical shape	Normal and pathological	9 ± 7 cm^{-1} MHz^{-1} x 10^{-3}
			Malignant tumours with productive fibrosis	17 ± 7 cm^{-1} MHz^{-1} x 10^{-3}
			Abnormal fibrosis	32 ± 5 cm^{-1} MHz^{-1} x 10^{-3}
			Normal fibrofatty parenchyma and fibrocystic disease	57 ± 12 cm^{-1} MHz^{-1} x 10^{-3}
Edmonds, Mortensen (12)	P.T., S.A., AET instead of transducer to prevent phase cancellations,3 – 8 MHz, 37 °C, tank with formalin, straight-line fits	Fresh biopsy specimens, manipulated in 37 °C buffered formalin to expel air, positioned in sample holder, thickness defined by chosen spacer of sample holder	Normal	1.96 ± 0.43 dB cm^{-1} MHz^{-1}
			Fatty parenchyma	2.00 ± 0.48 dB cm^{-1} MHz^{-1}
			Fat	2.00 ± 0.65 dB cm^{-1} MHz^{-1}
			Benign tumour	2.22 ± 0.68 dB cm^{-1} MHz^{-1}
			Malignant tumour	2.42 ± 0.48 dB cm^{-1} MHz^{-1}
Bamber (4)	P.E., S.A., 10 MHz, 20 or 37 °C	Excised, >60 years, entire breast cooled to 4 °C for 2 hours, sliced with thickness of 7 mm, stored in saline at 4 °C for 14 – 18 hours to remove air bubbles	Carcinoma (37°C, 1 - 7 MHz) Carcinoma (20°C, 1 - 7 MHz)	2.3 dB cm^{-1} MHz^{-1} [(c)] 2.7 dB cm^{-1} MHz^{-1} [(c)]
			Fat (37°C, 2 - 7 MHz) Fat (20°C, 1 - 8 MHz)	2.2 dB cm^{-1} MHz^{-1} [(c)] 1.7 dB cm^{-1} MHz^{-1} [(c)]
			Parenchyma (37°C, 1 - 6 MHz) Parenchyma (20°C, 1 - 7 MHz)	4.3 dB cm^{-1} MHz^{-1} [(c)] 3.7 dB cm^{-1} MHz^{-1} [(c)]
Foster, Strban (13)	P.E., scan 13 MHz, 37 °C, tank with distilled and degassed water	Excised, frozen, sliced with rotary meat slicer, samples placed between Quartz mirror and Mylar membrane	Carcinoma	8 ± 2.8
			Fat	11 ± 3
			Parenchyma	23 ± 8.3
			Skin	53 ± 11
D'Astous and Foster (14)	P.E., S.A., scan of sample, 5 MHz, 37 °C, tank with distilled and degassed water	Excised, frozen, cut into blocks of 3 cm x 3 cm x 4 or 8 mm, samples placed between Quartz mirror and Mylar membrane	Ductal Carcinoma	0.570 ± 0.14 dB cm^{-1} MHz$^{-1.3}$
			Fat	0.158 ± 0.03 dB cm^{-1} MHz$^{-1.7}$
			Parenchyma	0.870 ± 0.29 dB cm^{-1} MHz$^{-1.5}$

Article	Protocol	Samples	Tissue Type	Density [kg/m³]
Johns and Yaffe (22)	Buoyancy method	Frozen, stored, thawed, attenuation measurements are executed, the sample is stored in PBS again and then the volume density of mass is measured	Fat	928
Robinson, Richardson (20)	Archimedes' method	63 year old female, excision biopsies for malignant disease, stored in small dry airtight containers at 4 °C and measured 20 - 24 hours after excision	Fat	934
Lipkin and Hardy (23)	Radiation method	Tissues are stored in closed vessels in an icebox and maintained moist by a film of water in the bottom of the vessel.	Fat	920

Table S1: Overview of different articles that measured the speed of sound, attenuation or mass density of breast tissues in-vitro with fresh samples. (a): Ranges are estimated from Figure 3, Figure 4 and Figure 6 of Edmonds et al.(12), (b): Values are estimated from Figure 4 of Bamber (4), (c): Slopes are roughly estimated from Figure 5 of Bamber (4), *S.A.= Spectrum analysis, P.E.: Pulse echo, P.T.= Pulse transmission

Tissue Type	Age	Speed of Sound [m/s]		Frequency Dependent Attenuation		
		Left Breast	Right Breast	Model 1[(a)]		Model 2[(b)]
				α	a_0 [Np/m]	α
Fat	47	1469 (u=3.4)	1458 (u=4.5)	L: 4.9 Np/m MHz$^{-1.30}$ R: 7.7 Np/m MHz$^{-1.00}$	0.65 0.83	L:13.4 Np/m MHz$^{-1.14}$ R:10.4 Np/m MHz$^{-1.22}$
Fat	47	1453 (u=2.2)	1488 (u=5.5)	L: 4.8 Np/m MHz$^{-1.00}$ R: 6.4 Np/m MHz$^{-1.39}$	0.65 0.55	L: 17.4 Np/m MHz$^{-1.13}$ R: 23 Np/m MHz$^{-1.14}$
Fat	47	1453 (u=2.0)	1471 (u=3.5)	L: 4.5 Np/m MHz$^{-1.47}$ R: 6.7 Np/m MHz$^{-1.19}$	0.67 0.62	L:14.4 Np/m MHz$^{-1.18}$ R:17 Np/m MHz$^{-1.17}$
Fat	47	1451 (u=2.7)	1462 (u=4.1)	L: 5.3 Np/m MHz$^{-1.37}$ R: 5.6 Np/m MHz$^{-1.32}$	0.59 0.61	L:15.5 Np/m MHz$^{-1.16}$ R:19 Np/m MHz$^{-1.08}$
Fat	81		1403 (u=21.4)	5.3 Np/m MHz$^{-1.25}$	0.50	
Fat (formalin 24 hours)	81		1448 (u=22.1)	6.8 Np/m MHz$^{-1.47}$	0.80	
Skin	47	1590 (u=3.6)	1540 (u=3.1)	L: 4.0 Np/m MHz$^{-1.84}$ R: 5.5 Np/m MHz$^{-1.55}$	1.03 0.89	L: 6.5 Np/m MHz$^{-1.77}$ R:12 Np/m MHz$^{-1.47}$

Skin	81		1546 (u=26.1)	17.5 Np/m $MHz^{-1.42}$	1.07	
Skin (formalin 24 hours)	81		1557 (u=31.6)	31.6 Np/m $MHz^{-1.13}$	0.90	
Skin (formalin 24 hours)	81		1546 (u=26.5)	11.5 Np/m $MHz^{-1.58}$	0.64	
Glandular Tissue	47	1576 (u=5.9)	1574 (u=2.4)	L: 9.9 Np/m $MHz^{-1.50}$ R:11 Np/m $MHz^{-1.41}$	0.66 0.88	L:35 Np/m $MHz^{-1.13}$ R:14 Np/m $MHz^{-1.38}$
Glandular Tissue	51	1543 (u=19.8)		16.1 Np/m $MHz^{-1.46}$	1.23	
Nipple	47	1576 (u=5.9)	1574 (u=2.4)	L:3.0 Np/m $MHz^{-2.00}$ R: 6.2 Np/m $MHz^{-1.93}$	0.5 1.07	L:11 Np/m $MHz^{-1.33}$ R: 7.0 Np/m $MHz^{-1.89}$
Nipple	51	1582 (u=4.8)		11.1 Np/m $MHz^{-1.50}$	0.81	
Nipple	81		1565 (u=5.4)	6.6 Np/m $MHz^{-1.97}$	1.24	

Tissue Type	Age	Mass Density [kg/m³]	
		Left Breast	Right Breast
Fat	47	879 (IL), 881 (SL), 862 (SM), 851 (SM), 879 (SM)	901 (IM), 879 (IL), 892 (SL), 900 (SM)
Fat	51	840, 812	
Fat	81		876, 849
Skin	51	967	
Skin	81		973
Glandular Tissue	47	937	978
Glandular Tissue	51	801, 824	
Glandular Tissue	81		902, 907
Nipple	51	993	
Nipple	81		980

Table S2: Overview of results obtained using proposed measurement set-ups. (a) The following equation is used for Model 1; |A(x,y,f)/(A_0 (x,y,f))|=a_0 e^(-2αl), with l the sample thickness in [m]. (b) The following equation is used for Model 2; |A(x,y,f)/(A_0 (x,y,f))|=|(T_1 (f)R_2 (f)T_3 (f))/R_0 |e^(-2αl). * IL: Inferolateral quadrant, SL: Superolateral quadrant, SM: Superomedial quadrant, IM: Inferomedial quadrant.

The USCT reference database

N.V. Ruiter[1], M. Zapf[1], T. Hopp[1], H. Gemmeke[1], K.W.A. van Dongen[2], J. Camacho[3], C. Fritsch[3], J.F. Cruza[3], J.L. Herraiz[4], M. Perez Liva[4], J.M. Udías[4]

[1] *Karlsruhe Institute of Technology, Karlsruhe, Germany; E-mail: nicole.ruiter@kit.edu*
[2] *Delft University of Technology, Delft, The Netherlands*
[3] *Spanish National Research Council, Madrid, Spain*
[4] *Complutense University Madrid, Madrid, Spain*

Abstract

Ultrasound Computer Tomography (USCT) is an emerging technology mostly aimed at breast cancer imaging. Following the idea of open science a USCT reference database is established with open and easy to use data and code interfaces. The aim is to promote and facilitate the exchange of available reconstruction algorithms and raw data sets from different USCT devices throughout the growing USCT community. Additionally, the feedback about data and system architecture of the scientists working on reconstruction methods will be published online to help to drive further development of the various measurement setups.

Keywords: USCT, reference database, open science, open access, open source

1 Introduction

The Ultrasound Computer Tomography (USCT) reference database aims on applying available image reconstruction algorithms on provided USCT data in order to establish intercommunication and standards for an open data interface. The raw RF data sets and software for data access are available via the USCT database web page and the linked data and code repositories [1]. The long term goal of this work is to build a free and open licensed reference database which is available for the whole community. We expect this to enable reproducible comparison of image reconstruction algorithms and USCT systems. In addition, we aim to establish user friendly and easy to use interfaces, standards and data formats between the different USCT systems and their reconstruction algorithms, software and data formats.

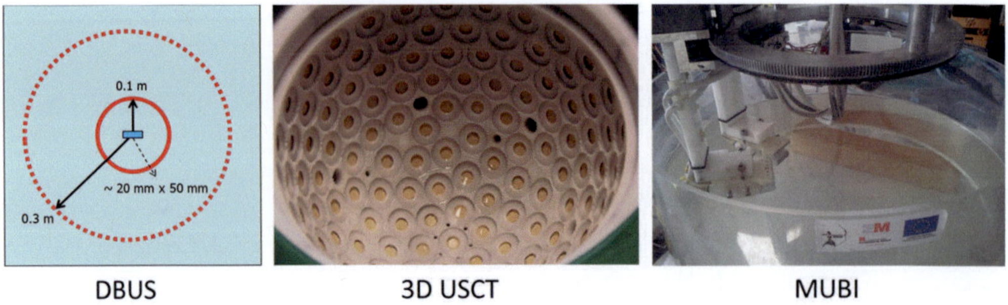

Figure 1: The three scanning systems of the USCT database; (left) Delft Breast Ultrasound Scanner (DBUS): 2D system, single transducers with 0.5 MHz center frequency, emitter radius 0.3 m and receiver radius 0.1 m; (center) 3D KIT USCT: 3D system, single transducers with 2.5 MHz center frequency, semi-elliptical aperture with 24 cm diameter and 17 cm height; (right) MUBI system: 2D system, two 3.5 MHz, 128 elements and 0.22 mm pitch arrays 95 mm radius, pulse-echo and through-transmission modes.

2 Reference database

Currently three systems with rather different transducer aperture and ultrasound frequency range provided raw data sets for the USCT database: Delft Breast Ultrasound Scanner (DBUS), KIT's 3D Ultrasound Computer Tomography system (3D USCT) [5] and Multimodal Ultrasound Breast Imaging System (MUBI) [6]. All data sets are provided with data access interface software. The source code is freely available and an issue tracker is provided at a Github repository. The materials of the USCT database are provided using a free and open license, i.e. the BSD 3-clause license for code and data, allowing free use and publication of results.

2.1 Delft Breast Ultrasound Scanner (DBUS)

The Delft Breast Ultrasound Scanner (DBUS) is depicted on the left-hand side of Figure 1. The system consists of a water tank with dimensions 0.75 m x 0.75 m x 0.65 m with a water level of 0.45 m. The temperature of the water is continuously monitored via thermocouples and kept constant within 1°C using heating mats and a temperature controller. On top of the system, two rotary stages (LG Motion LGR1090-PD), controlled by motor drivers (Parker), are mounted. The first rotary stage rotates the object, the second the receiver (0.5 MHz, Panametrics V318). The source, which is identical to the receiver, is mounted at a fixed position in the corner of the tank.

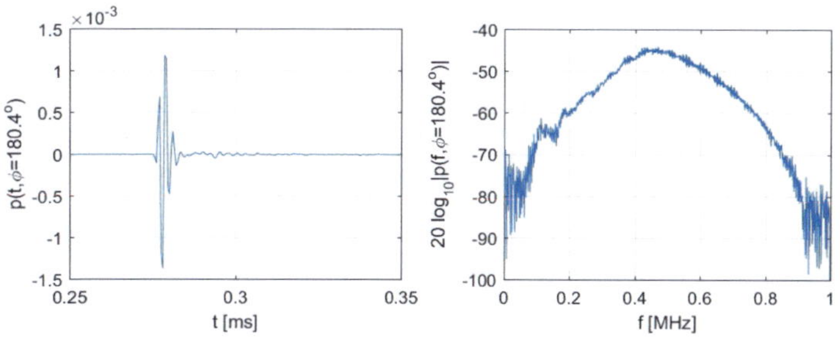

Figure 2: The RF data measured with the DBUS system in absence of an object; single A-scan in time (left) and frequency domain (right).

In this way a 2D tomographic scan of the object is obtained. For each A-scan, an electric pulse with a center frequency of approx. 0.5 MHz is generated by an arbitrary wave form generator (Agilent 33250A), amplified (Electronics and Innovation 210L 40 dB), and successively damped using a variable attenuator (JFW Industries, 50BR-036). The resulting wave field is measured using an identical transducer connected to a 14 bit A/D converter (Spectrum M3i.4142-exp - PCI) which is set to a sample rate of 400 MHz. For each A-scan, in addition to the raw (unfiltered) RF data, information such as temperature, source and receiver positions, etc. is stored. Together with a scan including an object, a scan in absence of an object, referred to as an empty scan, is made for reference. Figure 2 shows an example A-scan, presented in time and frequency domain, corresponding to a measurement with the source and receiver facing each other.

Two data sets are provided by the TU Delft. The first data set is made in absence of an object and can be used as reference measurement. It covers one source and 450 receiver positions equally distributed over 360°. The second data set is an agar based phantom with dimensions of 20 mm x 50 mm, and covers 45 source and 450 receiver positions, all equally distributed over 360°. The tissue mimicking phantom has a volume density of mass of approx. 1004 kg/m^3 and a speed of sound of approx. 1479 m/s. However, care has to be taken with these values as the conditions under which these values have been obtained may deviate from the actual scanning conditions. The three inclusions were generated by embedding drinking straws in the agar based phantom during curing. Prior to scanning the object, the straws were removed and the inclusions were filled with water.

2.2 KIT's 3D Ultrasound Computer Tomography system (3D USCT)

The KIT's 3D Ultrasound Computer Tomography system (3D USCT) is depicted in the center of Figure 1. The device has a semi-ellipsoidal 3D aperture. Approx. spherical wave fronts are generated by each emitter at 2.5 MHz and with a bandwidth of 1.5 MHz at -6 dB. The semi-elliptical aperture has a diameter of 26 cm and a height of 16 cm. Rotational and translational movements, so-called aperture positions, of the complete sensor system create additional virtual positions of the transducers.

The 2041 individual transducers are either operated as emitter (628) or receiver (1413). The transducers have opening angles of 38.2° (standard deviation ±1.5°) at -6 dB. Four emitters and nine receivers are grouped together including pre-amplifier and control electronics in so-called Transducer Array Systems (TAS). Each of the 157 TAS contains a temperature sensor for tracking the temperature distribution within the water basin and the shift at each TAS position during measurements. Additionally, two calibrated PT100 temperature sensors are embedded in the TAS holder to enable increased accuracy.

The data acquisition is carried out with an FPGA based system, which can store up to $80\ GByte$ of A-scans [4]. The digitalization is performed by 480 parallel channels ($12\ Bit$ at $20\ MHz$), enabling data acquisition at one aperture position in approx. ten seconds. After digitization, the parallel data streams are processed as follows: First, the data streams are bandpass filtered (1.67 to $3.33\ MHz$ at $-60\ dB$). Next, the data rate is reduced by a factor of six by performing bandpass undersampling. Finally, the reduced data is stored in the internal memory buffer. Using this approach up to 47 data sets at different aperture positions can be stored in one data acquisition step. A detailed description of the 3D USCT system can be found in [5].

The emitters are excited with a coded excitation signal, e.g. frequency coded chirps can be applied to increase the signal-to-noise ratio of the data. Also the gain of the receiving channels is set individually based on an initial measurement. The applied coded excitation, the individual gain, the temperature data and the spatial positions of the aperture are stored along with the A-scans for each measurement and can be used for signal (pre-) processing and image reconstruction.

Three data sets of different phantoms are provided, each with an empty scan acquired at the same day as the phantom and identical settings of the system's parameters. Figure 3 shows fotos of the phantoms and exemplary reconstructions.

Gelatin 3: The phantom consists of a gelatin phantom with diameter of approx. 0.07 m at the bottom and 0.10 m at the top, a height of approx. 0.13 m of which approx. 0.10 m where immersed into the USCT aperture. The speed of sound of the gelatin was approx. 1515 m/s. The gelatin was embedded in a plastic cup. Two inclusions were generated by embedding drinking straws with diameter 5 mm in the gelatin during curing. Prior to scanning the object, the straws were removed and the inclusions were filled with water. The phantom was positioned approx. centrally in the 3D USCT aperture.

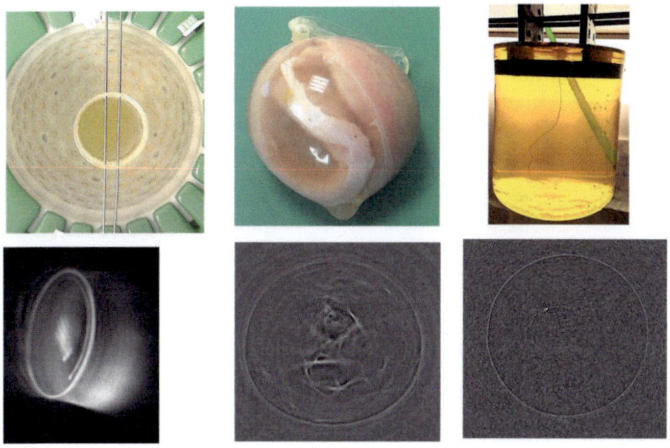

Figure 3: Phantoms scanned; (top) photo, (bottom) reconstruction using different reconstruction algorithms. From left to right: Gelatin 3 phantom reconstructed with SAFT in low resolution and displayed as maximum intensity projection to enhance the visibility of the bottom of the plastic cup, turkey phantom reconstructed with SAFT, and finally nylon thread phantom with speed of sound corrected SAFT reconstruction.

Turkey phantom: Two olives without stones where embedded into a turkey steak. This steak was then embedded in a condom and filled with gelatin. The resulting phantom has a diameter of approx. 9 cm. The phantom was positioned approx. centrally in the 3D USCT aperture. The turkey steak had an approximate sound speed of > 1550 m/s while the olives had a sound speed of approx. 1450 m/s.

Nylon threads: The phantom consists of a gelatin cylinder with both diameter and height of approx. 10 cm. In this cylinder a nylon thread of diameter 0.2 mm is embedded. The phantom was centrally positioned in the 3D USCT aperture.

2.3 Madrid's Multimodal Ultrasound Breast Imaging System (MUBI)

The Multimodal Ultrasound Breast Imaging System (MUBI) is a joint development of the Spanish National Research Council (CISC) and the Complutense University of Madrid (UCM), and it is intended to be a flexible platform for multi-modal ultrasound imaging research, mainly oriented to breast diagnosis [7].]. Up to know three imaging techniques were implemented: Phased-array, acoustic radiation force imaging [8] (both with full angle spatial compound), and ultrasound computed tomography [9].

The system is formed by two 3.5 MHz, 128 elements and 0.22 mm pitch arrays (P2-4/30EP, Prosonic, Korea) that rotate with 95 mm radius into a water tank, controlled by independent stepper motors with an angular resolution of 0.1°. A 128 channel full parallel ultrasound system (SITAU-112, Dasel, Spain) is used for excitation and signal acquisition.

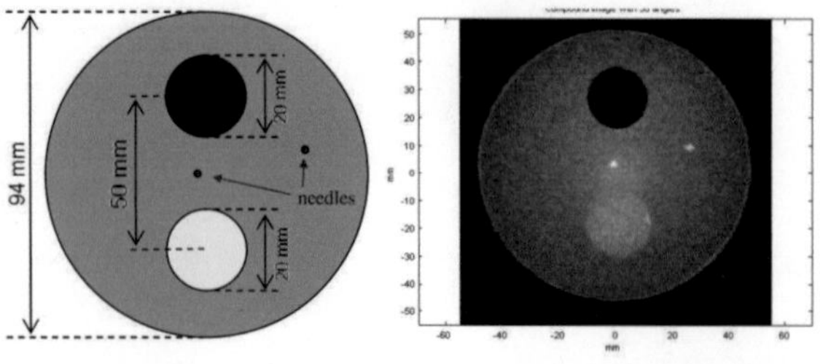

Figure 4: MUBI tissue mimicking phantom: technical drawing (left) and reconstructed with full angle spatial compounding (right).

While only one array can be used as emitter, both of them can act as receivers, allowing pulse-echo and through-transmission operation modes. The system is able to perform emission and reception beamforming in real-time implementing image compounding. It also gives access to the individual signals received by each array element for USCT reconstruction. The acquisition scheme for USCT follows the fan-beam approach of CT systems.

The 2D MUBI USCT data consists of two data sets. The provided phantom data set contains a circular scan of the tissue mimicking phantom, based on water, gelatin, graphite powder and alcohol. It includes a homogenous background with two cylindrical hollows: one filled with water and the other filled with a gelatin preparation with different proportions. Two 0.25 mm diameter steel needles were inserted in the approximate locations shown in Figure 4 left. Furthermore, a second dataset with the same acquisition parameters but without phantom (only water) is provided for calibration purposes. Figure 4 shows the phantom's technical drawing and a full angle spatial compounding reflectivity image.

3 Results of first release

As a result of the joint initiative, a database has been set up. In addition, a kick-off event for the USCT database took place at the USCT data challenge at SPIE Medical Imaging 2017 [3]. The aim of this event was to bring together experts from the USCT community to identify best practices, as well as to establish specifications for interfaces and to carry out a first comparison of reconstructed images. Six posters were presented and three detailed field reports of groups applying their image reconstruction to the provided data were submitted. The challenge hosted a two-hour panel discussion, where the panelists and the audience discussed the experiences on applying the currently available datasets and future directions.

As example the field report of the KIT team (main author Torsten Hopp) is summarized in the following paragraphs.

Both datasets of the 2D systems, i.e. the DBUS and the MUBI system, were tested with the KIT reconstruction software. For transmission tomography, a ray based algebraic reconstruction techniques (ART) [10] was used and for reflectivity imaging a 3D synthetic aperture focusing technique (SAFT) [11] including, if possible, sound speed correction.

For the DBUS dataset sound speed reconstructions performed with ART did not recover the rectangular shape of the imaged phantom. The imaged area appears nearly homogeneously with a sound speed of approx. 1491 - 1493 m/s.

The only contrast in the image seems to origin from the different water temperature at which the A-scans were acquired. Consequently the reflectivity reconstructions were performed with uncorrected SAFT using the average of the given water temperature to compute the sound speed. A-scans for reconstruction were selected by limiting the angle between emitter and receiver normal to 120°. Transmissions signals were removed in a preprocessing step. The pixel resolution was 0.2 mm leading to an image size of 996 x 996 pixels for the area reconstructed to cover the circle covered by the receiving transducer (Figure 5).

The computation time using a single NVidia GeForce GTX Titan GPU was approx. 8 s of which approx. 1 s was the computing time for the actual SAFT processing. A detail view of the phantom and its reconstruction is given in Figure 5.

For the MUBI system sound speed and attenuation images were reconstructed with an ART-based method using a CPU implementation.Figure 6 (top left) shows the result of the speed of sound reconstruction and attenuation reconstruction (top right). The phantom can be clearly distinguished from the water background. The water-filled hollow of the phantom can also be distinguished (lower sound speed area on the right).

Due to the limited resolution of the reconstruction method, the embedded needles are not visible. Subsequently we used the reconstructed sound speed maps to apply sound speed corrected SAFT. The results are given in Figure 6 bottom. The inner structures as well as the outline of the phantom are focused considerably better when applying the sound speed corrected SAFT algorithm. Both needles as well as the water-filled hollow are clearly visible, the second hollow with a different mixture of gelatine can be partly delineated in the lower part of the phantom.

The overall experience with the provided datasets was very positive. Using the interface software, the signal data and according metadata could be retrieved within minutes. For both datasets the KIT algorithm interfaces had to be adapted in order to apply reflectivity and transmission reconstruction, this adaption could be done in roughly one day per USCT system and modality. The images were mostly obtained with the basic parameter settings. Optimizing the parameters and methods to enhance the image quality would require additional time and insight into algorithms, systems and data.

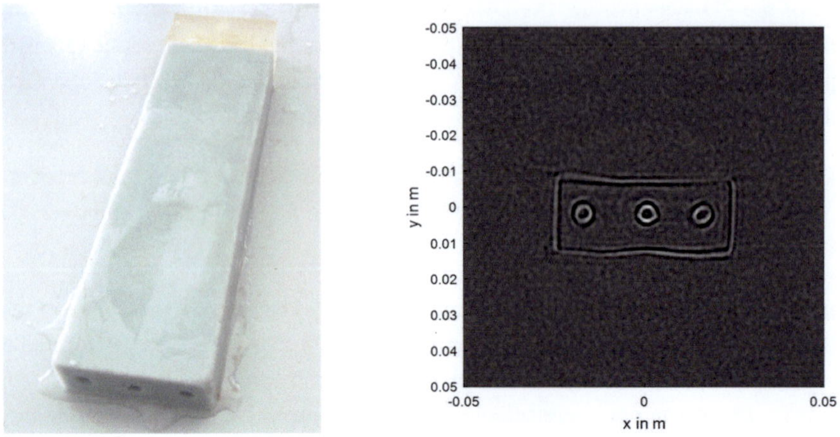

Figure 5: DBUS agar-based phantom: photo of the phantom (left) and reconstruction with 3D SAFT (right).

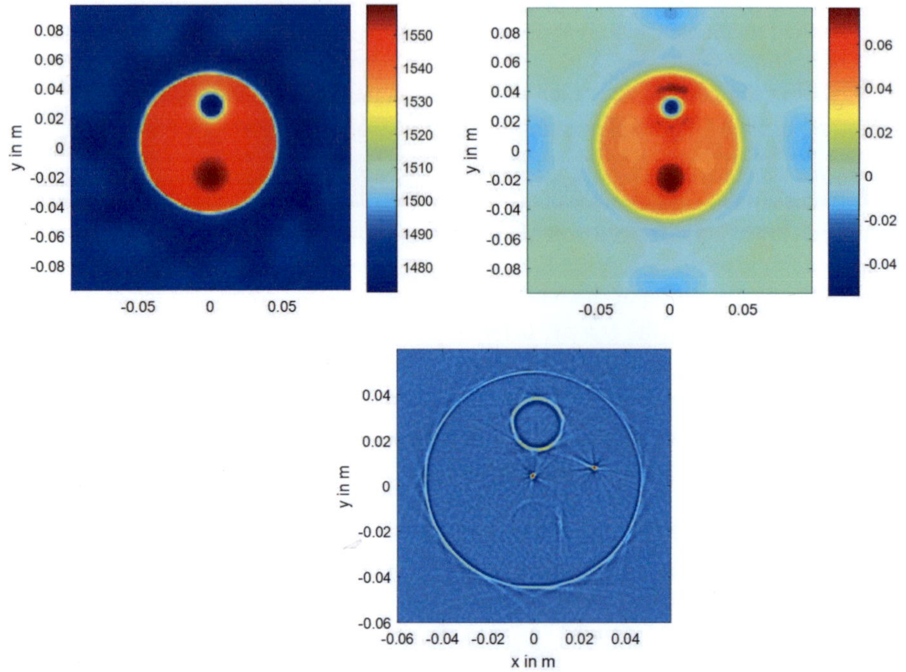

Figure 6: MUBI tissue mimicking phantom: speed of sound in m/s (top left) and attenuation reconstruction in dB/cm (top right); 3D SAFT corrected with reconstruced sound speed and attenuation map (bottom). Axes in m.

The reconstruced images are very promising. Sound speed and attenuation imaging was successfully applied to the MUBI data. Despite the ray approach, which comes with limited resolution, the reconstructed images were able to derive the phantom outline and both large inclusions. The rectangular shape of the DBUS phantom with the same algorithms could not be recovered. Further analysis is needed to identify the potential problems and/or limitations of the method or data. Additional metadata and knowledge about the system (e.g. excitation pulse, possible delays in the signal chain, temperature distribution in the water basin) could contribute to a deeper analysis.

For both systems, the phantoms could be reconstructed with the SAFT based reflectivity reconstruction. In case of the MUBI data, the data provided was not optimal for reflectivity imaging as there is only the 'fan beam' data provided. In consequence mostly the forward scattering is imaged, which limits the resolution and contrast of the reflectivity images.

Due to the GPU accelerated implementation of SAFT, sound speed corrected reflectivity images could be reconstructed in several seconds. Nevertheless there is still a large potential to speed up the reconstructions by optimizing data flows and parallelize data read-in and preprocessing.

4 Conclusion and future work

We expect the online database to enable reproducible comparison of image reconstruction algorithms and USCT systems. It should establish user friendly and easy to use interfaces, standards and data formats between the different USCT systems and their reconstruction algorithms, software and data formats. Further challenges are planned, e.g. comparing the image quality and/or computational performance obtained by different algorithms. Finally, other groups are invited to join in and participate.

References

[1] http://ipeusctdb1.ipe.kit.edu/~usct/challenge/

[2] https://opensource.org/licenses/BSD-3-Clause /, http://opendatacommons.org/licenses/by/

[3] Ruiter, N.V., Zapf, M., Hopp, T, and van Dongen, K.W., "USCT data challenge," in Proc. SPIE 10139, Medical Imaging 2017: Ultrasonic Imaging and Tomography, 101391N, 2017.

[4] https://github.com/KIT-3DUSCT/3DUSCT-data-access-script

[5] Kopmann, A., Bergmann, T., Gemmeke, H., et al. "FPGA-based DAQ system for multi-channel detectors," *Proc. IEEE NSS MIC,* 2008.

[6] Ruiter, N.V., Zapf, M., et al., "First Results of a Clinical Study with 3D Ultrasound Computer Tomography," *Proc. IEEE Internat. Ultrasonics Symp.,* 2013.

[7] Camacho, J., Medina, L., Cruza, J.F., Moreno, J.M., and Fritsch, C., "Multimodal ultrasonic imaging for breast cancer detection," Archives of Acoustics, 37(3), pp. 253-60, 2012.

[8] González-Salido, N., Medina, L., Camacho, J., "Full angle spatial compound of ARFI images for breast cancer detection", Ultrasonics, 71, pp. 161-171, 2016.

[9] Perez-Liva, M., Herraiz, J.L., Miller, E., Cox, B.T., Treeby, B.E., Udías, J.M., "Sound speed reconstruction in full wave ultrasound computer tomography for breast cancer detection," Radiotherapy and Oncology, 119, pp. S454-S455, 2016.

[10] Birk, M., Dapp, R., Ruiter, N.V., Becker, J., "GPU-based iterative transmission reconstruction in 3D Ultrasound Computer Tomography", Journal of Parallel and Distributed Computing 74(1), p. 1730-1743, 2014.

[11] Ruiter, N.V., Kretzek, E., Zapf, M., Hopp, T., Gemmeke, H., "Time of flight interpolated synthetic aperture focusing technique," Proc. SPIE Medical Imaging, 2017.

Object Classification and Localization with an Airborne Ultrasound Imaging System

Wei Yap Tan[1], Grischan Erbacher[1], Till Steiner[2], and Nicole V. Ruiter[1]

[1] *Karlsruhe Institute of Technology, Germany*
Email: wei.tan@kit.edu
[2] *Pepperl+Fuchs GmbH, Germany*

Abstract

An airborne ultrasound imaging system (ABUS) was developed at KIT for reflection tomography. The prototype system consists of sixteen ultrasonic transducers surrounding a region of interest (ROI) of defined shape with a diameter of 50 cm. The transducers have a center frequency of 200 kHz and a bandwidth of 20 kHz. The prototype aims to demonstrate possible industrial applications for object classification and localization with airborne ultrasound. This paper is a detailed version of the previous publication in IEEE Ultrasonics Symposium (IUS) 2017 [1].

Keywords: airborne ultrasound, reflection tomography, object classification, object localization

1 Introduction

An airborne ultrasound imaging system (ABUS) was developed at KIT for reflection tomography. The prototype system consists of sixteen ultrasonic transducers surrounding a region of interest (ROI) of defined shape with a diameter of 50 cm. The transducers have a center frequency of 200 kHz and a bandwidth of 20 kHz. The transducer distribution is optimized for a maximum coverage of the custom ROI and an homogeneous distribution of image quality using the optimization method described in [2]. In the current setup, each transducer sends an ultrasound pulse and the received signals, i.e. A-scans, at all transducers are sampled. In contrast to recent publications using linear ultrasound arrays [3, 4], this system is capable of imaging multiple objects from multiple angles around the ROI in a single acquisition using synthetic aperture focusing technique (SAFT)[5]. The reconstructed images allow recognition and localization of multiple objects simultaneously. Figure 1 shows the current system setup.

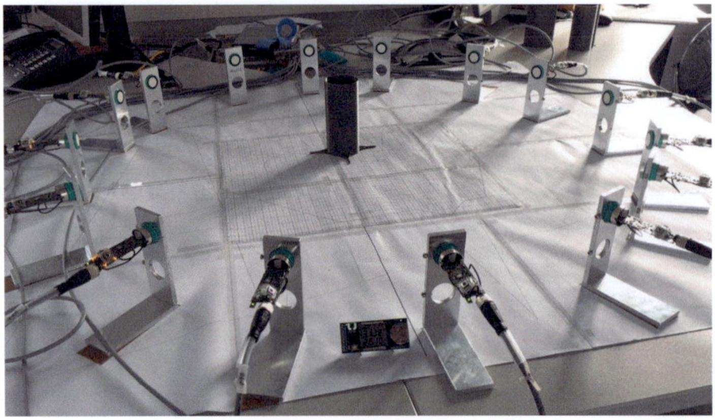

Figure 1: ABUS with sixteen ultrasonic transducers surrounding the ROI

In this work we aimed to automatically segment, classify and localize objects in the reconstructed image. The resulting workflow is essential in demonstrating possible applications for such airborne ultrasound imaging systems. For instance, ABUS can assist the localization of transparent objects, or objects of different colors with the same shape, where a camera solution faces difficulties. Figure 2 shows an example application of ABUS in industry, in which the robot arm can pick the desired objects based on the results from the proposed workflow.

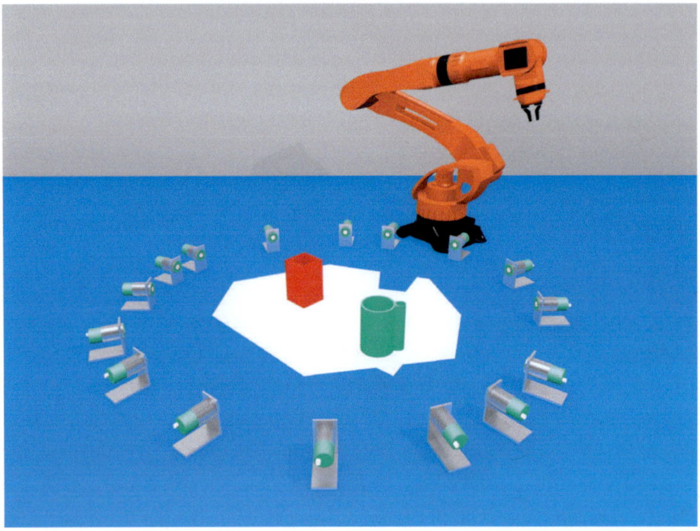

Figure 2: The figure shows a potential industrial application of ABUS for object recognition and localization.

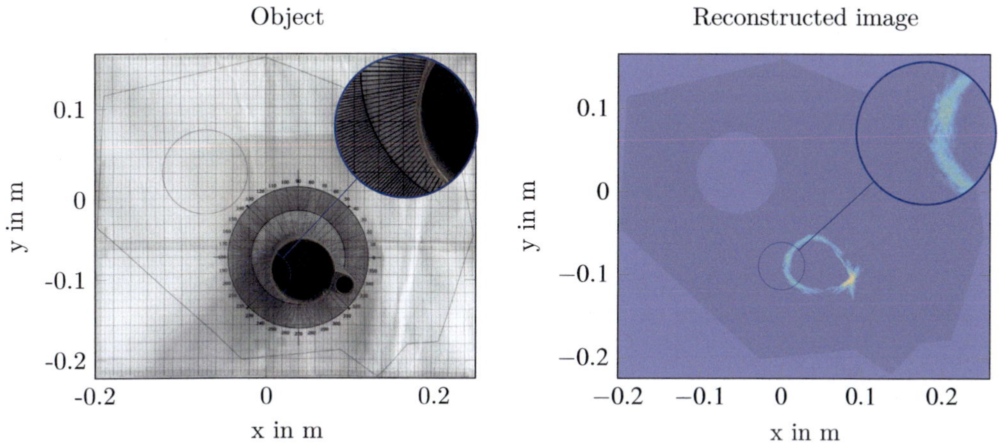

Figure 3: The images show the comparison between a camera image (left) and a reconstructed ultrasound image with ABUS (right).

2 Challenges and Objectives

Figure 3 shows an example reconstruction of an object with an asymmetrical feature. In the reconstructed image the object surfaces are depicted as edges with varying intensities. Besides that, the reconstructed edges contain spiky artifacts as shown in the magnified image. Due to the sparse transducer arrangement and the low bandwidth of our current setup, objects positioned closely to each other might not always be separable in the reconstructed images.

At the same time, large acoustic impedance between air and solid objects limits the transmission of the ultrasound wave through the objects. This leads to acoustic shadowing that results in incomplete reconstruction of objects despite multiple acquisition angles around the ROI. These image characteristics restrict the direct application of state of the art pixel oriented, edge and cluster based segmentation techniques, such as thresholding, active contours and region-growing methods.

Our objective is to develop an automatic workflow, which can be applied for the varying intensities of object edges to segment, classify and localize the objects. Our goal is to achieve a classification accuracy higher than 90 % and a localization accuracy comparable to the full width at half maximum (FWHM) of the point spread function (PSF) of 1.5 cm of the example system.

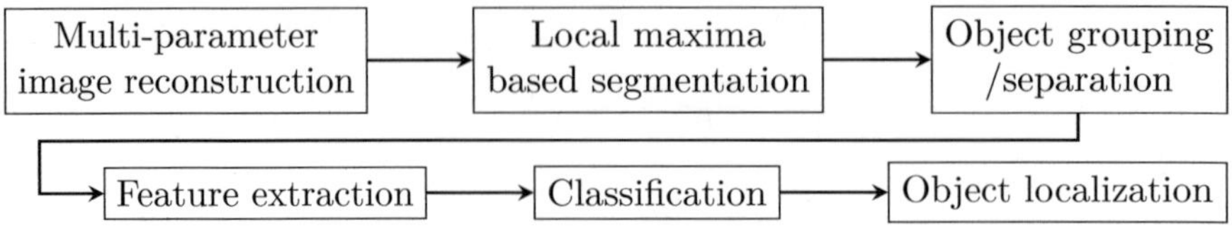

Figure 4: Workflow for automatic object segmentation and classification

3 Methods

Figure 4 shows the proposed workflow for automatic segmentation and object classification with ABUS. The workflow is a sequential process consisting of image reconstruction, image segmentation, post-processing of the segmentation results and classification and localization of the segmented objects.

3.1 Multi-Parameter Image Reconstruction

Before the SAFT reconstruction, we applied echo detection to the sampled A-scans and replaced the detected echoes with a sinc pulse with an equivalent FWHM of 1.7 mm, which is the wavelength of the ultrasound frequency used. Using SAFT, the intensity of each pixel is a sum of the signal amplitude in the A-scans for each selected sender-receiver-combination at the time equal to the time-of-flight for an ultrasound wave traveling from the sender to the pixel and to the receiver. In order to reduce grating-lobe artifacts, we extended our SAFT reconstruction algorithm with the sliding median filter introduced in [6].

According to this reconstruction method, the reconstructed image details and contrast can be influenced by changing the sets of sender and receivers and the width of the sliding median filter used. The two parameters are the angle ϕ, which limits the amount of receivers per sender and the median width k. The optimal values of these parameters are dependent on the size and surface curvature of the objects and their position and orientation in the ROI.

For example, a cylindrical object with a small radius reflects the ultrasound wave over a larger angle compared to a plane surface. The echoes will be received by more receivers nearby the sender, hence larger ϕ and k can be used. This settings are less suitable for reflection at plane surface, as the reflection will be treated as outliers by the median filter. Figure 5 demonstrates schematically the SAFT reconstruction with sliding median in ABUS.

The influence of ϕ and k on the image details is shown in Figure 6 with the same test object as in Figure 3. With a larger angle $\phi = 80°$ and median width $k = 5$, the spiky artifacts of the reconstructed object were reduced. However these parameters introduced an incomplete edge, as compared to the reconstruction with $\phi = 40°$ and $k = 3$. Since we have full access to the

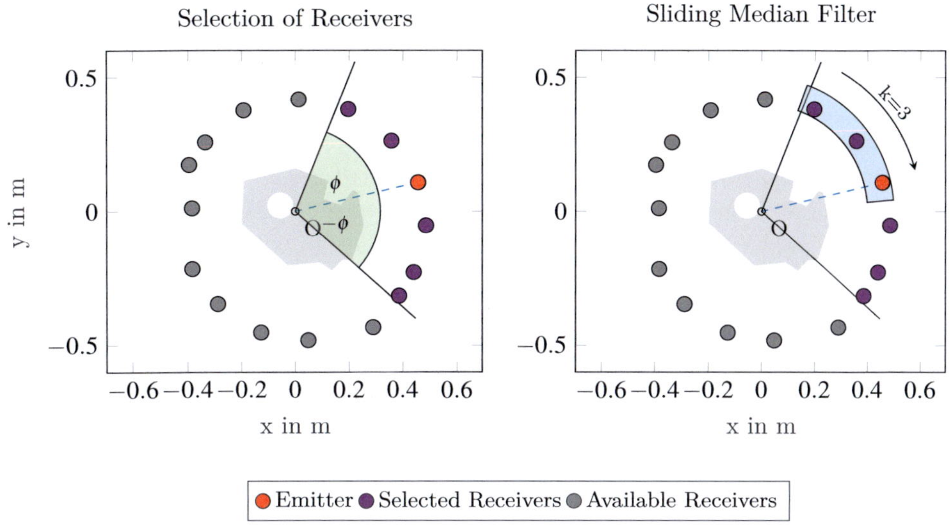

Figure 5: The figures show the selection of receivers for the Emitter S1 during the SAFT reconstruction with angle ϕ and the application of a sliding median for grating lobe reduction with a width of $k = 3$.

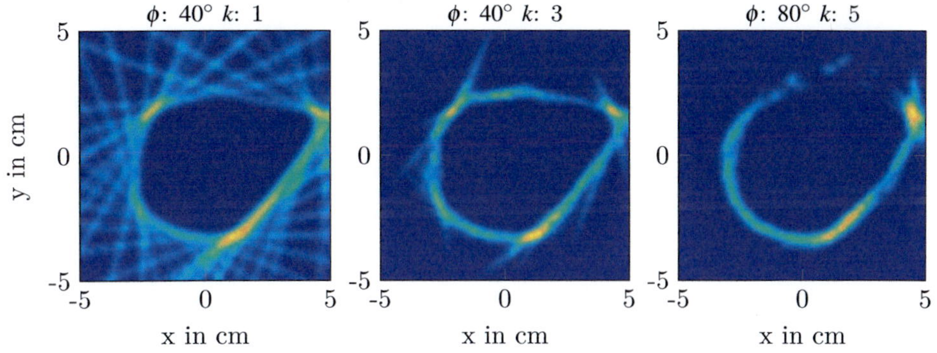

Figure 6: Influence of angle ϕ and median filter length k on the image details

A-scans, we propose the reconstruction of multiple images using different parameters to obtain better segmentation for objects with different sizes and surface curvatures.

3.2 Local Maxima based Segmentation

The varying intensity of the reconstructed objects limits the application of a global threshold to segment the image. Hence, the object segmentation applies local maximum detection using a sliding Gaussian window. The width of the Gaussian window can be set according to the measured point spread function (PSF) of the ultrasound imaging system.

In a separate matrix of the same size as the image, the frequency of a pixel being detected as a local maximum is recorded. Local maxima with occurrence frequencies lower than 3 were empirically found to be image artifacts and are discarded. Next, the remaining local maxima with intensities higher than the 98th percentile are selected, resulting in the image in Figure 6(b). It is generally assumed that higher intensity pixels are more likely to be part of the object edges and the object edges cover only a small amount of pixels in the images.

Local maxima extracted from the reconstructed images with different parameters are combined and morphological closing is applied to turn these local maxima into connected regions as shown in Figure 6(c). Lastly, the morphological skeletons of these regions are calculated to obtain the segmented object in Figure 6(d).

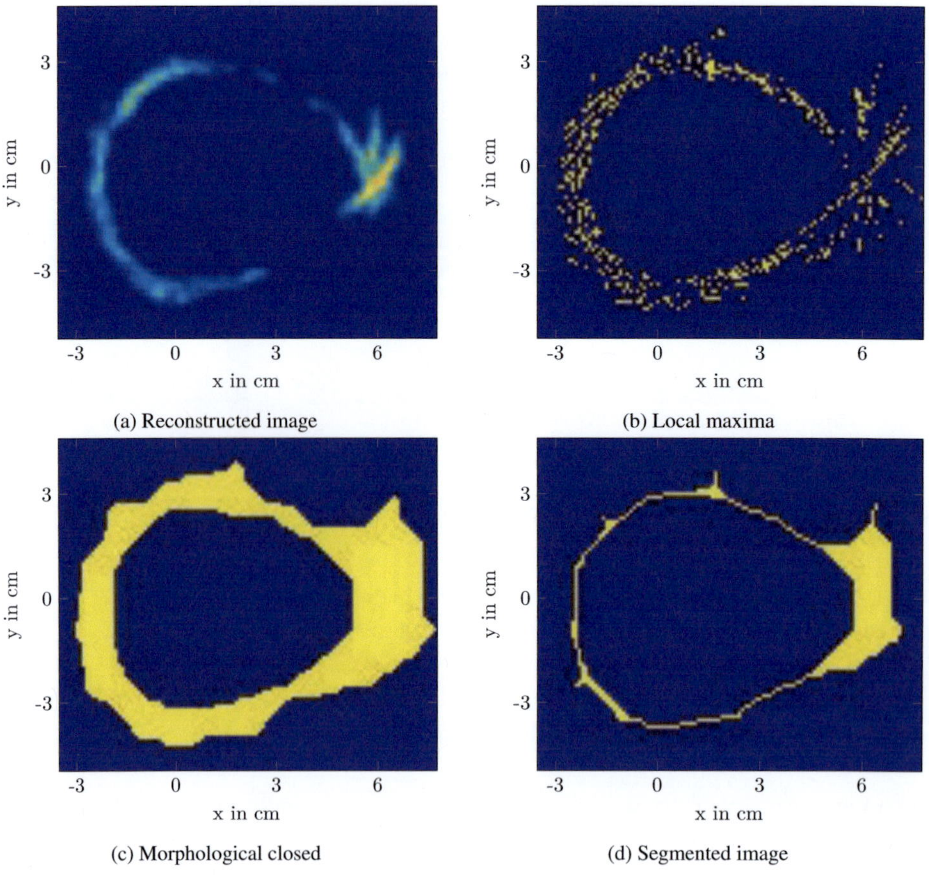

Figure 7: The figure shows the steps of an example segmentation.

3.3 Object Grouping or Separation

Due to the sparse transducer arrangement and shadowing effect of ultrasound at obstacles, an object may be reconstructed incompletely and segmented as separate regions. Post-processing of the segmentation results can be performed using prior knowledge about the imaging capability of the ultrasound system to join these regions to a single object.

In this work, we applied the Euclidean distance between pixels of each segmented region to group regions belonging to the same object. The maximum distance, in which two regions are grouped as a single object, can be set according to the PSF of the system or the minimum size of objects to be imaged.

3.4 Feature Extraction and Classification

The classification of the segmented object is implemented with a neural network for pattern recognition [7]. In this work, the following features are extracted from the segmented object as input values for the classification:

- Area
- Convex area
- Major axis length
- Minor axis length
- Eccentricity
- Perimeter
- Roundness metric
- Squareness metric
- Within clusters sum of point-to-centroid distances from *k*-means clustering [8].

The roundness metric R is calculated with

$$R = \frac{4 \cdot \pi \cdot \text{Area}}{\text{Perimeter}^2}. \qquad (1)$$

Whereas the squareness metric S is calculated as

$$S = \frac{\text{Area}}{16 \cdot \text{Perimeter}^2}. \qquad (2)$$

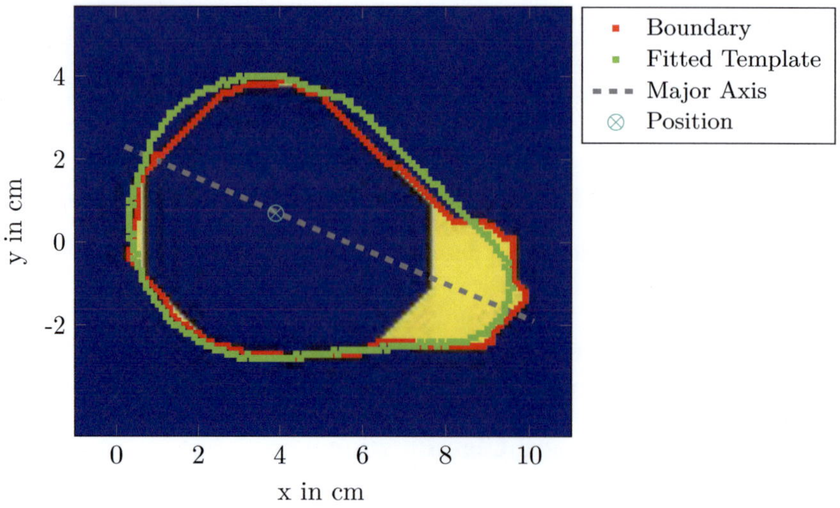

Figure 8: Object localization with Generalized Hough Transform

For a set of objects to be trained, we extract these features from reconstructions containing only one object and train the neural network under supervised learning with Bayesian Regularization Backpropagation, which prevents overfitting of the network [9].

3.5 Object Localization

The position and orientation of a segmented object can be determined by calculating the centroid and the major axis of the segmented region. For more complex objects with known geometry, template matching techniques such as Generalized Hough Transform (GHT) can be applied [10]. In our work, each object in the data set is assigned with a customized template, which is a binary image consisting of the outline of the object.

Figure 8 shows an example of the object localization with a template. The yellow area shows the segmented region with its outer boundary in red. The template is rotated during the application of GHT, in order to enable the detection of the object in different orientations. The position and angle of the template with the largest maximum point in the Hough space indicate the location and orientation of the object. In Figure 8, the fitted template is plotted with a green line.

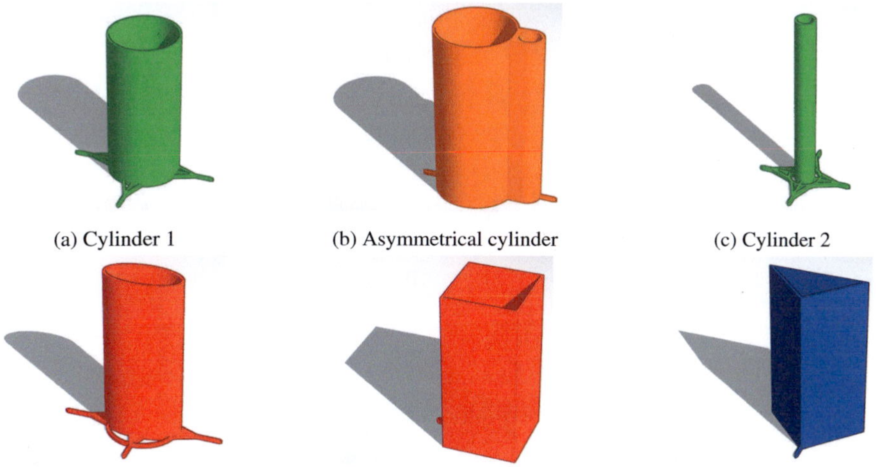

(a) Cylinder 1 (b) Asymmetrical cylinder (c) Cylinder 2

(d) Elliptic cylinder (e) Cuboid (f) Triangular prism

Figure 9: Test objects for evaluating the automatic segmentation, classification and localization of objects with ABUS

4 Evaluation

For the evaluation of the proposed workflow, six objects of different shapes and sizes were designed. These objects have in general a diameter of 6 cm and a height of 12 cm except for the smaller cylinder with a diameter of 1.5 cm (Cylinder 2 in Figure 9). The cross section of the objects are primitive shapes, such as circles, ellipses, rectangles, triangles and circles with an asymmetrical feature as shown in Figure 9. The shown CAD models were used for 3D printing of the test objects.

The multi-parameter image reconstruction was performed with angles $\phi = \{60°, 80°, 100°\}$ and $k = \{5, 6, 7\}$. For each object, forty measurements were performed at discrete positions and angles in the ROI. This data was divided into 70 % for the training of the neural network and 15 % each for validation and testing. The neural network has a hidden layer with fifteen neurons and an output layer with six neurons. The resulting overall confusion matrix after eighteen iterations is shown in Figure 10. A classification accuracy of 98.8 % was achieved in the training phase, 86.1 % in the validation phase and 88.9 % in the test. The overall classification accuracy was 95.4 %.

The asymmetrical cylinder was used as the test object in evaluating the localization accuracy. A total of sixty acquisitions was performed at discrete position and orientation and the ground truth values were recorded. We used the template as shown in Figure 8 for the GHT and obtained a positioning accuracy of 5 mm with a standard deviation of 2.7 mm and orientation accuracy of 2.8° with a standard deviation of 5.4°.

Output Class \ Target Class	Cylinder 1	Asymmetrical Cylinder	Elliptic cylinder	Cylinder 2	Cuboid	Triangular Prism	All
Cylinder 1	38 15.8%	0 0.0%	0 0.0%	0 0.0%	0 0.0%	0 0.0%	100% 0.0%
Asymmetrical Cylinder	0 0.0%	39 16.3%	0 0.0%	0 0.0%	2 0.8%	0 0.0%	95.1% 4.9%
Elliptic cylinder	0 0.0%	0 0.0%	40 16.7%	0 0.0%	0 0.0%	1 0.4%	97.6% 2.4%
Cylinder 2	0 0.0%	0 0.0%	0 0.0%	39 16.3%	0 0.0%	1 0.4%	97.5% 2.5%
Cuboid	2 0.8%	1 0.4%	0 0.0%	0 0.0%	37 15.4%	2 0.8%	88.1% 11.9%
Triangular Prism	0 0.0%	0 0.0%	0 0.0%	1 0.4%	1 0.4%	36 15.0%	94.7% 5.3%
All	95.0% 5.0%	97.5% 2.5%	100% 0.0%	97.5% 2.5%	92.5% 7.5%	90.0% 10.0%	95.4% 4.6%

Figure 10: Confusion matrix of the trained neural network for classifying the six test objects

5 Conclusion

In this work, we introduced an exemplary workflow for automatic object segmentation and classification for an airborne ultrasound imaging system. The local maxima based segmentation provides good results despite varying intensity and PSF in the reconstructed images. In combination with the multi-parameter SAFT, we were able to detect and classify objects of different sizes and surface curvature. Figure 11 shows the ability of the workflow in classifying and localizing two objects simultaneously with ABUS.

The evaluation results showed a overall classification accuracy higher than the required 90 % at 95.4 % with an accuracy of 88.9 % in the test phase. A localization accuracy of 5 mm was achieved, which is smaller than the measured FHWM of PSF of 1.5 cm. These results fulfilled the given objectives for our workflow.

Due to the sparse transducer arrangement and the limited bandwidth of the current prototype, the segmentation results cannot differentiate object features smaller than approximately 2 cm. This could be further improved with usage of more transducers or higher bandwidth of ultrasound transducers.

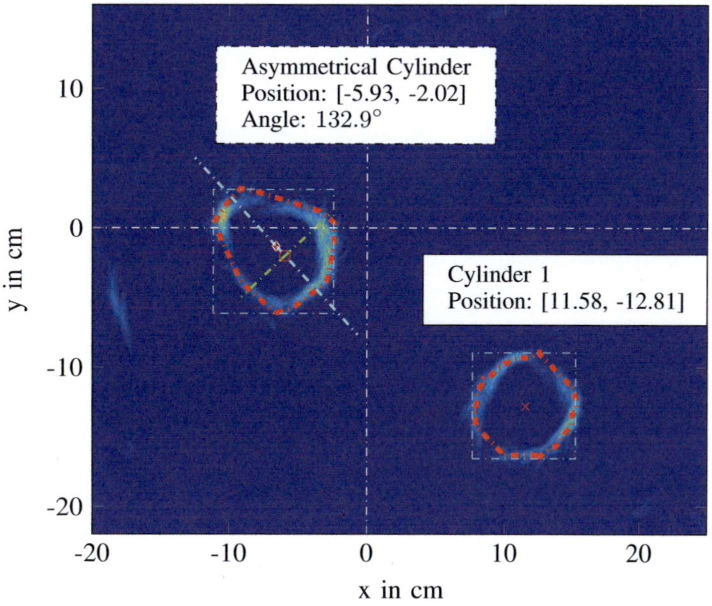

Figure 11: The figure demonstrates the ability of the workflow to classify and localize two objects simultaneously with ABUS.

References

[1] Tan, W. Y., Erbacher, G., Steiner, T., and Ruiter, N. V. Automatic segmentation and object classification with neural network for an airborne ultrasound imaging system. In *Ultrasonics Symposium (IUS), 2017 IEEE International* (2017).

[2] Tan, W. Y., Steiner, T., and Ruiter, N. V. Automatic optimization of sensor positioning for an airborne ultrasound imaging system. In *Ultrasonics Symposium (IUS), 2016 IEEE International* (10 2016).

[3] Brown, G., and Reilly, D. Proceedings of ultrasonics international 1995 ultrasonic tomographic imaging of solid objects in air using an array of fan-shaped-beam electrostatic transducers. *Ultrasonics 34*, 2 (1996), 111 – 115.

[4] Capineri, L., Bulletti, A., Calzolai, M., and Giannelli, P. An airborne ultrasonic imaging system based on 16 elements: 150 khz piezopolymer transducer arrays—preliminary simulated and experimental results for cylindrical targets detection. *Sensing and Imaging 17*, 1 (2016), 1–23.

[5] Stepinski, T. An implementation of synthetic aperture focusing technique in frequency domain. *IEEE Transactions on Ultrasonics, Ferroelectrics, and Frequency Control 54*, 7 (7 2007), 1399–1408.

[6] Ruiter, N. V., Dapp, R., Zapf, M., and Gemmeke, H. A new method for grating lobe reduction for 3d synthetic aperture imaging with ultrasound computer tomography. In *2010 IEEE International Ultrasonics Symposium* (10 2010), pp. 2372–2375.

[7] Bishop, C. *Neural Networks for Pattern Recognition*. Advanced Texts in Econometrics. Clarendon Press, 1995.

[8] Wu, J. *Advances in K-means Clustering: A Data Mining Thinking*. Springer Publishing Company, Incorporated, 2012.

[9] Burden, F., and Winkler, D. *Bayesian Regularization of Neural Networks*. Humana Press, 2009, pp. 23–42.

[10] Ballard, D. H. Readings in computer vision: Issues, problems, principles, and paradigms. Morgan Kaufmann Publishers Inc., San Francisco, CA, USA, 1987, ch. Generalizing the Hough Transform to Detect Arbitrary Shapes, pp. 714–725.